Public Health Skills
A Practical Guide for Nurses and Public Health Practitioners

Edited by

Lesley Coles
BA, RN, DN, RM, RHV, RNT, Cert Ed
Deputy Award Leader Pre Qualifying Nursing Programme
University of Southampton

and

Elizabeth Porter
BA MPhil, PGCEA, RN, RM, RHV, PT
Programme Leader for MSc/BSc (Hons) Public Health Practice
University of Southampton

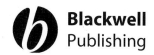

Blackwell
Publishing

© 2008 by Blackwell Publishing Ltd

Blackwell Publishing editorial offices:
Blackwell Publishing Ltd, 9600 Garsington Road, Oxford OX4 2DQ, UK
  Tel: +44 (0)1865 776868
Blackwell Publishing Inc., 350 Main Street, Malden, MA 02148-5020, USA
  Tel: +1 781 388 8250
Blackwell Publishing Asia Pty Ltd, 550 Swanston Street, Carlton, Victoria 3053, Australia
  Tel: +61 (0)3 8359 1011

First published 2008 by Blackwell Publishing Ltd

2   2009

ISBN-13: 978-1-4051-5519-9

Library of Congress Cataloging-in-Publication Data

Public health skills: a practical guide for nurses & public health practitioners / edited by Lesley Coles and Elizabeth Porter.
    p. ; cm.
  Includes bibliographical references and index.
  ISBN-13: 978-1-4051-5519-9 (pbk. : alk. paper)
  1. Public health nursing. 2. Public health personnel. 3. Public health. I. Coles, Lesley. II. Porter, Elizabeth, 1951-
  [DNLM: 1. Public Health Nursing—methods. 2. Community Health Services. 3. Needs Assessment. 4. Public Health Practice. WY 108 P977 2008]

RT97.P85 2008
610.73'4—dc22
                              2007032664

A catalogue record for this title is available from the British Library

Set in 9.5/11.5 Sabon by Newgen Imaging Systems Pvt Ltd, Chennai, India
Printed and bound in Singapore by Fabulous Printers Pte Ltd

The publisher's policy is to use permanent paper from mills that operate a sustainable forestry policy, and which has been manufactured from pulp processed using acid-free and elementary chlorine-free practices. Furthermore, the publisher ensures that the text paper and cover board used have met acceptable environmental accreditation standards.

For further information on Blackwell Publishing, visit our website:
www.blackwellnursing.com

4. Health and lifestyles – obesity/healthy eating, levels of physical activity (including considering safety), drugs and alcohol and links to antisocial behaviour, sexual health, and making healthier choices easier.

Together these discourses and frameworks form the four main sections of the book:

Section 1: Assessment of Public Health Needs.
Section 2: Management of Public Health Needs.
Section 3: Public Health Policies and their Impact on Practice.
Section 4: Facilitation of Public Health Activities.

To increase the book's practical usefulness, a large number of activities, exercises and case study examples are included to demonstrate how the ideas presented can be applied.

References

Cabinet Office (2006) *Reaching Out: an action plan on social exclusion.* www.cabinetoffice.gov.uk.

DH (Department of Health) (2004a) *Choosing Health: making healthier choices easier.* London: HM Stationery Office.

DH (Department of Health) (2004b) *The NHS Improvement Plan: putting people at the heart of public services.* London: HM Stationery Office.

DH (Department of Health) (2005) *Shaping the Future of Public Health: promoting health in the NHS.* www.dh.gov.uk.

Department of Health (2006) *Our Health, Our Care, Our Say: a new direction for community services.* HM Stationery Office.

Kelly A., Symonds A. (2003) *The Social Construction of Community Care.* London: Palgrave Macmillan.

Mossialos E., Dixon A. (2002) *Funding Health Care Options for Europe.* Maidenhead: Open University Press.

Skills for Health (2004) *National Occupational Standards for the Practice of Public Health Guide.* Bristol: Skills for Health. www.skillsforhealth.org.uk.

Skills for Health (2007). *Multidisciplinary/multi-agency/multi-professional Public Health Skills and Career Framework.* Bristol: Skills for Health. www.skillsforhealth.org.uk.

Wanless D. (2004) *Securing Good Health for the Whole Population.* London: HM Stationery Office.

WHO (World Health Organization) (2002) *The World Health Report 2002: reducing risks, promoting healthy life.* Geneva: World Health Organization.

How to Use this Book

Section introductions outline the key public health skills covered by the chapters in the section, for example:

Section 4 Introduction: Facilitation of Public Health Activities

Key Public Health Skills

- Developing quality and risk management within an evaluative culture
- Developing health programmes and services and reducing inequalities
- Ethically managing self, people and resources to improve health and wellbeing

Chapter introductions outline the specific public health skills covered in the chapter, for example, in Chapter 9:

Public Health Skills: strategic leadership

- Strategic analysis: SWOT analysis, PESTEL analysis, needs assessment and stakeholder analysis
- Strategic choice: revising the mission statement, identifying strategic options, and evaluating and selecting strategic options
- Strategic implementation: communicating the strategy, organizational structures in place, aligning culture and strategy, reviewing progress and amending the strategy

In the text, activity boxes help you understand and apply public health skills to your area of practice. They remind you of the key public health skills to take away with you from the areas you have just read about and to review how these can be applied to your everyday practice. For example, in Chapter 10:

Activity

As a public health nurse, what would your role be if a similar event to that in the case study occurred amongst your client group? Where could you obtain further information and guidance? What other agencies might be involved and do you know their contact details? Are there any health promotion activities you could initiate to prevent outbreaks such as this occurring? Reference For further information, see Hawker *et al.* (2005).

In the text, web activities help you access data and information from the world wide web. Using information technology to access, collect and manage data on health and wellbeing is an important key public health skill in the surveillance and assessment of the population's health and wellbeing. Some of these useful links have been developed into web activities, for example, in Chapter 14:

> **Activity**
>
> Visit the websites www.meetingwizard.org and www.effectivemeetings.com, and explore them to find out more about conducting meetings.

Case study examples help you review the use of specific public health skills and understand some of the decision-making skills involved, for example, in Chapter 6:

> **Case Study Example**
>
> Partnership working to improve health and wellbeing: detecting and managing postnatal depression in non-English speaking women
>
> A health visitor receives notification that a family have moved into the area of the city that she covers. The client is married with an 8-week baby. The health visitor determines that the mother may not be English given her name is Surjit Kaur and may well be a Sikh Punjabi. It is a policy expectation that health visitors meet families with children less than 5 years of age on at least on one occasion and to assess all women for postnatal depression within the first 3 months of delivery. A validated tool for screening women who speak Punjabi (Edinburgh Postnatal Depression Scale, EPDS) is available for health visitors (Werrett & Clifford 2006). Little empirical knowledge on how health visitors assess women who have a different ethnic and cultural background to their own is available.
>
> Figure 6.1 shows a flow chart outlining two ways the health visitor could respond. It describes some of the attitudes, skills and cultural knowledge that are required to successfully engage with women who do not have English as their primary language. This is a typical situation that health visitors are confronted with and although it is a hypothetical case it is drawn from research observations and interviews with health visitors assessing ethnic minority women for postnatal depression. However, it has been idealised to demonstrate a partnership approach to this aspect of health visiting. These idealizations are drawn from recommendations provided by participants in the equity project which is in progress. It is a fabricated description because a three-way partnership was not seen during either of the research projects. Due to limitations of space the case study is necessarily brief.

Reflective exercises enable you to examine your use of public health skills by drawing on interesting real life examples to help you explore how they relate to public health practice, for example, in Chapter 7:

> **Reflective exercise**
>
> Has there been a time when you have made a judgement about a family? You were sure you knew the reasons as to why they were experiencing problems and based on the assumptions made, you created a plan of action? Now use Table 7.4 as you reflect on that time.

Key terms are provided in a glossary that provides a brief explanation of each one:

Assessment of health need	A process that helps inform planning of health care for individuals and their families, communities and the wider population.
Community development	Work with people on a neighbourhood or community basis that promotes self-help, mutual support and collective action. The underlying idea is finding new and imaginative solutions to problems and better use of existing resources (PHEL).
Deprived areas	Areas characterised by significantly low social and economic levels measured on a range of indices such as unemployment and lower rates of income per head or agreed indices compared with the national average (PHEL).
Health improvement	The main function of health improvement is to find ways of preventing ill health, protecting good health and promoting better health – it is closely linked to the quality of life and the concept of wellbeing.

List of Abbreviations

ACORN	a classification of residential neighbourhood
AIDS	acquired immune deficiency syndrome
ASH	Action on Smoking and Health
BMI	body mass index
BNF	*British National Formulary*
CAF	common assessment framework
CAMHS	Child and Adolescent Mental Health Services
CDM	chronic diseases management
CMHN	community mental health nurse
CJD	Creutzfeldt-Jakob disease
COPD	chronic obstructive pulmonary disease
CPA	Child Protection Agency
CSCI	Commission for Social Care Inspection
DfES	Department for Education and Skills
EBP	evidence-based policy
EPP	Expert Patient Programme
EYFS	early years foundation stage
FASST	family and school support team
GP	general practitioner
HDA	Health Development Agency
HIV	human immunodeficiency virus
HNA	health needs assessment
HPA	Health Protection Agency
ICD	International Classification of Diseases
ICP	integrated care pathway
IMD	index of multiple deprivation
IVF	*in vitro* fertilization
KSF	Knowledge and Skills Framework
LA	local authority
MeSH	medical subject headings
MIU	minor injury unit
MMR	measles, mumps and rubella
NDC	'New deal for communities'
NESS	National Evaluation of Sure Start
NHS	National Health Service
NICE	National Institute for Health and Clinical Excellence
NLH	National Library for Health
NMC	Nursing and Midwifery Council
NMP	non-medical prescribing (nurse)
NPSA	National Patient Safety Agency
NSF	National Service Framework
NSPCC	National Society for the Prevention of Cruelty to Children
ONS	Office for National Statistics
OOH	out of hours

PACT   prescription analysis and cost
PALS   Patient Advisory Liaison Services
PCG   Primary Care Group
PCT   Primary Care Trust
PEST   political, economic, sociocultural and technological
PESTEL   political, economic, sociocultural, technological, environmental and legal
PGD   patient group direction
PHCR   personal child health record
PHEL   Public Health Electronic Library
PICO   population of problem, intervention, comparison and outcome
PRA   participatory rural appraisal
PREP   post-registration education and practice
RCA   root causes analysis
RCT   randomised controlled trial
RTA   road traffic accident
SAP   single assessment process
SARS   severe acute respiratory syndrome
SCPHN   specialist community public health nurse/nursing
SMR   standardised mortality ratio
SSLP   Sure Start local programme
STI   sexually transmitted infection
SWOTS   strengths, weaknesses, opportunities and threats
TB   tuberculosis
VCS   voluntary and community sector
WHO   World Health Organization
WiC   walk in centre

Section 1

Assessment of Public Health Needs

Section 1 Introduction:
Assessment of Public Health Needs

Key Public Health Skills

- Surveillance and assessment of the population's health and wellbeing

This first section of the book examines practitioners' contribution to surveillance and assessment of health need. The premise is that this is a purposeful activity focused on health and is expert and non-stigmatizing. Contact with the population in the home setting, primary care, acute setting or community offers opportunity for insight into individual's perception of their health and how they experience it. In developing profiles of the health and wellbeing of the population, practitioners bring together relevant epidemiological data, local information and needs as expressed by individuals and their local community. This information can be used to inform the local health plan and influence resource allocation to areas with the greatest health and social need, thus influencing the management of health needs.

Assessment of need involves the identification of threats to health and existing health problems as well as the positive factors that enable individuals, families and groups to remain healthy within situations of deprivation and vulnerability. Practitioners work in a variety of settings and are well placed to identify those who do not make appropriate use of services offered. They will include local marginalised and vulnerable individuals and groups who have limited access to services such as asylum seekers, homeless populations, new communities or travellers. Practitioners who successfully utilise public health skills are able to shed light on the nature of their difficulties including the inadequacy or inappropriateness of existing services or the lack of awareness of their own health needs.

The process of identification of health need is achieved in several ways and is examined within this section.

Introduction to Chapter 1

Public Health Skills: assessment

- How to assess: using frameworks, recognizing influences on health, profiling, and using identified criteria to systematically decide on health issues
- Analysing and interpreting health needs and target groups/individuals: screening, monitoring development through health, documenting and monitoring people, situations and the environment

Chapter 1 examines the skills required for identifying and assessing health needs. Theories are offered and frameworks for practice developed from these. The main focus of the chapter is on defining health, health needs assessment, its importance and the policy legislation to support it. The majority of the chapter is devoted to the various methods and tools used to assess and identify need within a defined population, including:

- skills required to address the competing concepts of need, demand and supply;
- three types of needs assessment: epidemiological, comparative and corporate;
- rapid appraisal;
- population, community, family and individual assessment and identification of need;
- the variety of assessment tools adopted by agencies;
- community health needs assessment and health profiling;
- the common assessment framework;
- screening programmes: population screening, systematic screening, opportunistic screening and screening for inherited disorders.

Introduction to Chapter 2

Public Health Skills: appraising and measuring

- Promoting self-esteem: encouraging self-determination and motivation
- Skills of analysis: interpretation and use of information, and methods of evaluating provision

Chapter 2 asks the question 'why understand health need?' and provides answers to this through examining issues around lifestyle and health and the economic cost of health. By debating the question of who takes responsibility for health improvement, the chapter explores the concept of informed choice and responsibility and uses examples of individual versus social responsibility in the case of *in vitro* fertilization and obese women. The importance of raising awareness of health need and the analyses, interpretation and use of information are proposed before the chapter concludes with discussion on promoting self-esteem, encouraging self-determination and evaluating provision, including:

- what is happening with health at societal and individual levels?
- responsibility for health – lifestyle, dilemmas, NHS to treat or not to treat?
- why raise awareness of health need? – access to health/social care/services.

Introduction to Chapter 3

Public Health Skills: surveillance

- How to measure health need: epidemiological needs assessment and community diagnoses
- How to collect and structure information in order to create a profile of the population
- Assessing the information collected: reading data, interpretation and analysis
- How to communicate data and information on the health and wellbeing and related needs of a defined population

Chapter 3 examines the contribution of epidemiology to the assessment of the health needs of a population. The author states that this approach is based on the natural history of disease and its interface with and entry to the health care system. The author uses the medical care model to explore the concepts of need, demand, resource and outcome before bringing in the dimensions of effectiveness and efficiency. How to undertake an epidemiological needs assessment is

1.1.2   Objectives

Stevens and Gillam (1998) highlighted five objectives of an HNA that flow from these aims:

1. Planning: this is the central objective of needs assessment, to help decide what services are required, for how many people; the effectiveness of these services; the benefits that will be expected; and at what cost.
2. Intelligence: gathering information to get an overview and an increased understanding of the existing health care service, the population it serves and the population's health needs – e.g. what is the baseline?
3. Target efficiency: having assessed needs, measuring whether or not resources have been appropriately directed – e.g. do those who need a service get it? Do those who get a service need it? This is related to audit.
4. Involvement of stakeholders: carrying out an HNA can stimulate the involvement and ownership of the various players in the process, for example the more members of the primary care team and others that are involved in the assessment, the more likely it is that attention will be paid to the findings of the assessment.
5. Equity: improving the spatial allocation of resources between and within different groups.

The economic and ethical principle underlying assessment of health needs is the equitable distribution of health care resources. Equity is a difficult concept to analyse. It may help to differentiate between horizontal and vertical equity:

1. *Horizontal equity* is concerned with the equal treatment of equal need irrespective of socioeconomic background. This means that to be horizontally equitable, the health care allocation system must treat two individuals with the same complaint in an identical way (Culyer 1995).
2. *Vertical equity*, on the other hand, is concerned with the extent to which individuals who are 'unequal' should be treated differently (Sutton 2002). In health care it can be reflected by the aim of unequal treatment for unequal need in order to achieve equal health status; for example, higher health care investment in areas of greatest socioeconomic need. An example of this concept in practice is the national development of Children's Centres, 'Healthy living' programmes and the provision of additional funding to 'spearhead' Primary Care Trusts in areas of greatest deprivation. These public health programmes are targeted to the areas of highest socioeconomic deprivation.

1.2   Why is Assessing Needs and Priorities Important?

Wilkinson and Murray (1998) state that historically much health service provision has been service-rather than needs-led, designed and developed at the convenience of the providers rather than the patients. In the light of this, government policies have increasingly emphasised the need to assess health need prior to planning and delivering services.

The NHS has been and continues to operate within a framework of finite resources with escalating financial pressures. This is due in part to the expansion of coverage and development of more expensive health technologies, set against a backdrop of higher public expectations of their health care services. The general public has increased access to information, particularly through the internet, which has led people to demand a wider range of services of high quality from health care practitioners.

However, it is also widely recognised that many people have inequitable access to adequate health care. For example, socially marginal and economically deprived groups have the greatest overall need for health care but are least likely to obtain it. This has been described by Tudor Hart as the 'inverse care law' (Hart 1971; Wright *et al.* 1998). Similarly, Anderson and Mooney (1990) report that there is a large variation in availability and use of health care by geographical area and point of provision. This inequity can only be addressed by a systematic approach to determining health care needs and these factors have triggered reforms of health services in both developed and developing countries.

It is anticipated that medical advances and demographic changes, particularly the ageing population, will continue the upward pressure on costs and health service demand. In the light of these factors, the challenge today and for the future is to make decisions that maximise benefit for the population, taking into account the resources available. Needs assessment facilitates decision making and has been widely supported and advocated by successive government White Papers and legislation.

1.3   National Policy and Legislation Supporting Health Needs Assessment

In the last decade, national health policies have strengthened links between HNA and service commissioning. *Saving Lives: our healthier nation* (DH 1999) stressed the importance of the community's role in the identification of health needs and priorities and set out a family-centred public health role for health visitors, working with individuals, families and communities to improve health and tackle inequality. This document also served to challenge the traditional 'medical model' approach to health care, proposing a more inclusive model incorporating sociocultural and economic influences on health outcomes.

The New NHS: modern, dependable (DH 1997) identified the assessment of population health needs as an imperative for the delivery of modern effective health care. *Shifting the Balance of Power within the NHS: securing delivery* (DH 2001) allotted specific responsibility for this to Primary Care Trusts for responding to local health needs and commissioning effective health care services, stressing the importance of collaboration and partnership while continuing to emphasise the role of health care needs assessment.

The Wanless report *Securing Good Health for the Whole Population* (Wanless 2004) also emphasised the importance of high levels of public engagement in order to achieve optimum gains in health outcomes, without which the NHS would not be sustainable based on public funding in the longer term. Two White Papers followed the Wanless report as the government's means of taking forward the implementation of the Wanless agenda. *Choosing Health: making healthy choices easier* (DH 2004) set a blueprint for tackling health inequalities, smoking, rising levels of physical inactivity and obesity, sexual health problems, mental health problems and alcohol misuse – all important determinants of disease and health care need. The White Paper, *Our Health, Our Care, and Our Say: a new direction for community services* (DH 2006) points toward a shift from secondary care predominance to increasing reliance (and investment) in community services, making health services accessible to patients closer to the point of need. The important point is made that 90 per cent of people's contacts with the health service take place outside hospital. The future is to:

> Create health and social services that genuinely focus on prevention and promoting health and well-being; that deliver care in more local settings ... and deliver services that are flexible, integrated and responsive to people's needs and wishes. (DH 2006, p. 3)

In 2005 the government embarked on the third major reorganization of the NHS in England since 1997, arguably the most ambitious with far-reaching consequences for those working in the NHS and on the receiving end of its services. *Commissioning a Patient-led NHS* (DH 2005) outlined significant changes to the structure of the NHS and identified how the Department of Health should develop commissioning throughout the whole NHS system, with some changes in function for Primary Care Trusts and Strategic Health Authorities.

The current overall policy context is dominated by payment by results, practice-based commissioning, and patient choice. *Practice-based commissioning* is intended to liberate the talents of GPs and other front-line staff. It is designed to stimulate services that are more local, providing services that are based on the identified health needs of the local community and tailored to these needs. Choice is part of a cultural change within the NHS and one of the core principles of the NHS plan (DH 2000), advocating a far greater involvement of patients and the public in determining how their health care should be delivered. Chapter 5 provides further discussion on how to engage users in public health to improve health and wellbeing. Arguably, these aspirations can only be achieved through systematic HNAs to identify local health priorities and the involvement of local people and communities in these processes.

In the light of these changes and the drive to deliver more localised, needs-led health services, health care practitioners need to understand the complexities of the changing health care system in England, the impact it will have on how they work, and the context in which they will deliver health care services in the future. Practitioners will need to adopt a more collective view on health and consider the wider and complex needs of the community in collaboration and partnership with local people. HNA can be a useful tool in this process as a systematic methodology to target services and support toward the most disadvantaged groups in society.

1.4 Health, Health Need and Health Care Need

It is commonly accepted that the social and economic conditions under which people live impact on the health status of a population. However, the predominance of the medical model in British health care may have reduced awareness of factors that contribute to good health. Hall and Elliman (2003) assert that in the 21st century social, economic and environmental factors are more important than biological disorders as causes of ill health. 'Health needs' incorporates these wider social and environmental determinants of health.

1.4.1 Health

The World Health Organization's definition of health is often used as a holistic approach to health:

> Health is a state of complete physical, psychological, and social wellbeing and not simply the absence of disease or infirmity. (WHO 1999)

The World Health Organization defined the determinants of health as: social gradient, stress, early life, social exclusion, work, unemployment, social support, addiction, food and transportation. Consequently, analysis of deprivation in relation to health outcomes (i.e. mortality and health service utilization) is a major part of the HNA.

The socialization aspects of health should not be underestimated and typically reflect the wide variations within communities where both young and old live. People's ideas and perceptions about health will be mediated by their own experiences, learnt patterns of behaviour and the varying influences of key figures from their lives through the home, family, school and work environments. Housing, income, employment and access to goods and services, including health services, have all been recognised as important components of health. The preferred model of the determinants of health, states Beaglehole (1986), is dynamic and interactive, adopting a life course approach to health status, recognizing the complexity of the interplay between antenatal, early and later life influences on the development and maintenance of health and disease. Dahlgren and Whitehead (1991) have described the factors affecting health in a 'rainbow model' (Figure 1.1).

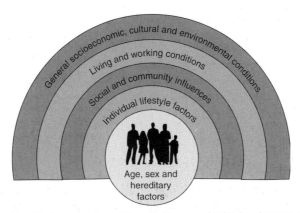

Figure 1.1 Determinants of health. *Source:* Adapted from Dahlgren and Whitehead (1991). Reproduced with permission.

The factors affecting health status are complex and multilayered. At the core of the diagram are age, sex and hereditary factors, which are key contributors to health, and are essentially fixed. Individual lifestyle factors such as whether a person smokes or exercises are choices made by the individual, but are also influenced by wider social, cultural, environmental and socioeconomic factors.

1.4.2   Health needs and health care needs

This wider definition allows us to look beyond the confines of the medical model based on health service provision, to the wider influences on health. The health needs of a population will be constantly changing, and many will not be amenable to medical intervention.

Meeting health need is not the exclusive responsibility of the health sector, but is rather the responsibility of multiple sectors and involves ongoing collaboration between health, education, housing, employment and welfare sectors. Nurses may need to advocate for patients where multiple external factors are impacting on their health – for example a health visitor may advocate for a family living in substandard accommodation which is impacting on the physical health of the children; or a nurse may need to advocate for a patient's need to be cared for at home. This is explored further in Chapter 16.

There is currently a significant debate around the responsibility of the individual to make 'healthy' choices. In July 2006, Tony Blair urged the nation to take more responsibility for its own health. In the second of a series of major speeches on domestic policy, the then prime minister argued that the government cannot make decisions for people in a bid to improve their wellbeing:

> The government can't be the only one with the responsibility if it's not the only one with the power. The responsibility must be shared and the individual helped but with an obligation also to help themselves. (Tony Blair, Nottingham, July 2006)

Blair also stated that:

> Our public health problems are not, strictly speaking, public health questions at all. They are questions of individual lifestyle – obesity, smoking, alcohol abuse, diabetes, sexually transmitted disease. They are the results of millions of individual decisions, at millions of points in time.

The issue of individual responsibility has become a topic of national debate and is likely to continue to be so into the future.

1.5   Need, Demand and Supply

Need is a critical concept in the pursuit of efficient health care and is equally critical to the development of services that are equitable (Mooney *et al.* 2004). In health care, need has a variety of meanings that may change over time, so it is not surprising that different groups of health professionals refer to 'needs assessment' in very different ways (Jordan & Wright 1997). It is important to recognise the different perspectives illuminating the relationship between the concepts of *need*, and *health care needs* (Asardi-Lari *et al.* 2003)

1.5.1   Need

In a sociological environment, Bradshaw (1972) divided 'need' into four types:

- normative need – distinguished by professionals, such as vaccination;
- felt need – wants, wishes and desires;
- expressed need – vocalised needs or how people use services;
- comparative need –needs arising in one location may be similar for people with similar sociodemo-graphic characteristics living in another location.

Bradshaw's taxonomy of need creates a definition which is more practical for health service research workers, although it does acknowledge the concept of cost containment. Bradshaw (1994) argued that his taxonomy of need was constrained because of inherent problems with the concept of need. This issue is yet to be resolved as there is still no consensus as to what constitutes 'need'.

The most widely presented definition of need favoured by economists is 'the ability of people to benefit from health care provision' (Stevens & Gillam 1998); in other words, 'need' exists only if there is a 'capacity to benefit' from a particular health care service. As such it is differentiated from demand, which arises when someone with a need for care expresses it.

1.5.2 Supply and demand

Wright *et al.* (1998) state that in recognition of the scarcity of resources available to meet these needs, health needs are often differentiated as needs, demands and supply:

- Need is defined as the ability to benefit from health care, i.e. a measurable change in health status attributable to the intervention.
- Demand is what people ask for. It is not necessarily what they need, i.e. they may not benefit or may not meet NHS eligibility criteria. GPs and consultants have a key role as gatekeepers in controlling demand, and waiting lists become a surrogate marker for and an influence on it.
- Supply, that is the health care interventions and services that are available to the population, including the resources that are made available by the NHS. This will depend on the interests of health professionals, the priorities of politicians and the amount of money available.

Need, demand and supply overlap and this relation is important to consider when assessing health needs (Figure 1.2).

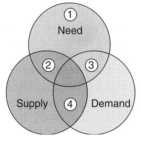

Examples:

① Treatment of child abusers
② Health promotion, some screening
③ Terminations of pregnancy, waiting lists
④ Antibiotics for viral upper respiratory tract infections

Figure 1.2   Relation between need, supply and demand – central area shows ideal relation. *Source:* Modified from Stevens and Raftery (1994). Reproduced with permission from the BMJ Publishing Group Ltd.

1.5.3 Health care need

The term 'health care need', according to Wright *et al.* (1998), can be used to describe a population's need for the provision of particular health care services and those that can benefit from health care (health education, disease prevention, diagnosis, treatment, rehabilitation, end of life care). Most doctors will consider needs in terms of the health care services that they can supply. Patients, however, may have a different view of what would make them healthier – for example, a job, decent housing or access to affordable leisure facilities.

In an analysis of the resources necessary for the effective provision of health care, health care needs assessment not only reflects the prevalence or incidence of the condition or disease state concerned, but the number of individuals likely to benefit from treatment and for whom treatment is generally regarded as a reasonable investment for a publicly funded treatment. An example of this is the much debated (2006) issue of Herceptin prescribing for women with early breast cancer.

There needs to be some consideration of the effectiveness, including cost-effectiveness, of services in which an investment is being considered. Because available resources in all health care systems are finite, and demand will always outstrip supply, prioritization of health service purchasing is necessary.

1.6 Approaches to Health Needs Assessment

Wright *et al.* (1998) state that a comprehensive HNA involves an epidemiological (quantitative) and qualitative approach to determining priorities, and should incorporate clinical and cost-effectiveness and patients' perspectives. This approach must also balance clinical, ethical and economic considerations of need – that is, what should be done, what can be done and what can be afforded (Black 1994).

In practice three types of needs assessment have been described: epidemiological, comparative and corporate (Stevens & Raftery 1994).

1. *Epidemiological* statistics measure the total amount of ill health in the community, for example mortality and morbidity statistics. Indicators of deprivation are used to identify groups of people who may experience social and economic disadvantage, for example unemployment rates. Such quantitative measures have been used to underpin government health policy and to enable the government to target resources to those most in need. An example of this is the development of Children's Centres, which local authorities are tasked with developing, initially in the 20 per cent most socially and economically deprived areas.

   The epidemiological approach to HNA has three elements:

   - determining the incidence and/or prevalence of the health problem;
   - identifying the effectiveness (and cost-effectiveness) of existing interventions for the problem;
   - identifying the current level of service provision.

This combination of epidemiological (health status assessments) and evidence (effectiveness/cost-effectiveness) has also been described as an *evidence-based approach* to HNA. Chapter 3 offers a detailed analysis of how to undertake a HNA using the epidemiological approach.

2. *Comparative* need is defined as existing where the population of one area has a lower uptake of a particular intervention than that of another area, after adjustment for any differences in age or other population characteristics. These could be cross-national comparisons, for example comparing England with other countries in Europe, or comparisons at a more local level or comparing the service provision in one town or locality with another that has similar demography. A common approach is to compare a GP practice with evidence-based guidance such as the National Service Framework or those from NICE.
3. The *corporate* approach involves the systematic collection of the expert knowledge and views of informants on health care services and needs. Valuable information is often available from health authority staff, provider clinicians and GPs, as well as from local people. Ideally, some system of formal consensus development should be used (Stevens *et al.* 1998). In the context of the NHS, this corporate approach has been widely used, and was encouraged in the 1989 health reforms and the emphasis on partnership and collaboration in the 1997 White Paper (DH 1997).

Each of these approaches requires a considerable amount of resources and can be time intensive. A comprehensive needs assessment usually involves a combination of all three approaches.

An alternative model, *rapid appraisal*, offers certain advantages in such circumstances (Rikkin 1992). This is a multidisciplinary approach that incorporates flexibility and innovation and which draws extensively on the views of the local community (Murray 1999). It is quick, as its name indicates, and it emphasises timely insights and 'best bets' rather than final truths. It involves using key informants to build up a community health profile. This approach has been used to enhance community involvement in developed countries (Ong *et al.* 1991). Information is collected on nine issues, in an 'information pyramid' (Figure 1.3).

The bottom layer defines the structure and composition of the community and how it is organised. The second layer is concerned with socioeconomic influences on health. The third layer looks at resources in the community, including their accessibility and acceptability. The top layer looks at national, regional and local health policies (Brown *et al.* 2006). This information, taken together, can then inform current service provision, identify the views of local residents and stakeholders, and make recommendations for health improvements.

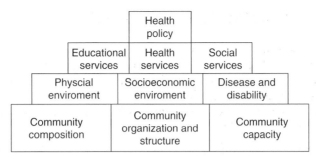

Figure 1.3 Rapid appraisal information pyramid. *Source:* Brown, Lloyd and Murray (2006).

There are other contemporary approaches to service-related assessment of need; these include social services assessments, individual health care needs assessment, and population and client group surveys, for example.

In the light of the limitations of these approaches to HNA, Stevens and Raftery (1994) have developed what has been described as the *pragmatic approach* to assessment of need. This draws on the data from a variety of sources. Information on the epidemiology of the condition in question is given concisely, the range of possible interventions is defined, and evidence for the effectiveness of each one is summarised. This is reflected in the literature as there is an increasing focus on strategies for assessing needs which allow the use of multiple data sources to interpret the diverse and wide ranging needs that are found within the community (Carey 1999). Assessment of need for health care, using whichever of these models is appropriate, is a prerequisite for the optimal allocation of resources. The advantages and disadvantages of these approaches are summarised in Table 1.1. A combination approach is more likely to reflect reality, however, than using one method alone (Figure 1.4).

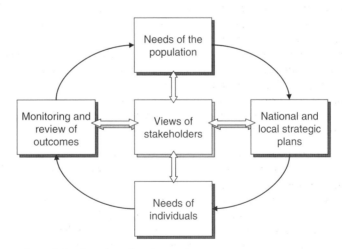

Figure 1.4 The process of population based needs assessment.

1. 7 Health Needs Assessment: Practical Approaches

There is no single best way of assessing the needs of a particular target population in a local area. The methods that you use will be completely dependent upon who your target population is, and what you want to find out about that population.

Table 1.1 Advantages and disadvantages in approaches to health needs assessment.

Needs assessment approach	Advantages	Disadvantages	Source of information
Epidemiology	Gives overall figures of numbers likely to have specific problems (e.g. cancer, depression, hypertension) Relatively quick and easy, can be done from a desk top Identifies the broad range of clinical conditions and their likely prevalence Systematic and objective	Assumes uniform prevalence, although can be weighted (crudely) for known risk factors, e.g. deprivation. Can tend toward medical rather than social needs This approach is only possible for some conditions, where there is straightforward means of identifying those with clinical indications Frequent lack of existing local epidemiological data and lack of evidence for certain interventions Carrying out new epidemiological work is also costly and time consuming	ONS surveys of morbidity/ mortality Hospital episode statistics Compendium of clinical and health indicators Census data Screening data Public health observatories, www.swpho.org.uk National statistics, www.statistics.gov.uk Neighbourhood statistics, www.statistics.gov.uk
Comparative	Sets local service provision against national norms Good for identifying inequalities. Uses existing data and multiple sources of information	Relationship unclear between provision, utilization of services and actual need Assumes that the intervention rate in the area where it is higher is the correct one – fails to take account of differences in disease prevalence rates or of previous treatment	Prescribing data GP practice based data (disease registers) Hospital activity data Screening uptake data/ vaccination uptake Car ownership, employment, age profiles, housing tenure, self-reported limited illness Indices of deprivation 2000
Corporative	Involves local health care providers and local people Responsive to local concerns and fosters local ownership of the issues	If carried out in isolation may determine demands rather than needs and stakeholder concerns may be influenced by the political agenda Risks legitimizing existing patterns of care that may have little rational basis	Sources of information for this methodology can be drawn from any of the other three approaches – using local/ national quantitative data and qualitative data such as focus groups/interview and surveys
Rapid Appraisal	Good for community profiling Highly participative Good qualitative information	Does not generate statistics for planning purposes Subjective May raise local expectations	Local informants Local information/ reports – practice profiles, community directories Semistructured interviews Questionnaires Focus groups Observation of community

ONS, Office for National Statistics.

The HDA (2005) suggests that the HNA population can be identified as people sharing:

- geographic location – e.g. living in deprived neighbourhoods or housing estates;
- settings – e.g. schools, prisons, workplaces;
- social experience – e.g. asylum seekers, specific age groups, ethnicity, sexuality, homelessness, drug/alcohol use;
- experience of a particular medical condition – e.g. mental illness, coronary heart disease, cancer.

A target population can also be identified through a combination of main and subcategory groups, e.g. children under 5 years living in a deprived neighbourhood. Levels of HNA range from individual contact between the health care professional and the client, to local, national and international assessment (e.g. by the World Health Organization) of population health needs (Wilkinson & Murray 1998).

1.7.1 Criteria for choosing priorities

Four explicit criteria are at the core of the HNA process (Hooper & Longworth 2002), and are used throughout this chapter to help clarify thinking and lead to changes that will improve health.

1. What are the conditions/factors that have the most significant *impact*, in terms of severity and size, in health functioning?
2. Can the most significant conditions/factors be effectively *changed* by those involved in the assessment?
3. What are the most *acceptable* changes required for the maximum positive impact?
4. Are the resource implications of these changes *feasible*?

It is important that the practitioner considers the principles and criteria for HNA when deciding whether to embark on a formal health needs assessment project.

1.7.2 The HNA project team

Before you begin a needs assessment it is important to determine who needs to be involved in the process and that there is sign-up to the project from senior managers and local policy makers (if appropriate). As the assessment is likely to involve other agencies it is useful to consider the need to involve partners from the local authority (e.g. social services, education), local voluntary agencies, community groups and the police.

It is essential to appoint a team leader who will take responsibility for the overall management of the project and to set up a steering group whose remit is to lead the needs assessment. The project manager then reports to the steering group. It is the task of this group to ensure that the process is done properly, that it is completed within a reasonable timescale, and that the findings result in action. The team must have established a need for the project and have clear aims and objectives for what they want to achieve that are realistic and deliverable.

Hooper and Longworth (2002) suggest that those involved in the process should comprise:

- those who know about the issues relating to the target population: service providers or practitioners, and people with research expertise in the area;
- those who care about those issues: representatives from the target population, from family or carer groups, or from the wider community;
- those who can make changes happen: managers of appropriate partner organizations/agencies, service planners and commissioners.

The benefits of undertaking an HNA from a multidisciplinary team perspective include:

- improved team and partnership working;
- professional development of skills and experience of HNA;
- improved communication with other agencies;
- strengthened community involvement in decision making;
- identification of local health need and inequalities within the target population;
- improved patient care with better use of health resources (Hooper & Longworth 2002).

The primary outcomes of an HNA are a set of recommendations, an action strategy based on the evidence gathered about the population, and the identification of effective and acceptable interventions. These should be used to influence policy and service delivery in order to improve health outcomes.

1.8 A Framework for Assessing the Health Needs of a Population

Various tools and guides have been produced by individuals and organizations in recent years to assist practitioners undertaking HNAs. Cavanagh and Chadwick (2005) have produced a revised practical guide *Health Needs Assessment* based on the work of Hooper and Longworth (2002) outlining a five-step process to undertake an HNA.

This framework has been recognised as a flexible, systematic process that has been well tried, tested and refined over several years and provides practitioners with a consistent process for undertaking an HNA (Cavanagh & Chadwick 2005). However, it needs to be noted that health profiling alone is not HNA, nor is undertaking a rapid appraisal exercise, but both can contribute.

Table 1.2 summarises the questions or steps involved in a formal HNA project and can be used as a guide for practitioners in undertaking an HNA. It is important to recognise that the process seldom follows a linear path through the steps and, in essence, an HNA can be approached in much the same way as doing a jigsaw, so that different pieces are put together to give a complete picture of local health (Figure 1.5). Practitioners can follow these steps to systematically develop a local HNA within an area

Table 1.2 Steps involved in a formal health needs assessment project. *Source:* NICE (2005). Reproduced with permission.

	Aim	Outcome
Step 1: getting started	What population? What are you trying to achieve? Who needs to be involved? What resources are required? What are the risks?	A clear definition of the population you are going to assess and a clear rationale for the assessment and its boundaries Agreement to proceed with allocation of resources required for the project Project lead and steering group identified Project plan in place with timescales for each task
Step 2: identifying health priorities	Population profiling Gathering data Perceptions of needs Identifying and assessing health conditions and determinant factors	A short list of health priorities identified for the profiled population with a profile of these issues Using the first two explicit criteria: Impact Changeability A limited number of overall health priorities determined; check these with the steering group and other stakeholders
Step 3: assessing a health priority for action	Assessment of a specific health priority for action Determining effective and acceptable interventions and actions	Health conditions/determinant factors selected that have the most significant impact on health functioning for the selected health priority Be sure the action is focused on reducing health inequalities for that health priority Acceptable and cost-efficient actions to improve the selected health priority are identified
Step 4: planning for change	Clarifying aims of intervention Action planning Monitoring and evaluation strategy Risk management strategy	A clear set of aims, objectives, indicators and targets agreed Set out the actions and tasks you need to undertake to achieve these Agreement on how to evaluate your programme Key risks to the success of the programme are identified and how they will be managed
Step 5: moving on/review	Learning from the project Measuring impact Choosing the next priority	What went well, and why? What did not go well, and why? Is any further action required? Identify further action to be taken

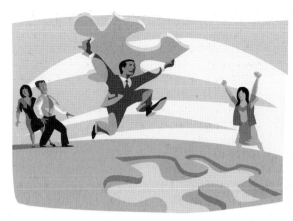

Figure 1.5　Completing the 'Local Picture'.

of practice. Examples of HNAs undertaken using this framework in a variety of settings can be found in *Health Needs Assessment: a practical guide* (Cavanagh & Chadwick 2005).

1.9　Community Health Needs Assessment and Health Profiling

1.9.1　Community health needs assessment

Community HNA is a process that:

- describes the state of health of local people;
- enables the identification of the major risk factors and causes of ill health;
- enables the identification of the actions needed to address these.

A community HNA may not be a one-off activity but can be a developmental process that is added to and amended over time. It should not be an end in itself but a way of using information to plan health care and public health programmes in the future. The steps of a community HNA are as follow.

1. Profiling: the collection of relevant information that will inform the community HNA about the state of health and health needs of the population, and analysis of this information to identify the major health issues.
2. Deciding on priorities for action.
3. Planning public health and health care programmes to address the priority issues.
4. Implementing the planned activities.
5. Evaluation of health outcomes.

These stages correspond to the Cavanagh and Chadwick (2005) five-step process.

1.9.2　Health profiling

Health profiling is a method by which needs are assessed and uses mainly quantitative data, such as statistical information. Within the five-step process described by Cavanagh and Chadwick (2005) this is step 2. Qualitative health data such as individual assessments and client perceptions can also be incorporated to give a more holistic assessment. On completion of the profiling the community HNA will be in a position to:

- describe the state of health of local people;
- identify the major risk factors and causes of ill health;
- identify the actions needed to address these.

An example of this can be found in the case study presented in Box 1.1.

BOX 1.1

Profile information

1 *Characteristics of the population*
  - Geography
  - Numbers
  - Age distribution
  - Gender distribution
  - Ethnicity and religion
  - Population trends
  - Educational factors

2 *Health status of the population* (measures of health)
  - Mortality
  - Morbidity
  - Low birth weight
  - Disease prevalence
  - Health behaviours – smoking/alcohol/drug use
  - Use of local health services

3 *Local factors affecting health*
  - Work and employment
  - Poverty and income
  - Environment
  - Transport
  - Access to leisure services

4 *Health concerns and priorities of the local community*
  - Interviews
  - Focus groups
  - Community/residents survey

5 *Local and national priorities and targets*

Health profiling for nurses and multiagency teams can take place in four key areas:

1. *Community* – assessment of need with a neighbourhood or district.
2. *Practice* – an assessment of need within a registered GP population.
3. *Caseload* – an assessment of need within a specific caseload of a nurse/health visitor/allied health professional.
4. *School health profile* – a framework to encourage and support school-based partnerships, establish the health profile of the school community, identify priorities for action, and agree the most effective way forward.

Each of these profiles may contribute to another – for example a GP practice profile or school health profile may contribute to the wider community profile. Once the health profile is complete, steps 3–5 (see Table 1.2) need to be progressed through to determine the priorities for action, to plan the intervention to address the priority, and to implement the service and evaluate the effectiveness of the intervention, making appropriate changes as required.

The framework offered by the health profile with its multiple data sources allows a comprehensive picture of health needs to emerge. Nurses and public health practitioners are now in a unique position to effectively contribute to a health profile and can use this tool in any area of their work to identify health needs. It is then about translating identified needs into service provision. An example of an HNA can be seen in Table 1.3. Further examples can be found in the *Health Needs Assessment Workbook* (Hooper & Longworth 2002).

1.10 Individual/Patient Health Status and Health Needs Assessment

The distinction between individual needs and the wider needs of the community is important to consider when assessing needs. Commonly, the health status of patients is evaluated according to clinical tests, for example blood tests, scans and X-rays. In recent years there has been an increasing interest in evaluating the health status of patients through self-completed responses to questions about health status. There are also general or generic measures (often referred to as 'quality of life' measures) designed to evaluate the 'overall' health status of individuals or groups. These are intended to be equally applicable to all irrespective of health status, gender or ethnicity and give an indication as to the 'felt' needs of the respondents.

There are important contributions that the individual health assessment record can make to two important population-based tasks (National Architecture Design Board Health Information Service for Wales 2006):

1. The management of groups of individuals in a population in order to provide care directly to each individual, such as chronic disease management and screening.
2. The management of information about a population in order to understand the population itself for purposes such as epidemiology, health services management and planning.

Table 1.3 Health needs assessment in action. Source: Bournemouth Teaching Primary Care Trust, Clinical Services and Public Health Directorates (2005).

Step	Outcome
Target population	Drug-using adults (18 years and over) accessing a local drop-in drug support service
Why chosen?	There is an acknowledged drug/substance misuse problem in the area, which is centred on one part of the town. An estimated 1 in 44 of the local population are presenting to substance misuse treatment services, compared to 1 in 75 in the county It was recognised by the local drop-in drug service that there was an unmet need for access to health services, particularly for hepatitis C screening and hepatitis B vaccination
Aims and objectives	To improve the health and wellbeing of people who are actively using drugs and reduce inequalities in access to local health services; to determine the need for a blood-borne virus service to this particular vulnerable group
Project team	A multiagency steering group was established with representatives from the PCT (public health, clinical services, pharmacy advisor), hospital staff (consultant gastroenterologist, nurse specialist for blood-borne viruses), local GPs, project manager from the drop-in drug service and other local providers of drug services. A project lead was designated to manage the process
Identifying health priorities	Information was gathered from a variety of sources including national, regional and local data re prevalence of hepatitis B and C; referral data from GPs to hospital services re GP attendances within the geographical location; data from local drug service providers re health status of the service users and numbers registered with a local GP The views of the service users and their families were elicited using interviews and focus groups The views of local GPs and primary care practitioners were included and the views of the specialist hospital services
Key issues identified	The key concerns from health service providers and the target population were the lack of access to advice, screening, counselling and support in relation to the transmission of blood-borne viruses – namely HBV and HCV and to accessing hepatitis B immunization

(Continued)

Table 1.3   (Continued)

Step	Outcome
Assessing a health priority for action	The health priority for action was determined as being the need to develop a blood-borne virus service to the local drug- using population. This approach to providing targeted health services to this group is supported by the government's 10-year strategy for tackling drug misuse *Tackling Drugs to Build a Better Britain*, and is informed by a number of guidance documents The steering group developed a plan to: ● develop an access site for serological testing for blood- borne viruses (HBV, HCV, HIV) for current drug users ● provide a programme for hepatitis B immunization ● provide hepatitis A immunization as appropriate ● provide education, harm minimization services and raise awareness of blood-borne viruses through health promotion ● advise on accessing services and referral pathways ● to involve service users in the planning, implementation and evaluation of this project The expansion of opportunities for voluntary HCV testing and proactive targeted testing and immunization for hepatitis B, accompanied by appropriate counselling and support, has been recommended by the Advisory Council for the Misuse of Drugs and the National Treatment Agency
Resource Implications	Funding required to develop a new service. The National Treatment Agency provided £21 000 and the local drug action team £14 000. Total budget for this service £35 000
Planning for change	The steering group, led by the project manager, developed a full business proposal for the blood-borne virus project within the financial envelope available. This included identifying clear health outcomes and measurable targets, full costing for implementation, clinical governance and risk management issues The business plan was then consulted on through the PCT, Hospital Trust, local drug service providers and local service users. It was then agreed and signed off by the PCT and Hospital Trust who would deliver the service The plan identified the tasks and designated lead managers to implement the service
Moving on/ review	The service went live in May 2005 and is now an established outreach service targeting current injecting drug users and those clients who are in early recovery. This is a difficult group of clients to reach as they are unlikely to access traditional health care services via a GP and often have chaotic lifestyles
What was achieved?	The service offers HIV, HCV and HBV testing and HAV and HBV immunization. Clients also seek advice on sexual health issues and general health concerns which need to be addressed
How did it contribute to reducing inequalities?	The service operates from four sites across the town, accessible to the target population. There is joint working between primary and secondary care and opportunity for referral into secondary care. It also offers continuity and increases access to services In the first 6 months of the service 62 sessions were held seeing a total of 378 clients; of these 28 were diagnosed with chronic hepatitis C infection; 2 with chronic hepatitis B infection (and 9 with a previous infection and acquired immunity). The results were shared with the registered GP and 11 were then referred to secondary care services
Next steps	This service was set up with a finite financial resource allocation. The plan is to embed this service as part of the PCT service provision to drug-using clients by securing ongoing funding A new service is being developed at the Big Issue offices in the town. The PCT also hope to expand the sessions at this new location to target the homeless. The service has been approached by staff from The Soup Kitchen based in the town that are keen for the service to expand and offer testing at this location A significant percentage of the females seen by the service are 'working girls' and sexual health advice is also an important part of the information offered to this group. There may be a need to offer testing for Syphilis as well as the main blood-borne viruses. This will need further assessment

HAV, hepatitis A virus; HBV, hepatitis B virus; HCV, hepatitis C virus; HIV, human immunodeficiency virus; PCT, Primary Care Trust.

The individual health assessment is now being designed to bring together information from many sources and incorporate it into a consistent single record. Examples of this are seen in the elderly services with the *single assessment process* (SAP) and in children's services with the *common assessment framework* (CAF). Such single assessment processes are well positioned to provide information and to identify circumstances requiring action that spans providers. Furthermore, the information can also be used collectively to give health and social care information regarding neighbourhoods and communities and to assist in community needs assessment and health care planning.

Within the context of children's services, it has been recognised that a number of factors will impinge on the health and wellbeing of children and young people and their families that can also have a significant impact on physical and emotional health. Capturing the health and social care needs of children and families can play an important part in determining the health needs of local communities and in determining local interventions to meet identified needs.

To assist this process an assessment tool – the common assessment framework (DfES 2006) – has been developed and is currently being implemented in practice. Chapter 13 looks specifically at this assessment as a means of identifying needs and how it can be effectively used in practice.

1.10.1   The common assessment framework

The CAF for children and young people as outlined in the 'Every child matters' agenda (DfES 2006) is a key part of the strategy to shift the focus from dealing with the consequences of difficulties in children's lives to preventing things from going wrong in the first place. The CAF enables the implementation of a common approach to needs assessment that can be used by the whole children's workforce, whether they are in universal or specialist services, for any child in need of support. The key aims of CAF are to:

- make it easier and quicker for children and young people who have additional needs to get extra help;
- reduce the number of times that children and families are assessed or asked for the same information;
- improve the way people working with the same child or young person work together and share information.

The CAF will promote more effective, earlier identification of children's additional needs and improve multiagency working. It will also facilitate the resource management of children's health and social services to areas of greatest need by identifying communities/neighbourhoods with children and young people requiring additional services.

There are three stages in the CAF process which have assessment forms to support the stages.

Activity

Why not visit www.ecm.gov.uk/caf and explore the assessment tools used in this process? To help with this, the stages in the CAF process can be seen in Figure 1.6, and the following is a brief summary of the main steps.

---

1. *Preparation.* The practitioner recognises a potential unmet need for a child; information already known about the child and family is gathered and considered with the involvement and consent of the child (if age allows) and the parent/carer. Once this is completed a decision is made by the practitioner, in partnership with the child and parent/carer, whether or not to undertake a CAF.
2. *Discussion.* The practitioner completes the assessment, involving others as appropriate – for example, other family members and other professionals involved with the family. The assessment will identify areas of unmet need and what may help improve the outcomes for the child.
3. *Delivery.* This involves implementing the agreed action plan with the cooperation of the child and family, and monitoring and evaluating the impact of the plan on the child and family.

An example of how this assessment process has been used in practice through a multidisciplinary team approach is demonstrated through a case study in Box 1.2.

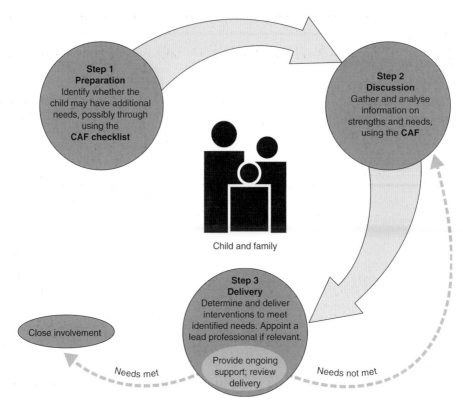

Figure 1.6   The common assessment framework in practice. *Source:* DfES (2006). Reproduced with permission.

1.11   Population Screening

A method of determining the health needs of the population is through screening programmes. Population screening is a significant departure from the clinical model of care, because it involves apparently healthy individuals being approached proactively or opportunistically by the health service. In the UK, screening programmes are approved by the National Screening Committee (NSC). The NSC defines screening as:

> [A] public health service in which members of a defined population, who do not necessarily perceive they are at risk of, or are already affected by a disease or its complications, are asked a question or offered a test, to identify those individuals who are more likely to be helped than harmed by further tests or treatment to reduce the risk of a disease or its complications. (www.nsc.nhs.uk)

Many screening programmes (both systematic and opportunistic) are currently available in England with further programmes under review, for example the Diabetes, Heart Disease and Stroke Pilot Programme (www.nelh.nhs.uk/screening/diabetesproject(England)).

It is important to note that screening is not appropriate for all conditions. The decision to screen healthy people for a disease depends on many factors, including the test's ability to accurately detect or rule out the condition, the nature of the disease, the characteristics of the population and the ability of the health care system to cope with diagnosis, treatment and follow-up (BMA 2005). There are strict criteria in place to determine whether a programme should be considered. These are based on the classic criteria first promulgated by the World Health Organization in the 1960s, but take into account both the more rigorous standards of evidence required to improve effectiveness and the greater concern about the adverse effects of health care.

BOX 1.2

Case study example: early intervention. Source: Bournemouth Teaching Primary Care Trust (2005)

Joint working to identify needs

Tim is a 10-year-old boy who was experiencing ongoing behavioural difficulties at home and school; poor personal hygiene; social isolation / no friends; emotional preoccupation with symptoms of obsessive compulsive disorder (strong family history of mental health problems); and a poor relationship with his parent. Tim lives in a single parent family and is the only child. He has had no contact with his father since the age of 4 years.

Multiagency approach

Common assessment framework (CAF) presentation and discussion at the team meeting. Core group invited: special educational needs coordination officer (SENCO), teaching assistant, social worker, learning support advisory teacher, behaviour support advisory teacher, educational psychologist, child care and family support manager, family resources manager, and primary mental health worker for children.

Action plan

- Social worker to make referral to family support team to facilitate improvements in relationship between mother and child. Explore resources available for out of school activities
- Mental health assessment; home visit planned and individual sessions with Tim in school. Short-term work planned for joint sessions with Tim and his mother with a view to informing assessment and joint parent/child work required
- Additional support in school from behaviour support service; introduction of 'Circle of friends' and additional training for teaching staff re behavioural management
- Involvement of school nurse to address issues of personal hygiene through class work rather than single Tim out

Lead professional

SENCO identified as he has had the most involvement with Tim (all those involved in case to report progress to lead professional).

Outcomes

- Improving relationship with mother through supportive family work and individual sessions with Tim
- Greater self-awareness regarding his symptoms of repetitive behaviour; acknowledging that he was not mentally ill should serve to diminish this behaviour
- Increased confidence in himself and establishing his own identity through direct work with the primary mental health worker; evidenced by his interactions in school and improved behaviour at home
- Increased integration with his peers in school through 'Circle of friends' and nurturing group
- Noticeable improvement in his personal presentation; paying more attention to his appearance with the support from his mother

---

The NSC recognises four major age categories of testing: (i) antenatal; (ii) child; (iii) adult; and (iv) old age. The details of the screening programmes within each area, current policies, and timetables for reconsidering current practice and considering new screening programmes can be viewed at the NSC website, www.nsc.nhs.uk.

Activity

Visit the www.nsc.nhs.uk website and explore more about national screening

---

1.11.1   Systematic screening programmes

These are formal programmes that invite all members of a certain population to take a test, for example the breast screening programme where all women between 50 and 70 years routinely receive invitations to have a breast examination, the cervical screening programme targeting women between the ages of 24 and 50 years, and more recently the bowel screening programme initiated in April 2006.

Activity

Visit the www.cancerscreening.nhs.uk website and develop your knowledge of screening and identify your risk of disease.

1.11.2 Opportunistic screening programmes

These programmes are aimed more at individuals who are at risk, although these people may be reluctant to admit their eligibility for screening. An example of this is sexually transmitted infection (STI) screening where the test is offered to the target population as and when they are in contact with the health service at the primary care level, e.g. all pregnant women are offered HIV testing as part of their antenatal care. Chlamydia screening is another example of an opportunistic screening programme aimed at young people aged 16–24 years that is currently being extended across England.

Activity

Visit the www.dh.gov.uk website and explore policies and guidance on the National Chlamydia Screening Programme.

1.11.3 Screening for inherited disorders

Newborn screening is the only population-based type of screening for inherited disorders. One public health benefit of population-based screening means that everyone is tested. This is especially useful for studying inherited disorders, since it permits scientists to determine with great accuracy how frequently some inherited disorders occur in the general population.

1.11.4 Uptake of the national screening programmes

As with other areas of the NHS, there are issues around equity of access to screening programmes. Independent assessment of screening programmes has revealed significant variation in access to services by geography, socioeconomic status and ethnicity (BMA 2005). For example, there is poorer uptake of breast and cervical cancer screening among women from black and ethnic minority groups. It is also recognised that people with learning disabilities often do not have suitable information and support to help them to decide whether to attend screening. There are measures set out in the Department of Health 2004 White Paper, *Choosing Health*, to tackle these inequalities; these include specific measures to increase screening uptake. It is recommended practice that Primary Care Trusts in England should use tools such as health equity audits to gain an understanding as to why some groups are less likely to attend screening, and use this information to implement ways of improving access.

Activity

For more information on health equity audits see HDA (2005) *Clarifying Approaches to: Health Needs Assessment, Health Impact Assessment, Integrated Impact Assessment, Health Equity Audit, and Race Equality Impact Assessment*. Visit www.screening.nhs.uk to view more information for health professionals in the UK.

Activity

Visit the websites below and see if you can identify which programmes represent systematic screening and which ones represent opportunistic screening:

- www.nehl.uk/screening/diabetesproject(England)
- www.cancerscreening.nhs.uk(England)
- www.dh.gov.uk.

Activity

Before reading the conclusion, why not review the case study example in Box 1.2 on early intervention and what it can achieve.

Conclusion

This chapter is but the start of the journey for nurses to understand the complexities of health and health care needs assessment. We have seen health needs assessment aims to ensure that health services are provided in an equitable and effective way to the target population. The challenge for health practitioners in achieving this is firstly to understand the practicalities of health needs assessment and the tools and skills required to undertake this systematic process. Secondly, the practitioner needs to ensure that the results of the needs assessment are integrated into local health care planning and commissioning of services to achieve effective change.

Nurses working in the community are in the unique position to be able to combine accessibility and acceptability of health care, health skills, knowledge of health and social care systems, and understanding of health determinants in their day to day work. They are also able to work at individual and population levels. Arguably this combination offers a huge potential for health improvement work and in contributing effectively to both the individual and wider health needs assessments of local communities and targeted groups.

References

Anderson T.V., Mooney, G. (1990) *The Challenge of Medical Practice Variations*. London: Macmillan.

Asadi-Lari M., Packham C., Gray D. (2003) Need for redefining needs. *Health and Quality of Life Outcome* 1, 34.

Beaglehole R. (1986) Medical management and the decline in mortality from coronary heart disease. *British Medical Journal* 292, 33.

Billings J. (1996) *Profiling for Health: the process and the practice*. London: Health Visitors Association.

Billings J. (1999) *Profiling Health Needs* In: *Profiling Health Needs in Public Health in Policy and Practice – a sourcebook for health visitors and community nurses* (ed. Cowley S). London: Bailliere Tindall.

Billings J., Cowley S. (1995) Approaches to community needs assessment: a literature review. *Journal of Advanced Nursing* 22, 721–30.

Black D. (1994) *A doctor looks at health economics*. Office of Health Economics Annual Lecture. London: Office of Health Economics.

BMA (British Medical Association) (2005) *Population Screening and Genetic Testing – a briefing on current programmes and technologies*. London: Board of Science.

Bournemouth Teaching Primary Care Trust (2005) *Profile Tool*. Bournemouth: Clinical Services and Public Health Directorate, Bournemouth PCT.

Bradshaw J. (1972) The concept of social need. *New Society* 30, 640–3.

Bradshaw J. (1994) The contextualisation and measurement of need: a social policy perspective. In: *Researching the People's Health* (eds Popay J., Williams G.). London: Routledge.

Brown C.S., Lloyd S., Murray S.A. (2006) Using consecutive rapid participatory appraisal studies to assess facilitate and evaluate health and social change in community settings. *BMC Public Health* 6, 68.

Carey L. (1999) Using health profiling as a tool for needs assessment. Supplement: learning curve. *Nursing Times* 95 (5), S6–S7.

Cavanagh S., Chadwick K. (2005) *Health Needs Assessment: a practical guide*. London: Health Development Agency.

Culyer A.J. (1995) Need: the idea won't do – but we still need it. *Social Science and Medicine* 40, 727–30.

Dahlgren G., Whitehead M. (1991) *Policies and Strategies to Promote Social Equity in Health*. Stockholm: Stockholm Institute of Future Studies.

DfES (Department for Education and Skills) (2006) *Common Assessment Framework for Children and Young People: a manager's guide*. London: Department for Education and Skills.

DH (Department of Health) (1997) *The New NHS: modern, dependable*. London: HM Stationery Office.

DH (Department of Health) (1999) *Saving Lives: our healthier nation*. London: HM Stationery Office.

DH (Department of Health) (2000) *The NHS Plan: a plan for investment, a plan for reform*. London: HM Stationery Office.

DH (Department of Health) (2001) *Shifting the Balance of Power within the NHS: securing delivery*. London: HM Stationery Office.

DH (Department of Health) (2004) *Choosing Health: making healthy choices easier*. London: HM Stationery Office.

DH (Department of Health) (2005) *Commissioning a Patient-led NHS (CPLNHS)*. London: Department of Health, Stationery Office.

DH (Department of Health) (2006) *Our Health, Our Care, and Our Say: a new direction for community services*. London: Department of Health, HM Stationery Office.

Hall D., Elliman D. (eds) (2003) *Health for All Children*, 4th edn. Oxford: Oxford University Press.

Hart T. (1971) The inverse care law. *Lancet* i, 405–12.

HDA (Health Development Agency) (2005) *Clarifying Approaches to: Health Needs Assessment, Health Impact Assessment, Integrated Impact Assessment, Health Equity Audit, and Race Equality Impact Assessment*. London: Health Development Agency.

Hooper J., Longworth P. (2002) *Health Needs Assessment Workbook*. London: Health Development Agency. www.hda.nhs.uk/publications.

Jordan J., Wright J. (1997) Making sense of health needs assessment. *British Journal of General Practice* 47 (424), 695–6.

McKee M., Figueras J. (2004) Strategies for health services. In: *Oxford Textbook of Public Health*, 4th edn (eds Detels R., McEwen J., Beaglehole R., Tanaka H.). Oxford: Oxford University Press.

Mooney G. (1994) *Key Issues in Health Economics*. Hemel Hempstead: Harvester Wheatsheaf.

Mooney G., Jan S., Wiseman V. (2004) Measuring health needs. In: *Oxford Textbook of Public Health*, 4th edn (eds Detels R., McEwen J., Beaglehole R., Tanaka H.). Oxford: Oxford University Press

Murray S.A. (1999). Experiences with 'rapid appraisal' in primary care: involving the public in assessing health needs, orientating staff, and educating medical students. *British Medical Journal* 318, 440–4.

National Architecture Design Board Health Information Service for Wales (2006) *Extended Individual Health Record Design Brief, Populations and Agents*. Cardiff: National Architecture and Design Board Wales.

NICE (National Institute for Health and Clinical Excellence) (2005) *Health Needs Assessment: a practical guide*. London: National Institute for Health and Clinical Excellence.

Ong B., Humphries S.G., Arnett H., Rikkin S. (1991) Rapid appraisal in an urban setting: an example from the developed world. *Social Science and Medicine* 32, 909–12.

Rikkin S. (1992) Rapid appraisal for health. *Rapid Appraisal Notes* July, 7–12.

Stevens A., Gillam S. (1998) Needs assessment: from theory to practice. *British Medical Journal* 316, 1448–52.

Stevens A., Raftery J. (eds) (1994) *Health Care Needs Assessment – the epidemiologically based needs assessment reviews*. Oxford: Radcliffe Medical Press.

Stevens A., Gillam S., Spiegal M., *et al.*, *Health Needs Assessment from Theory to Practice*, London Kings Fund.

Sutton M. (2002) Vertical and horizontal aspects of socio-economic inequity in general practitioner contacts in Scotland. *Health Economics* 11 (6), 537–49.

Wanless D. (2004) *Securing Good Health for the Whole Population*. London: HM Stationery Office.

Wilkinson J., Murray S. (1998) Assessment in primary care: practical issues and possible approaches. *British Medical Journal* 316, 1524–8.

WHO (World Health Organization) (1999) *Basic Documents*. Geneva: World Health Organization.

Wright J., Williams R., Wilkinson J. (1998) Development and importance of health needs assessment. *British Medical Journal* 316 (7140), 1310–13.

CHAPTER 2

Health Needs Assessment: Appraising and Measuring Need

Cindy Carlson

Public Health Skill: Appraising and measuring skills

- Promoting self-esteem: encouraging self-determination and motivation
- Skills of analysis: interpretation and use of information, and methods of evaluating provision

Introduction

The health of the population has been a subject of personal, social and political concern for at least 150 years in the UK. From the studies and actions of the great Victorian reformers, such as Chadwick, to the current debates around teenage pregnancy, binge drinking and obesity, the public's health in the UK has been a matter of intense interest and debate.

The politics of health continue to swing from a discourse of societal responsibility to one of individual responsibility. At the time of writing this chapter, the UK media are in the midst of arguing whether the now recognised 'obesity epidemic' should be tackled at individual or societal level. In the more measured discussions, it is clear that the answer is that health remains both an individual and societal responsibility.

This chapter therefore explores how health needs assessment can be used to build both momentum for individual action as well as to help inform programmes that can provide support at community and wider levels.

2.1 Background

During the early stages of public health awareness in the 19th century, infectious diseases were the primary cause of ill health. Killer infections were especially severe amongst the poorest populations, and public health leaders like Chadwick and John Snow were able to link the wretched living conditions of poor people to their poor health status, even though the agents of infection (bacteria, viruses, etc.) had not yet been discovered (Young 1999).

As the UK population has become wealthier, and infectious diseases more easily treated through antibiotics, chronic illnesses – and the causes of chronic illness – have come to dominate the public health agenda. Despite the changes in the types and causes of disease in the late 20th/early 21st century, the least well off in the UK still suffer a disproportionate amount of ill health (Wanless 2004).

Table 2.1 provides an indication of what illnesses patients consulted their GPs about in 1991/92, as a ratio, by their social class. Assuming 100 is the 'normal' consultation rate, then any figure above 100 means an above-average rate, while any number below 100 is a below-average rate. Social class categories run from professional (I and II) to semiskilled and unemployed (IV and V). As can be seen in Table 2.1, both men and women from poorer social classes were more likely to consult their GP for mental illness, respiratory and digestive problems, and accidental illness. Higher ratios for infectious diseases amongst professional classes appear to be an anomaly, and might be explained by things such as more people in professional classes travel more often. The information in Table 2.1 allows practitioners to ask more penetrating questions to understand why these disease patterns exist in this way. Thus health statistics are a useful starting point for any health needs assessment.

2.1.1   Lifestyle and health

In the last few years the main government health priorities have focused on what might be called 'lifestyle' health problems, and include over-consumption of alcohol, effects of elicit drugs, obesity, teenage pregnancy, diabetes and problems related to smoking tobacco. The prioritization of these different problems is based on solid epidemiological and economic grounds. Table 2.2 shows what the growing trend has been in these health problems.

However, Table 2.2 provides a mixed picture of trends in health-related behaviours and problems. While the percentage of people smoking and of teenagers becoming pregnant appears to be decreasing over time, the percentage of people who are obese or who are diabetic is increasing. The Wanless report (Wanless 2004) put particular emphasis on the fact that obesity in children rose alarmingly between 1995 and 2002, from 24.6 to 31.6 per cent of all children aged 6–15 years, or a 7 per cent increase. The same report also found that there were stark differences in high-risk behaviours and social classes, exacerbating health inequalities. The main outcome of these inequalities is that there is a large difference in life expectancy between the professional classes and those who are unskilled or unemployed. Wanless (2004) calculated that while 22 per cent of men in professional classes die before they reach the age of 70, 48 per cent of men in the unskilled/unemployed classes are dead before the same age. The compilers of the Wanless report went on to calculate that 15 per cent of this difference could be attributed to smoking cigarettes.

2.1.2   Economic costs of health

The economic costs of ill health are also being more regularly calculated in the UK as health care costs continue inexorably to rise. The economic value of health, or cost of ill health, is of concern to decision makers in both state-funded health systems, such as the UK NHS, and privately funded health systems, such as the US system. Not only are politicians and health managers worried about the direct costs of ill health, in the form of treatment and care, but also indirect costs, in terms of loss of productive labour to illness. Rising levels of pre-conditions for illness, such as smoking and obesity, therefore set alarm bells ringing.

In the last few years, various economic analyses have been done to calculate the costs of a variety of major illnesses to the UK. Levels of coronary vascular disease in the UK were calculated to cost the health system around £14 750 million in 2003, while coronary heart disease was calculated to have cost around £3500 million that same year. Productivity costs of both diseases combined for 2003 were estimated to be around £9300 million, most of this cost due to the death of someone of working age (British Heart Foundation 2003). Mental illness is another major health issue in the UK, with over a third of the burden of illness in the UK attributed to mental ill health (LSE 2006). The Sainsbury Centre for Mental Health (2003) estimated that mental illness in England alone cost £12.5 billion, when taking into account treatment and care provided by the NHS, local authorities, private providers, family and friends. Productivity costs came to around £23.1 billion in lost output from those no longer able to work. Alcohol misuse is another area that has come under economic scrutiny. A UK government paper (Cabinet Office 2003) found that the costs of treating and caring for inpatients whose illness was either partially or wholly alcohol misuse related came to £526 million in 2003. Outpatient costs ranged from

Table 2.1 Patient consulting ratios (age-standardised) by ICD-9 chapter, social class and sex in England and Wales. *Source:* Bajekal et al. (2006).

	Men					Women				
	I&II	IIIN	IIIM	IV & V	Other	I&II	IIIN	IIIM	IV & V	Other
I Infectious and parasitic diseases	103	104	99	99	93	101	98	104	105	93
II Neoplasms	115	102	92	84	112	109	104	96	91	89
III Endocrine, nutritional and metabolic diseases and immunity disorders	97	104	98	108	92	83	94	117	118	107
IV Diseases of blood and blood-forming organs	89	104	102	111	111	84	99	113	116	96
V Mental disorders	78	101	99	128	144	83	92	109	122	110
VI Diseases of the nervous system and sense organs	98	99	99	103	109	95	99	102	104	103
VII Diseases of the circulatory system	90	101	103	111	110	87	95	110	115	103
VIII Diseases of the respiratory system	99	102	99	102	98	96	97	105	109	97
IX Diseases of the digestive system	87	93	107	115	90	86	98	108	115	100
X Diseases of the gentiourinary system	96	102	99	108	100	95	99	106	108	93
XI Complications of pregnancy, childbirth and the puerperium	–	–	–	–	–	107	97	112	103	83
XII Diseases of the skin and subcutaneous tissue	100	101	99	98	106	91	100	103	106	104
XIII Diseases of the musculoskeletal system and connective tissue	80	93	113	118	87	89	94	114	118	93
XIV Congenital anomalies	99	97	81	112	162	95	93	73	112	121
XV Certain conditions originating in the perinatal period	146	–	149	–	–	127	82	196	96	48
XVI Symptoms, signs and ill-defined conditions	89	100	104	114	93	88	99	105	117	93
XVII Injury and poisoning	80	92	114	119	82	92	95	113	116	92

Indicates significantly raised ratios.

Indicates significantly lowered ratios.

Table 2.2 Trends in illness rates in the UK.

Health-related behaviour	Women		Men	
	1994	2004	1994	2004
Alcohol consumption* (>14 units women/21 units men)	14%	18% (2002)	30%	30% (2002)
Diabetes*	1.9%	3.4%	2.9%	4.3% (2003)
Mental Illness†	20% (1993)	20% (2003)	12.6% (1993)	14% (2003)
Obesity* (BMI >30)	17.3%	23.2%	13.8%	22.7%
Smoking*	27%	23%	28%	24%
Teenage pregnancy‡	45.4/1000 (1998–2001)	42.2/1000 (2002–2004)		

* From DH (2004) Health Survey for England; 2004 results, http://www.ic.nhs.uk/pubs/hlthsvyeng2004upd/04TrendTabs.xls/file.
† Office of National Statistics (2000) www.statistics.gov.uk/downloads/theme_health/psychmorb_sumrep.pdf.
‡ From EMPHO (2006) Under 18 Conception Rates, England and Wales Local Authorities, http://www.empho.org.uk/THEMES/ teenagepregnancy/teenagepregnancy.aspx. BMI, body mass index.

£222 million to £445.6 million. All health care related costs combined together ranged from £1.2 to £1.7 billion per year. The indirect costs of alcohol misuse, including loss of work productivity and alcohol-related crime, came to another £18 billion.

With just these three examples alone, it is no wonder that the UK government is so interested in the health of its population. The question then becomes, whose responsibility is it to take the necessary steps to reduce the burden of illness in the UK?

2.2 Who Takes Responsibility for Health Improvement?

The debates around health responsibility are not new, even though the patterns of disease in the UK have changed dramatically in the last 150 years. Public health legislation in the 19th century, such as the Public Health Acts of 1848, 1872 and 1875, sought to legislate and enforce better environmental conditions and the introduction of medical officers into local councils. These social reforms began to make a large impact on the health of poor people as water supplies, sewage and rubbish were all brought under the responsibility of local government. Biomedical models of health started to become prominent towards the end of the 19th century after the discovery of bacteria, accompanied by views that individual treatment could stop the tide of infectious disease. However, social models of health improvement continued to dominate into the early 20th century as further legislation sought to protect the health of children (e.g. the 1906 School Meals Act) and workers (e.g. the 1911 National Insurance Act). The 2004 public health White Paper for England, *Choosing Health: making healthy choices easier* (DH 2004), updates government policy on public health, emphasizing the need for a balance between government and individual responsibility. The core principles laid out in *Choosing Health* include:

- informed choice;
- personalization;
- working together.

2.2.1 Informed choice

Informed choice refers to people's expectation that they have access to all the information they need to make their own decisions about lifestyle factors, while also expecting government to provide an enabling environment that allows them to exercise the choices they have made. *Personalization* refers to providing targeted support to ensure that information and assistance is contextualised and provided in a meaningful way. Finally, *working together* refers to the fact that enabling healthy choices needs to done by a combination of government, individuals and local/community bodies working in partnership.

Critique of the White Paper has included a perception that it lays too much responsibility for health at the feet of individuals and not enough at government's door (Ashton 2005). Specific campaign groups, such as ASH (Action on Smoking and Health), felt that policy was not going to go far enough in key areas, such as a blanket ban of smoking in public places (ASH 2005). In some cases sustained lobbying has led to key public health legislation such as the smoking ban in England and Wales since July 2007. Others have cited the fact that financial and human resources are not sufficient to implement fully the recommendations of *Choosing Health*, and that the government needs to put its money where its policy mouth is (Marks & Hunter 2005).

There is no doubt that the rise of chronic illness, often due to lifestyle choices, has created a dilemma for public health professionals who must work at both individual and community/area levels to support health improvement. Halting infectious diseases through supplying clean water or introducing safe waste disposal can be easily seen as a government responsibility as there is both a direct collective cost and benefit. However, great debates are arising over how much individuals need to change their health behaviours and take responsibility for this. While there is no doubt that individuals must have some measure of responsibility for what they eat, how much they exercise, how much alcohol they drink, etc., health behaviour models also demonstrate that the behaviours people engage in are the product of complex interactions. Social determinants, such as income, education, occupation, gender and ethnicity have been shown to correlate positively with health status (Gwatkin 2000). There are genuine concerns that too much focus on individual health and responsibility will in the long run exacerbate already high levels of health inequalities. *Saving Lives: our healthier nation* (DH 1999) places a greater emphasis on a broad strategic approach to tackling health inequalities. This corresponds with proposals for new approaches that move away from the disease model towards the promotion of social support and the development of family and community strengths (Wilkinson 1997; Campbell & Aggleton 1999). It is further confirmed by authors such as Tessa Davies (1996, p. 139) whose own research indicates that there is strong 'evidence to show that living on a very low income not only affects mental and physical health, but also may provoke families into adopting unhealthy behaviour (smoking, poor diet, etc.).'.

The UK's policy approach reflects a wider international agenda as well. The World Health Organization formally adopted a programme to address health inequalities within the 'Health for all 2000' programme (WHO 1985).

Case Study Example

Individual versus social responsibility: the case of IVF and obese women

In August 2006, the British Fertility Society recommended that women whose body mass index (BMI) was greater than 30 should not be given fertility treatment on the NHS unless they committed themselves to a programme of weight reduction. The grounds for this recommendation are that women who are very severely overweight (BMI > 30) or obese (BMI > 36) have a lower success rate with fertility treatment, as well as enduring more complications with their pregnancies. The recommendations would appear to make sense on both clinical as well as economic grounds. However, critics quickly pointed out that this recommendation will impact disproportionately on women from lower classes and from ethnic minorities, since women in the lowest classes are twice as likely to be obese than those in social class I, while 19.5 per cent of black Caribbean women aged 16–34 are obese, compared to only 12.7 per cent of women of the same age in the general population (Cochrane 2006). The National Food Alliance (1997) studied the degree to which low income impacts on family diets and found that poor people make rational choices about how to spend their limited income, which includes purchasing less expensive, less healthy food (e.g. foods high in fat and sugar and low in fibre). The same report found that there are also less healthy food options available in deprived communities, and that food shops in deprived areas tend to be more expensive than supermarkets, which are inaccessible to many poorer families.

So while on the surface saying women must lose weight if they wish to qualify for IVF on the NHS seems sensible, if there are not other government policies and programmes in place that make healthy eating and more exercise accessible then this recommendation is also highly discriminatory.

Overall, it is clear that while individuals can and should take on responsibility for how their own lifestyle choices impact on their health, it is also clear that there remain important areas of intervention for government and communities, especially where individuals lack the means, information and motivation to make healthy choices. The focus of much of this debate is on local areas and communities with a strong emphasis on collaboration and participation. Health needs assessment is an important tool for public health practitioners who need to begin untangling at what level interventions need to take place.

2.3   Raising Awareness of Health Need: Motivation for Action

As mentioned previously, health needs assessment occurs on different levels, depending on what the ultimate purpose of the needs assessment is. Each level requires some similar public health skills, as well as unique skills. For example, working with individuals on helping them to assess their own health needs as a precursor to more long-term health promotion and behaviour change requires different tools from undertaking a community or local area health needs assessment that feeds into programme planning. Chapters 4–7 explore different features of measuring population need, working with communities and in partnership, etc. and the public health skills required to approach each of these facets of needs assessment. The focus in this section, and this chapter, is on individual needs assessment, how it is done and why it is important.

2.3.1   Individual health needs assessment

Individual health needs assessment is important as it allows both the practitioner and the user/patient to examine the causes and effects of ill health or poor health behaviours, and to consider appropriate interventions for improving the individual's health. Part of this analysis and consideration is introducing patients or users to services that they might not have known existed, or helping them to find ways of accessing services that previously seemed inaccessible.

Different authors of health promotion texts recognise that a good starting point for assessing individual and population health needs is to first analyse whether the need is normative, felt, expressed or comparative (Bradshaw, cited in Ewles & Simnett 1999; Naidoo & Wills 2000). Bradshaw's (1972) definition of needs (as defined in Chapter 1 here) is as follows:

- *normative needs* as defined by experts or professional groups;
- *felt needs* as defined by clients, patients, relatives or service users;
- *expressed needs* when felt needs become a demand;
- *comparative needs* identified when people, groups or areas fall short of an established standard.

The public health skills needed to work with individuals and to help them make healthy choices include: analysis, interpretation and use of information, promoting self-esteem, encouraging self-determination, and evaluating provision.

2.4   Analysis, Interpretation and Use of Information

Resources are limited in most health settings, and particularly for work deemed non-clinical. It is therefore important for public health practitioners to be able to target individuals and settings to ensure that they are addressing the most pressing needs of specific groups. A starting point is to look first at the normative needs of the population the practitioner works with. For school children this could be looking at diet or risky sexual behaviours; for cardiac patients this could be looking at diet and exercise regimes; and for the elderly this could be assessing potential risks of falling. To illustrate how to use information to help define possible interventions let us use the tricky issue of adolescent health as an example.

Case Study Example

Experiences from Bodyzone: analysing, interpreting and using data

In the late 1990s, staff in the family planning service of Oxfordshire's Community Health Trust found that there appeared to be increasing gaps in provision of health services for young people in rural areas. The service was running clinics for young people in Oxford City that were fairly well attended, but with clients almost exclusively from Oxford itself or towns and villages close by the city. In examining this problem more closely, they discovered that young people found going to their GP for advice on health issues that concerned them most (e.g. bullying, sex, substance misuse) very difficult, due to the close knit nature of rural communities and lack of anonymity and the dearth of public transport to take them from their villages to nearby towns. Teenage pregnancy rates in Oxfordshire were slightly lower than the national average (conception rates in under 18-year-olds: 31.4 per 1000 in Oxfordshire), while school nurses were reporting problems with binge drinking in many of the schools they worked in (Greenhall 2000).

Staff then looked at what evidence existed of best practice models for improving young people's health services. They found a fairly strong evidence base from the USA indicating that school-based programmes were a good way of reaching adolescents who would not use mainstream health services. A few programmes in the UK were showing similar results. The Family Planning Service therefore decided to pilot a scheme aiming to bring adolescent-appropriate health services into places where young people congregate, including schools and youth centres.

Public health practitioners need to know where to access local area data that come from both routine data collection (e.g. from hospital and GP surgery reports) and from occasional surveys undertaken by either their Primary Care Trust or by researchers in their area. Public health information analysts can be very helpful in explaining and interpreting data. Practitioners also need to know how to find evidence of what interventions have proven effective and be able to interpret research results to ensure they are receiving as objective a view as possible.

2.5   Promoting Self-Esteem and Encouraging Self-Determination

Having examined health risks and determinants in a population, it is then important to get a sense of felt and expressed needs. As all behaviour change models indicate, individuals need to recognise the need for change before they will begin the often arduous road to changing behaviours. While almost everyone has some awareness of what is or is not a healthy behaviour, due to both government information and mass media, this information often remains abstract or unrelated to individual circumstances. People can easily ignore exhortations to quit smoking or to eat five portions of fruit and vegetables a day until the effects of unhealthy lifestyles are personalised. The trick is to help people become aware of how these behaviours impact on their health without creating the view that they are in some way 'bad' people. It is therefore critical to find ways to raise awareness and help individuals to identify steps they feel they can take themselves to improve their own health, rather than overwhelming them with a sense that they are hopeless cases.

Coveney (1998), in exploring the ethics of nutrition promotion, found that while practitioners wield a certain power over patients or communities merely by the fact of choosing nutrition as the object of change, individuals can also be challenged to be more self-reflective, leading to a greater ability to solve their own health problems. In some areas in the UK, for example, healthy eating programmes do not rely just on the promotion of good nutrition, they also work with deprived communities to create food banks or co-operative stores that ensure residents have affordable access to the means of a healthy diet (Food Access Network, http://www.sustainweb.org/page.php?id=50).

Activity

Explore the Food Poverty website, http://www.sustainweb.org/page.php?id=50, for yourself and consider how those running the project have synchronised individual and community-level response to health needs. When considering normative needs, felt needs, expressed needs and comparative needs, what do you think some of the strengths of the Food Access Network are? Which needs do you think have more emphasis, and which less?

Case Study Example

Bodyzone: promoting self-esteem and self-motivation

Having recognised that young people were having difficulty in accessing services, Family Planning Service staff then approached secondary schools in some of the larger market towns in Oxfordshire to explore whether they could work together to bring health services to students. Having received the go-ahead from school staff and governors, health service staff then consulted with students to find out what sort of services they would like from a health clinic geared at their needs, and where the clinic should be based (e.g. within the school limits or outside). In this instance, staff were operating under a set of normative needs (e.g. what services they felt students should have) while also tempering these with students' felt needs. At the first school where services were set up, students had clearly indicated that the clinic should be within the school and operate during school lunch time so that they could easily access the services.

The first Bodyzone was set up in 1997 and was staffed by a school health nurse, a family planning nurse and a youth worker, with a local GP on call in case medical input was needed. Each member of staff had a specific role to play when meeting young people: the youth worker talked to students who were having social problems such as family concerns or bullying; the school nurse met with students who were concerned about health problems such as diet, smoking, stress, etc.; and the family planning nurse provided information on contraception, sexually transmitted infections and sexual relations more generally, while also providing contraceptives when deemed appropriate. Each student who attended a Bodyzone session was able to indicate what type of service they needed and then saw the most appropriate member of staff. The staff would explore in some detail with each student how they could make best use of their time at the Bodyzone clinic, what their alternatives were for acting on their own problems, whether they needed to be seen on an ongoing basis, and whether they needed referring to other services out in the community. Students interviewed as part of an initial evaluation of the programme indicated that they felt that Bodyzone staff were empowering as they offered non-judgemental advice and assistance (Carlson & Peckham 2001).

The Bodyzone project shows how relatively simple interventions, when made convenient and personalised can improve a 'hard to reach' group's health-related knowledge, and help affect their health decisions. These programmes require extra resourcing as spending time in schools or youth clubs is not often in the job description of most community nurses or health staff. On the other hand, these types of initiatives do show that with imagination and resources much can be done to empower people with knowledge and help them to make more informed decisions about their lifestyles.

2.6   Evaluating Provision

Public health practitioners need to be able to incorporate evaluation methodologies into their needs assessment work, as planning–evaluation cycles can help to keep health needs assessment alive and ensure that services that arise out of an initial needs assessment remain relevant to a target group's felt or expressed needs, as well as conforming to the latest evidence on how best to meet specific types of health needs. To ensure that evaluation is effective the object being evaluated, whether a service or programme, needs to have a clearly stated aim, objectives and indicators that provide measurable points of reference. UK government targets have provided health professionals with some ways of measuring how well their services are operating, though these targets are highly normative and do not necessarily reflect local health needs.

2.6.1 Teenage pregnancy in the UK

Using teenage pregnancy as an example, most areas in the UK have had to develop local, multisectoral teenage pregnancy strategies that are clearly connected to targets that have been set for England and Wales, but which are grounded in local contexts and needs. The Department of Health funded a programme of evaluation training for teenage pregnancy coordinators in England in 2002, which provided broad guidance for what elements coordinators needed to ensure were in place to allow them to evaluate the implementation of their strategies. A worked example of aim, objectives and indicators provided to coordinators, based on needs expressed by teenagers, can be found in Table 2.3.

Health needs assessments imply that a certain degree of consultation has taken place with the groups whose needs are being assessed. It therefore follows that setting aims, objectives and indicators for programmes to address people's needs should also be done in consultation with these same groups. Participatory evaluation or programme reviews, using action research methods, can be very empowering in themselves – whether it is working with individuals to set their own individual goals or whether it is working with groups in the community to determine the aims and objectives of their programmes (Stringer 1999).

Practitioners also need to recognise the limitations of evaluation findings. Besides having to struggle with determining what and how to evaluate, it can also be very difficult to attribute the outcomes uncovered in evaluations to the programme interventions being evaluated. The many texts written about evaluation, research and evidence-based practice (Muir Gray 1996; Ovretveit 1998; Perkins *et al.* 1999) all suggest that evaluation is complex and can consume time and resources that might otherwise be devoted to programme interventions. On the other hand, it is vital to continue working on informing the evidence base of the effectiveness of public health practice, and it is therefore critical to strive for a balance between gathering solid evidence through evaluations and the use of scarce resources.

Table 2.3 Teenage pregnancy. *Source:* Carlson (2002).

Project structure	Indicators	Means of measurement
Wider aim: reduce rate of teenage pregnancy by 50%	Teenage conceptions reduced to 5% in Neatshire	Hospital record; PCT records
Objectives:		
1 Increased access to contraceptive supplies	75% of at risk teenagers visiting some form of health service for contraceptives	PCT/GP and family planning records
2 Improved, appropriate advice provided to teenagers	90% of teenagers satisfied with advice received	Surveys of teenage service users
Activities:		
1 Identify appropriate facilities for a teen-focused health clinic		
2 Upgrade these facilities		
3 Provide specific training to staff		
4 Increase the amount of free and low cost contraceptive methods		
GP, general practitioner; PCT, Primary Care Trust.		

Case Study Example

Bodyzone: evaluating provision

The Family Planning Service realised that they were receiving more and more requests from around Oxfordshire to set up Bodyzones in more secondary schools. Before embarking on an expansion of the Bodyzone clinics, staff felt it was important to evaluate existing services to get a picture of what was working well and what needed improving. A local university was asked to help with evaluating the service.

The evaluation used both quantitative and qualitative methods to assess how well the programme was being implemented and whether it was achieving its stated objectives. The focus groups with students, school staff and Bodyzone staff were particularly enlightening. Participatory methods were used with students and Bodyzone users in order to ensure that young people were able to express what their main concerns and views were, rather than being lead by researcher questions.

The evaluation of the pilot phase of the programme found that the service was highly appreciated by students and school staff. While a relatively small proportion of students made use of the services, those that did tended to come from vulnerable backgrounds, and many had been referred by their teachers who felt the Bodyzone staff were more competent to handle some of the problems facing these particular students. The evaluation also found that more young women than young men were accessing Bodyzone and suggested that having a male nurse or youth worker might help to attract more young men to the weekly clinics.

The evaluation team also found that the programme's objectives were too ambitious for the scale of services that Bodyzone was able to offer. As these objectives had not been quantified through indicators, it was left to the evaluation team to interpret how well the objectives were being met. It was therefore recommended that the programme team reconsider their programme objectives and set them at a more realistic level for what could be achieved in a clinic that provided services only once a week for 1 hour (Carlson & Peckham 2001).

Conclusion

Health needs assessment and the skills required to be effective in assessing and responding to need, are key to the toolkit of any public health practitioner. Appropriate and accurate assessment of health needs, including contextualizing these needs, is an important first step to being able to help individuals and communities to participate in improving their own health. It is therefore critical to consider both the process of health needs assessment itself, as well as planning interventions, and how best to involve individuals and community groups in assessment and planning exercises. The next chapter explores the medical care model of health needs assessment.

References

ASH (Action on Smoking and Health) (2005) *Choosing Health: making healthy choices easier*. Evidence to the House of Commons Health Select Committee. London: Action on Smoking and Health. http://www.ash.org.uk/html/policy/choosinghealthevidence05.html.

Ashton J. (2005) Delivering choosing health through settings. *Healthy Settings*, Special edition, June 2005. University of Central Lancashire, http://www.uclan.ac.uk/facs/health/hsdu/publications/newsletter/newsletter_se_1.pdf#search=%22Choosing%20Health%20Ashton%22.

Bajekal M.I., Osborne V., Yar M., Meltzer H. (2006) *Focus on Health*. London: UK Office of National Statistics/Palgrave Macmillan.

Bradshaw J. (1972) The concept of social need. *New Society* 30, 640–3.

British Heart Foundation (2003) *Economic Costs of CHD and CVD*. http://www.heartstats.org/datapage.asp?id=101.

Cabinet Office (2003) *Alcohol Misuse: how much does it cost?* London: Cabinet Office, Strategy Unit. http://www.strategy.gov.uk/downloads/files/econ.pdf#search=%22economic%20cost%20illness%20UK%22.

Campbell C., Aggleton P. (1999) Young people's sexual health: a framework for policy debate. *Canadian Journal of Human Sexuality* 8 (4), 249–63.

Carlson C. (2002) *Preparing for Evaluation: understanding what it is you want to evaluate!* Oxford: Health Development Agency/Teenage Pregnancy Unit Evaluation Training Team.

Carlson C., Peckham S. (2001) *Bodyzone Programme: evaluation report phase 1.* Oxford: Oxfordshire Community Health Trust, Family Planning Service.

Cochrane K. (2006) Too fat for a family? *Guardian* 31 Aug 2006, G2, 10–11.

Coveney J. (1998) The government and ethics of health promotion: the importance of Michel Foucault. *Health Education Research* 13 (3), 459–68.

Davies T. (1996) The politics of 'lifestyle': government policies and the health of the poor. In: *Community Health Nursing* (eds Gastrell P., Edwards J.). London: Balliere Tindall.

DH (Department of Health) (1999) *Saving Lives: our healthier nation.* London: HM Stationery Office.

DH (Department of Health) (2004) *Choosing Health: making healthy choices easier.* London: HM Stationery Office.

Ewles L., Simnett I. (1999) *Promoting Health: a practical guide.* London: Balliere Tindall.

Greenhall E. (2000) *Bodyzone Clinics – young people's services in Oxfordshire.* Oxford: Oxfordshire Community Health Trust, Family Planning Service.

Gwatkin D. (2000) Health inequalities and the health of the poor: what do we know? What can we do? *Bulletin of the WHO* 78 (1), 3–18.

LSE (London School of Economics) (2006) *The Depression Report: a new deal for depression and anxiety disorders.* London: London School of Economics, Centre for Economic Performance's Mental Health Group. http://cep.lse.ac.uk/textonly/research/mentalhealth/DEPRESSION_REPORT_LAYARD.pdf#search=%22mental%20illness%20economic%20cost%20LSE%22.

Marks L., Hunters D. (2005) Moving upstream or muddying the waters: incentives for managing health. *Public Health* 119, 974–80.

Muir Gray J.A. (1996) *Evidence-based Health Care.* London: Churchill Livingstone.

Naidoo J., Wills J. (2000) *Health Promotion: foundations for practice.* London: Balliere Tindall.

National Food Alliance (1997) *Myths about Food and Low Income.* http://www.sustainweb.org/publications/downloads/pov_myths.pdf.

Ovretveit J. (1998) *Evaluating Health Interventions.* Milton Keynes: Open University Press.

Perkins E.R., Simnett I., Wright L. (1999) *Evidence-based Health Promotion.* London: John Wiley.

Sainsbury Centre for Mental Health (2003) *Economic and Social Costs of Mental Illness in England.* http://www.scmh.org.uk/80256FBD004F6342/vWeb/pcPCHN6FRLCM.

Stringer E.T. (1999) *Action Research*, 2nd edn. Thousand Oaks, CA: Sage Publications.

Wanless D. (2004) *Securing Good Health for the Whole Population.* London: HM Treasury Office. http://www.hm-treasury.gov.uk/consultations_and_legislation/wanless/consult_wanless04_final.cfm.

Wilkinson R. (1997) Health inequalities: relative or absolute material standards? *British Medical Journal* 314, 591–5.

WHO (World Health Organization) (1985) *Targets for Health for All: targets in support of the European Regional Strategy for Health for All by the year 2000.* Copenhagen: WHO European Regional Office.

Young T.K. (1999) *Population Health: concepts and methods*, 2nd edn. Oxford: Oxford University Press.

CHAPTER 3
Needs Assessment
John Acres

Public Health Skills: Surveillance

- How to measure health need: epidemiological needs assessment and community diagnoses
- How to collect and structure information in order to create a profile of the population
- Assessing the information collected: reading data, interpretation and analysis
- How to communicate data and information on the health and wellbeing and related needs of a defined population

Introduction

This chapter examines the contribution that epidemiology can make to assessing the health needs of a population. It is based on the natural history of disease and its interface with and entry to the health care system. The chapter aims to provide:

- a conceptual framework;
- the measurement of health need;
- assessing the information collected;
- some tools to structure a community profile: classic/descriptive epidemiology.

3.1 A Conceptual Framework

Nurses make judgements about situations all the time and assessing the needs of clients is nothing new. What is different about the assessment of the needs of groups of people in public health? The answer is there is very little difference, groups being made up of individuals. We use similar techniques for groups as we do for individuals.

Case Study Example

She summed up the situation in a moment – the door ajar, a pale sad looking 4-year-old girl on her own in the kitchen clambering from a chair up onto the crowded work surface (was that bruise on her arm from an adult's thumb?), the unwashed cutlery in the basin, the empty cans of beer in the waste bin, mother next door, the games show blaring from the unwatched TV. Where should she begin?

3.1.1 Why assess need? Balancing resources with needs

The purpose of assessing need is to identify the resources that will be effective in meeting the need and so improve health. If the resources are not effective, then they are wasted and could have been used for someone else. Resources such as time and money will always be limited, so the continuing challenge is to find the best balance between the needs we find and the effective resources available. Figure 3.1 illustrates this.

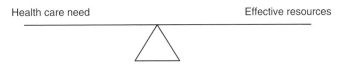

Health care need   Effective resources

Figure 3.1   The balancing act.

> **Activity**
>
> Explore this concept further by reading the chapter 'Epidemiologically based needs assessment' by Andrew Stevens and Mike Sadler in *Needs to Know: a guide to needs assessment for primary care* edited by Andrew Harries (1997).

3.1.2 The context of needs assessment: the health care pathway

When someone feels unwell they will usually do something about it. The next case study example illustrates this and the health care pathway (model) that is followed.

> **Case Study Example**
>
> A man calls his GP complaining of a pain in his abdomen. The story sounds like an acute appendicitis, he is referred to the hospital where he is operated on and his inflamed appendix is removed. He is discharged feeling better and makes an uneventful recovery.

In this case a man recognises that he has a need for health care and he goes to the GP, i.e. he converts a *need* into a *demand*. As a result he uses health care resources and the outcome is cure and uneventful recovery. This is represented in Figure 3.2. However, there can be two responses to demand – demand may be met or unmet:

- *met demand* is, in effect, a measure of the use of resources – e.g. the number of patients admitted or bed days used in a year;
- *unmet demand* is a measure of people waiting to use resources – e.g. number on the waiting list or waiting time until admission.

Both of these are routinely measured by the health service. Outcomes, however, are often assumed but not measured routinely.

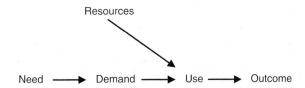

Resources

Need ⟶ Demand ⟶ Use ⟶ Outcome

Figure 3.2   Simple medical care pathway.

The translation of need into demand

Need is not always translated into demand and demand does not always mean there is a health care need (Figure 3.3). Here are three situations in which this may occur.

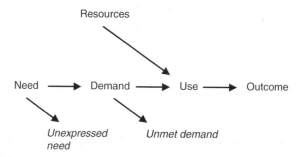

Figure 3.3   Medical care pathway – need–outcome.

Situation 1 People do not always realise they have a health care need and, as a consequence, do not convert it into demand. This may be because they just do not realise the significance of their symptoms. For example, a man, who is a smoker, has a cough that he puts down to a 'smoker's cough'. He does not go to his GP as he does not realise that the symptoms are coming from an early lung cancer.

Situation 2 People may realise they have a health problem but are afraid or embarrassed to go to the doctor. As a response to this they do not convert their need into demand. For example, a woman with a lump in the breast may not go to her GP because she is frightened she will be told it is breast cancer; some women with stress incontinence may not go to their GP because they are embarrassed by it or they may not know that there are treatments that can help.

Situation 3 There may be situations where someone places a demand on the health service, but does not actually have a health need. An extreme example of this might be that someone wants a lift into town to go shopping and telephones for an ambulance. Although this sounds unbelievable, it has been known to happen.

Need and demand are different. It is not just helpful to distinguish between the different elements of the medical care model, it is *essential* if we want to have a true picture of what is happening. Unless we have this true picture we cannot tackle the real problems.

Can demand ever be used as a surrogate for need?

Measuring need is more difficult than measuring demand. Sometimes, in the absence of any other information, demand can be used as a surrogate for need. For example, in severe acute conditions like acute heart attack, admissions to hospital might be a 'near enough' measure of the number of people surviving an acute heart attack. For other situations, however, it can be very misleading. Where no resource exists, then there can be no use of that resource. There will also be no waiting list kept for a resource that does not exist. We saw earlier that resource use (met demand) and waiting lists (unmet demand) are measures of overall demand. The key point here is that if there is no met demand (use of services) and no waiting list, then there is nothing to tell us that there might be a need for the service. An important message here is that the level of resource or service available will always influence demand for that resource or service.

3.1.3   Efficiency and effectiveness

Effectiveness and efficiency are about the use of resources:

- *efficiency* is about how much resources are used to achieve the outcome you want – can you achieve what you want more quickly or more cheaply?
- *effectiveness* is about how good the resources are at achieving the outcome you want – does what you do achieve what you want?

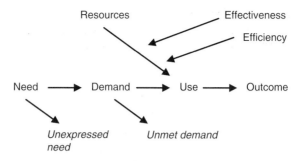

Figure 3.4   Medical care pathway – effectiveness and efficiency.

Both of these are key questions that need to be asked whenever resources are being used. Figure 3.4 is the same as Figure 3.3 but has the dimensions of effectiveness and efficiency added.

3.1.4   Effectiveness: how do we know what works?

There are several research approaches used to assess how effectively something works. Nowadays, most of these are intervention studies, where a drug is given to one group and the results compared to another very similar group that does not receive the drug. One of the best types of study is the randomised controlled trial (RCT).

Randomised controlled trials look forward in time and patients to be studied are selected from a larger number of patients with the condition of interest. They are then divided randomly into two groups. One group (experimental or treated) is exposed to an intervention that is thought to be helpful. The other group (control or comparison) is treated the same in all ways except that members are *not* exposed to the intervention. The groups are followed and any differences found are attributed to the intervention. Historically, the first RCT carried out was on streptomycin for the treatment of tuberculosis (TB), which at the time was a massive public health issue.

There are other types of study that can be used to assess effectiveness and these can also be used to identify the causes of disease. The main ones are case control studies and cohort studies.

Case control studies look back in time and involve patients who have the disease and a group of otherwise similar people who do not have the disease. Researchers look back in time to determine the frequency of exposure of the two groups to a particular treatment or risk factors.

Cohort studies look forward in time and are also called longitudinal or prospective studies. In this case a group of people is assembled, none of whom have experienced the outcome of interest, but all of them could experience it. They are observed over time to see which of them experiences the outcome of interest. It is then possible to see how initial characteristics (including a treatment they may have been on) relate to subsequent outcome events.

Each of these types of approach has their pros and cons, but some are better than others in the confidence you can have in the results. Box 3.1 is an example of how they have been ranked in terms of confidence.

Case Study Example

Why it is worth knowing about the interplay between need, demand, use, resource level and effectiveness

In 2004/5 there was a wide variation in the rate of surgical revascularization for coronary heart disease across England (Chief Medical Officer 2005). Can we conclude that this was reflecting different levels of coronary heart disease in these areas? From our knowledge of the health care pathway we know we cannot jump to that conclusion. It could reflect differences in need, demand or level of resources, as well as the effectiveness of other resources being used for coronary heart disease in these areas.

BOX 3.1

Heirachy of study designs for studies of effectiveness. *Source:* **Adapted from: University of York: Centre for Reviews and Dissemination (2001).**

Best   Experimental studies (e.g RCT with concealed allocation)

Quasi-experimental studies (e.g. experimental study without randomisation)

Controlled observational studies
          Cohort studies
          Case control studies

Observational studies without control groups

Expert opinion based on pathophysiology, bench research or consensus

---

Activity

Explore these issues further by reading the chapter 'Waste not, want not'. *The Annual Report of the Chief Medical Office on the State of Public Health* (Donaldson 2005).

3.1.5   What is missing from this health care model? Where is prevention?

What is missing from the health care model described so far is any mention of prevention or health promotion. However, exactly the same decision process is required to decide how to use resources most efficiently and effectively to reduce need. Figure 3.5 shows the inclusion and development of this within the pathway.

By taking obesity as an example we can see from the health care model where the problems are going to arise and where we need to intervene in order to improve health. If we simply respond to demand, then as time goes by there will be an inexorable increase in demand from the complications of obesity (e.g. diabetes, coronary heart disease, blindness). This will result in more admissions to hospital, more hospital bed days used, more consultants needed and more NHS resources used. Overall we may be ameliorating people's health problems created by the obesity, but we have not improved people's health. Examining the model with this thinking in mind points very clearly to the need for the prevention of obesity and the way to make best use of the resources we have available.

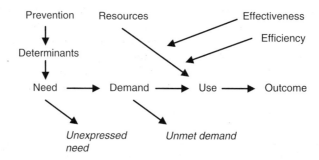

Figure 3.5   Medical Care Pathway – prevention.

3.2   Measurement of Health Need

3.2.1   Epidemiological needs assessment

All public health practitioners need to know that there are different types of need. For example there is expressed need, felt need, comparative need, normative need (Bradshaw 1972) and medically determined need. In an ideal world we would put all these together to form an overall assessment. For the purposes of this chapter, the focus is on the contribution that an epidemiological needs assessment makes to this. To see how to start doing this, it might be helpful to go back to the basic question of why we are measuring health need at all.

A community diagnosis

When a patient goes to the doctor or GP, the aim of the GP is to find out what is making that person unwell so that the doctor can do something to improve the patient's health. The GP makes a diagnosis. Decisions about treatment are based on the diagnosis. In public health practice the public health specialist is doing the same as the GP but for a population rather than for a single patient. In effect, the public health specialist is making a community diagnosis in order to provide effective resources to improve the community's health.

What to measure

This divides into two main groups:

1. The population in which you are interested.
2. Measures of poor health and their determinants.

3.2.2 Measuring the population

Examples of populations you could be dealing with include, amongst many others:

- a geographical area, e.g. a town or an electoral ward;
- a general medical practice;
- an institution such as a school, nursing home or prison;
- children in a playgroup;
- mothers under the age of 16 in a specific geographical area.

As you will see later, this population forms the denominator for rates, and the events (e.g. deaths) you are looking at form the numerator.

Populations in geographical areas

Geographically based populations are the ones you are likely to be interested in if you are creating a community health profile. Within the United Kingdom of Great Britain and Northern Ireland, the country is divided up into units of administration varying from parishes to regions. They all have their reasons for being there. Politics is one of them, as in order to be a member of parliament you needed to define the people who could vote for you – your electorate. The main boundaries that have been used over time for defining units of population have, therefore, been electoral wards. Today these wards can be grouped together to form unitary, district or borough council areas and these council areas can be further grouped into counties all of which have elected representatives.

Activity

Search for information on your local council's website and visit the following website for details of information provided: www.communities.gov.uk.

Health administration boundaries have been changed frequently to match changing fashions in NHS administration. They do not normally cut across electoral ward boundaries, though they may cut across district or borough council boundaries. The reorganization of health boundaries under the NHS Act 2006 sees more co-terminosity between NHS and local authority boundaries.

The government keeps track of the population through a 10-yearly census. With the exception of 1941, there has been a census every 10 years since 1801. It contains a large amount of very valuable information, but there is so much of it that it can take 3 years or more to be published. A year or so before the census takes place those responsible for carrying it out advertise part-time, short-term jobs for people to deliver the census forms and then make sure they are collected after the day of the census. These people are the 'enumerators' and the area they cover is the 'enumeration district'. This is the area that one person can reasonably cover in a day. In a rural area the geographical size of the area may be large, though the population may be small. In an inner city area, the geographical size may be small, but the population covered large. The enumeration district is the building block for all the other levels of aggregation of population, up to that of the whole country.

Activity

Have a look at the local census in your reference library or visit www.statistics.gov.uk and identify your enumeration district.

The term *estimates* is usually used to describe what is calculated to be the present or past population size – you can never be absolute in this. *Projections* is the term used to describe what is expected in the future. Because the census is only carried out once every 10 years, local authorities make predictions about what is happening in the meantime so that they can plan services. The predictions are based partly on the expected births and expected deaths that will occur. However, the most important change factor affecting both losses and new arrivals is *migration*. Migration (inward or outward) is the most significant factor in creating population change.

Planners will make use of all types of information available to them including electoral registers (for those entitled to vote), school roles, planning applications, development plans, changes in the economy, etc. Public health information analysts keep information about local populations and may well make this available on a local website. There is also a wealth of statistics about local areas through the government website.

Activity

Visit the following website and explore your local population: http://neighbourhood.statistics.gov.uk/dissemination/. Information is also available through regional Public Health Observatories and your local one can be accessed through http://www.apho.org.uk/apho/.

3.2.3   Measures of health and poor health

Health itself is difficult to measure and public health specialists usually measure the absence of health rather than health itself. A benefit of this is that it immediately tells us where the problems are. The following are used as measures of this:

- death – mortality;
- illness – morbidity;
- disability.

When it comes to measuring mortality, morbidity and disability it is important to understand their strengths and weaknesses (Fletcher *et al.* 1996). This is demonstrated in Table 3.1.

3.2.4   Definitions of diseases: the International Classification of Disease and Reid Codes

A key feature in comparisons is the necessity to compare like with like – apples with apples. If care is not taken in doing this, false conclusions can be drawn. A classification system for disease is a necessary

Table 3.1   Sources of information – their strengths and weakness.

Mortality	In the mid-1800s there was a hunger both to learn about the causes of health of the population, and to take steps to tackle these causes. The General Registration Act 1837 made it a legal requirement to register deaths and the opportunity was taken to include cause of death as part of this registration.
	Included on the death certificate is cause of death, age, gender, where the person lived and their occupation. Although people do not always get the cause right, it is the best dataset we have and it goes back over a long period of time so that time trends can be seen. Linking, for example, occupation to deaths has allowed people to discover occupational causes of disease
Morbidity (illness)	Routine measures of illness are usually measures of demand (expressed need) that have been met. It requires surveys to obtain information about unexpressed need
	Hospital use and inpatients: during the 1970s and early 1980s information about inpatient hospital use was collected using a system called Hospital Activity Analysis. Although it was not designed for public health, it could be used for epidemiological purposes. With NHS reorganizations, collection of these data stopped and was subsequently replaced by information collected for health authority purchasing services from hospitals. The motive was financial, but again the information could be used for epidemiological purposes. The same type of information continues to be collected by Primary Care Trusts. It is possible to look both at the diseases leading to admission to individual hospitals and the referral patterns of practices and individual GPs. It is also possible to combine hospital data to describe the diseases leading to hospital admission from populations in geographical areas
	Outpatients: there is information collected about patient numbers attending different types of clinic, (e.g. medical, surgical) but this does not include the diagnosis, age, gender, residence or occupation of those attending. It is currently of very little value in assessing need or use of services
	GP data: the introduction of GP computers in the 1980s began to make it possible to collect information about illness systematically, though issues of definition prevented comparisons to be made between practices locally. Although a few practices made a point of collecting morbidity data, it is only since the introduction of the new GP contract in 2003 that information on certain chronic diseases (e.g. coronary heart disease, diabetes, chronic obstructive pulmonary disease) has been collected routinely. This will enable practices to measure the levels of these conditions among the population registered with their practice. Although the data is postcoded, there is still work to be done to combine information from several practices to provide information about the morbidity of the population in a geographical area
	Quite separate from this, GP data from a sample of practices around the country have been collected every 10 years since 1970/71. These provide valuable information about the types of conditions presenting to general practice and how this has changed over time. See www.dh.gov.uk/en/Publicationsand statistics/Publishedhealth surveyfor England/index.htm
Disability	There is no systematic information collected about disability and what is available tends to have only crude definitions of the type and level of disability. What information there is tends also to be held discretely by different departments. Unfortunately, it is not, therefore, of great use in assessing need

prerequisite for this. The most widely used one is the International Classification of Diseases (ICD) and the one used mainly in general practice is that based on the Reid Codes (WHO 2004).

The International Classification of Diseases

After the General Registration Act required the registering of births, deaths and marriages in 1837 it was realised that there was no single classification of diseases in general use. In the 1850s a meeting of statisticians agreed to undertake the task of setting such a classification up. It took several years, but by the turn of the century a single classification of the causes of death was agreed and the ICD was born. This meant that a disease was called the same everywhere. Since the disease was classified the same in different countries, it meant that information from different countries could now be compared. Without the ICD these vital comparisons would not be possible.

Because new diseases are being found all the time (AIDS, for example, was unheard of 30 years ago), the ICD is revised and updated. The current edition is now the 10th revision (Silman & Macfarlane 2002).

Reid Codes

Mortality statistics are generally complete and there has been a standard system for their collection and collation for more than a century. However, in general medical practice the position is completely different. It was not until the 1980s that a classification system (the Reid Codes) more suited to the general medical practice setting (where symptoms cannot always be classified into a disease) began to be more widely used. Initially there was no requirement to collect and collate the information and the computer systems introduced at that time were to improve practice management rather than help in epidemiological needs assessment. As a result not all practices used the system. This is now changing. Reid Codes are linked to the ICD and computer systems are now in place that will enable the number of cases of a particular diagnosis to be counted. So, within general medical practice (though not yet a geographical population), rates of a disease can now be collected using GP data. There are also a great deal of prescribing data available. These changes now make it possible to use GP data in a reliable way.

Types of information and their sources

There are two main forms of information, systematic information and surveys, as well as other local sources of information collected by groups of staff.

Systematic information is information collected routinely all the time. It should normally be of good quality and is often published in reports and your local public health information analyst is a good source of advice on this. You will see later in the chapter that much of the information used to describe the causes of mortality and morbidity in a population are from systematically collected data.

Surveys are carried out periodically for specific reasons to find information that is not routinely available. National surveys are usually carried out through questionnaires and there needs to be a high level of return of these for the information to be reliable. They are costly and need to be done well by people who specialise in this type of work. To be able to look at time trends the survey has to be repeated asking exactly the same questions. National surveys will usually only give a broad indication of what is going on in a small area. There are techniques, however, for using national information and predicting what would be the position in a small local population if the local population were similar to the national population.

Other local information is often kept by people such as community nurses. This information is often kept either in paper form or on handheld computers. These can sometimes be used to provide more information about the patient or client group. It can also sometimes be quite easy to do a small survey locally of patients or clients to find out other information that may be useful.

Activity

Do not imagine that you are the first person to look for information about your area. Others may have done this before you. So, if you want to save time and resources, it is important to check that this information has not already been collected before starting to search for it. Annual reports of the Director of Public Health are good sources of information and there may be other pieces of work in public health departments that have not been published. Your local public health information analyst is also a good person to ask. Find out as much as you can about local information sources by locating annual reports, searching local websites and generally asking around.

3.2.5   The determinants of health

The Dahlgren and Whitehead (1991) model is a helpful reminder of factors that are important in determining good health and is shown in Figure 3.6. Broadly speaking, the model encompasses environmental and behavioural factors including:

- health-related behaviours (e.g. smoking);
- social environment (e.g. education, employment) and physical environment (e.g. atmospheric pollution, housing conditions).

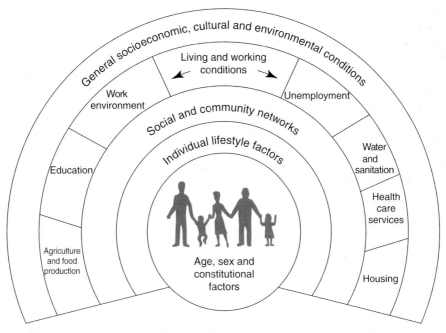

Figure 3.6 Health and influences on levels of health Dahlgren: and Whitehead (1991) model. *Source:* WHO (1992).

3.2.6 Health-related behaviour

Local surveys are expensive to carry out, take a lot of time and are rarely repeated. Most information about health behaviours, for example smoking or physical activity, comes from surveys done at a national level, for example the Health and Lifestyle Survey (Johnson 2000). These surveys do not provide detailed information about a small geographical area, but they are of good quality and can be used for predicting what is likely to be the position locally. More recently general medical practices have started to collect data about smoking and obesity routinely and in a standardised way, so it should now be possible to obtain smoking rates and obesity for practice populations. In due course it will be possible to combine data from individual general medical practices to give a geographical perspective.

3.2.7 Social and physical environment: the index of multiple deprivation

Various factors are used to measure how deprived populations in geographical areas are. Taken together these form the index of multiple deprivation (IMD) (Shaw *et al.* 1999). The IMD includes measures of:

- educational attainment, skills and training;
- income;
- employment;
- health and disability;
- living environment – indoor and outdoors;
- barriers to housing (including overcrowding);
- crime and disorder.

It is well known that poor levels of these factors contribute to poor health (Barker *et al.* 1998; Acheson 2000; DH 2004, 2006; Institute of Fiscal Studies 2006). As a consequence we can use the overall IMD to identify which areas are likely to have poor levels of health and, therefore, need more resources.

However, we can be more specific about this. For example, we can look at each of the measures (domains) that make up the overall index and identify which of the determinants are really creating the problems. It may be, for example, that housing conditions in an area are good, but unemployment is high and income levels are low. This would point to the need for agencies designed to promote employment and to ensure that the take up of benefits are high (Department of Trade and Industry 2006; Department of Works and Pensions 2006). This approach can provide a focus for collaborative working.

Figure 3.7 demonstrates how in one electoral ward being studied it is educational attainment that is the factor that stands out as being particularly poor. The focus for effort here, therefore, needs to be around educational attainment. This might involve work by health visitors on parenting, and the involvement of pre-school playgroups, schools and community development and other groups. Taking this a step further, improvements in educational attainment would have many health benefits and would be one plank in approaches to, for example, reducing teenage pregnancies (Figure 3.8).

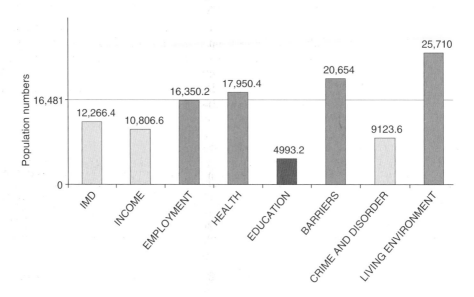

Figure 3.7   Ranking of the domains of the index of multiple deprivation (IMD) in Alamein Ward compared to the rest of the UK.

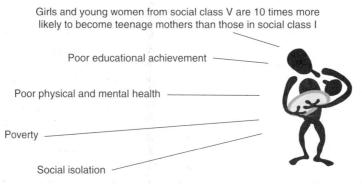

Figure 3.8   Predisposing factors for teenage pregnancy.

Activity

Why not explore the teenage pregnancy strategy of the Department for Education and Skills (DfES 2006); for more information see the website http://www.teensandtoddlers.org/.

3.2.8   Predicting where health problems are likely to be

This can be done simply by using population and deprivation information. When it comes to allocating resources, we can make some good judgements based simply on our knowledge of the characteristics of the population itself. This information is easily available through the census and IMD. Using this information it is now easy to design a table where, if we assume that the electoral wards have the same size populations, it is possible to make predictions about their predominant health needs.

Activity

Try this yourself using the information in Table 3.2 on predicting health needs in two electoral wards.

From this simple activity using Table 3.2, it is clear that Alamein ward, which has more children, will have a higher volume of children's illnesses and create a higher demand for services. However, it is more than that. Having read the evidence, we know that children living in deprived areas are more likely to have more accidents, are more likely to miss out on immunizations, are more likely to have problems of low self-esteem, are more likely to become teenage parents, and are generally more likely to experience a range of other problems (DfES 2006).

Table 3.2   Predicting health needs in two electoral wards.

Electoral ward	Population under 15 years	Population over 75 years	Index of multiple deprivation
Alamein	25%	3%	29.9
St Bartholemew	12%	17%	14.6

3.3   Assessing the Information Collected: Some Tools of the Trade

3.3.1   Numbers

Case Study Example

You are a funeral director who has moved to a new area to set up business. There are no other funeral directors around. There are two towns, Feeling under Par and Generally Overwhelmed. You want to locate your main business in the town that will provide most work. You look up the number of deaths that are occuring in each of the towns and what you find is shown in Table 3.3. Clearly the place to locate the business is in the town with the larger number of deaths, i.e. Feeling under Par.

You might adopt a similar type of approach if, for example, you were a children's service manager. Instead of using deaths you would use the number of children. If the number in one area was twice that in another area, then you would expect the demand for health visiting and school nursing to be around twice as high. This would give you a rough guide as to the volume of resources you need to put in.

Table 3.3   Number of deaths in the last year.

Feeling under par	Generally overwhelmed
400	200

Table 3.4 Number of deaths last year and population size.

	Feeling under par	**Generally overwhelmed**
Number of deaths	400	200
Population	400 000	200 000
Death rate	1/1000	1/1000

3.3.2   Rates

If you want to compare two areas or populations in order to decide which is the more needy (i.e. less healthy), then you need something different. You need to find out which has the higher proportion of its population that is less well. Table 3.4 shows the information you would be looking for and how, when the two towns are compared, it can be seen that the death *rates* are exactly the same.

Calculating rates

A rate is the number of events (e.g. number of deaths) divided by the population in which these events took place (e.g. men aged 45 years of age and over in the Primary Care Trust) multiplied by, for example, 1000, 10 000 or some other convenient round number.

Rates are effectively the proportion of the population that experience something. For example, one-quarter (0.25) of the population might have condition A. However, it is usually more convenient to show this proportion as a whole number. So, for example, by multiplying the proportion 0.25 by 100, we can say that 25 in 100 (25%) of the population have condition A. Often we need to multiply the proportion by 1000 or 10 000 or more in order to arrive at whole numbers. In this example, the rate might be expressed as 250/1000 or 2500/10 000.

Different types of rates

1. *Incidence rates.* Incidence is the number of new cases of something that occur in a defined population over a defined period of time.
2. *Prevalence rates.* Prevalence is the number of cases of something that exist in a defined population over a defined period of time (Farmer *et al.* 1996).

Case Study Example

To get an idea of the difference between these, consider rheumatoid arthritis. The number of new cases of rheumatoid arthritis that are diagnosed in a year is not high, but because this disease usually lasts a lifetime, the prevalence (i.e. the number of new cases that have occurred in the past year plus all the cases that already exist) will be much higher.

---

3. *Crude rates.* A key to success when comparing rates is knowing where the traps might be and how to get round them, so this section is aimed at helping you to understand some of these. When a rate is calculated by dividing the total number of deaths that occur in a population by the total population, it is a simple exercise and the rate produced is called a crude rate.

   There are a number of limitations of crude rates. Crude rates take no account of the age structure of a population and the fact that the death rates at different ages (the *age-specific death rates*) vary and generally increase with increasing age. The more people you have in a particular age group, the more the rates in this age group will affect the overall result. It is a bit like mixing paints of different colour. The more blue paint you add to red paint, the more blue the resultant purple mixture becomes. The more elderly people you have in a population (with higher death rates), the higher the overall crude death rate tends to be.

Table 3.5 Effect of different age structures on crude rates.

Age group (years)	New Town			Old Town		
	Population	Death rate/1000	No. of deaths	Population	Death rate/1000	No. of deaths
0–4	4000	1/1000	4	1000	1/1000	1
5–14	5000	2/1000	10	3000	2/1000	6
15–24	4000	5/1000	20	3000	5/1000	15
25–44	3000	10/1000	30	4000	10/1000	40
45–64	3000	20/1000	60	5000	20/1000	100
65+	1000	30/1000	30	4000	30/1000	120
Total	20000	7.7/1000	154	20000	14.7/1000	282

Case Study Example

In Table 3.5 there are two towns – New Town and Old Town – with exactly the same numbers (20000) in their total populations. Not only that, the death rates in the different age groups (the age-specific death rates) in the two populations are exactly the same. You might expect, therefore, that their overall crude death rates would be the same. But they are not. The crude death rate in Old Town is nearly twice that of New Town. The reason for this is simply that the numbers of people in each age group are different and this has caused the dramatic differences in the results of the crude death rates.

From Table 3.5 it is easy to see that the crude death rate has to be accepted for what it is – it is useful, but it is an unsophisticated crude measure.

---

4. *Standardised rates.* See the following section for details of standardised rates.

3.3.3 Standardization: correcting for differences in the structures of populations being compared

Standardised rates

Standardization is the white knight on a galloping charger used to overcome the difficulties that arise when comparing populations with different age structures. Standardizing the death rate is a method by which the differences in the age structures of a population are cancelled out. (Rates can also be standardised for other differences in the populations, e.g. gender or social class, but the most commonly used standardization is for age.) When we compare the death rates for two places using standardised rates we know that any differences that we find are not caused by differences in the age structures of these two places.

Activity

To develop your understanding of the mathematics of this, look at *Essential Public Health* by Donaldson and Donaldson (2003). Also have a look at http://www.nchod.nhs.uk/, which has simple explanations of statistical methods used in its compendium of clinical and health outcomes.

Standardised mortality ratio

The job of the standardised mortality ratio (SMR) is also to compare the mortality experience of one place with the mortality experience of another in a way that neutralises the effect that any differences in age structure may have. In other words, it does pretty much the same as standardised rates. However, there are two main differences:

1. It manages to show the difference using just one final figure (as compared to having to put the standardised rate of one place beside the standardised rate of another in order to see any difference between them).
2. It gives the ratio of the number of deaths (not rates) that *actually* occurred locally with the number of deaths that *would have* occurred locally if the age-specific death rates in another 'standard' population somewhere else (often the population of England) had applied locally. (This is then normally expressed as a percentage by multiplying by 100.)

So, if the number of occurring deaths locally was 400 and the number of deaths that would have occurred locally would have been 800 if the age-specific death rates of a standard population elsewhere had applied, then the SMR would be:

400/800 = 0.5 multiplied by 100 to give 50.

In another example, if the number of occurring deaths locally was 400 and the number of deaths that would have occurred locally would have been 400 if the age-specific death rates of a standard population elsewhere had applied, then the SMR would be:

400/400 = 1 multiplied by 100 to give 100.

In another example, if the number of occurring deaths locally was 800 and the number of deaths that would have occurred locally would have been 400 if the age-specific death rates of a standard population elsewhere had applied, then the SMR would be:

800/400 = 2 multiplied by 100 to give 200.

The key things to remember about the SMR are:

1. It takes account of differences in age structure.
2. If the SMR is under 100, then the mortality experience of the population you are looking at is better than the standard population.
3. If the SMR is above 100, then the mortality experience is worse. (If the SMR, for example, were 200, then the population you are looking at is twice as 'bad' as the standard population you are comparing yourself with, which is always 100.)
4. The standard population used in this country is often England or England and Wales. More recently, an artificial European population has been used so that people can compare SMRs across Europe (Silman & Macfarlane 2002).

Activity

To help you understand the maths behind this, have a look at Chapter 1 of *Essential Public Health* by Donaldson and Donaldson (2003).

Comparing rates and the International Classification of Disease

You need rates if you are going to compare things. This applies to health as much it does to holidays (cost per week with one travel company compared with cost per week with another). The important thing to remember, however, is that you need to compare like with like – apples with apples, and pears with pears – room-only rates with room-only rates, bed and breakfast rates with bed and breakfast rates. This is where the ICD (WHO 2004) comes into its own. If everyone uses the definitions in the ICD, then we know that we can make proper comparisons.

3.3.4 Confidence intervals: how confident can you be in the results gained from small numbers?

As a general rule, the smaller the number of events that occur, the less confident you can be that what is found is typical of the general picture. An example of this might be deaths from road traffic accidents (RTAs), where death rates from road traffic accidents are relatively low in England and Wales as a whole (www.gov.mu/portal/sites/ncb/cso/report/natacc/road04/index.htm).

Case Study Example

For a population living in a small town, the chances are that several years may go by without there being any deaths from RTAs at all. The death rate from RTAs would be zero in each of these years. However, if one year a family of five people went on holiday and were involved in an RTA that killed them all, then the death rate from RTAs in the population in that town would suddenly appear to be very high. Neither 'no deaths' nor 'five deaths' would give a very representative picture for the town overall.

The picture presented in this case study example contrasts with what the picture might be with deaths from coronary heart disease. These are high in England and Wales as a whole. This means that for a population living in a small town, the chances are that a fair number of people will die from coronary heart disease in any one year. If, in any one year, the number went up by five or down by five, this would not affect the rate very much and would not be very noticeable when compared to the overall number dying (Barker *et al.* 1998).

How public health practitioners get round the problem of small numbers

One way of getting round the problem of small numbers is to cluster years together (e.g. cluster 3 or 5 years), which increases the number involved. You can then take an average.

Another way is to show the range within which you are confident that, if you were to take several measurements over time, 95 per cent of the results would fall within this range (the *confidence interval*). So, in the example of the RTA deaths above, where the number of events is so small and any one result is not very representative, there would be quite a wide confidence interval. In contrast, where there is a high mortality from something, e.g. coronary heart disease, the numbers would be much higher, the uncertainty would be much lower and the confidence interval would be much smaller.

Figure 3.9 shows a typical example of how confidence intervals are shown on a bar chart. Although towns B and D have lower rates than town A, the confidence intervals for them overlap with the confidence interval of town A. This means that the death rates, although appearing lower on this occasion, were not really significantly different from the death rates in town A. In contrast, town C has the lowest death rate and the confidence interval does not overlap those of the other towns. This means that the death rate in this town is significantly lower than the others.

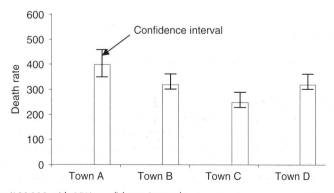

Figure 3.9　Death rates/100 000 with 95% confidence intervals.

3.4   Some Tools to Use When Constructing a Community Profile: Classical/ Descriptive Epidemiology

The information you have collected about the population and the determinants of health will form part of the profile you put together. The question arises, however, as to how best to structure this and the information you have on the rates of the health problems you find, e.g. heart disease or cancers. One answer is to use the tools offered by classical (descriptive) epidemiology. These have been used for a long time as a way of describing the health problems of a population.

The tools of classical epidemiology are much the same as you would use in clinical practice. When you summarise a patient's history you usually describe more than just the symptoms and signs; it should also include information on:

- time;
- place;
- person.

The summary may elaborate on the situation of the patient, as shown in the following case study example.

Case Study Example

Mrs Smith is a 35-year-old married Indian mother of two who is a non-smoker and works part time in a local chemical factory. She presents with a history of a cough that began when she first took up part-time work as a cleaner in the local chemical factory. The cough is worse during the week but seems to be better at weekends.

Her story is important as it gives us the following information about:

1. When she has the problem – *time*.
2. Where she has the problem – *place*.
3. Characteristics of who she is – *person* – including:
   - gender;
   - ethnic background;
   - marital status;
   - parity;
   - occupation (and, therefore, social class);
   - place where the problem occurs;
   - health behaviour.

These tools can be helpful when trying to predict what a diagnosis is likely to be if one does not yet have enough information to be absolutely precise about what it is. This applies as much to a community diagnosis as it does to an individual diagnosis. For example, Table 3.6 shows how this might help in clinical work.

The tools of time, place and person used to help make a community diagnosis in clinical work are the same as those used in classical (descriptive) epidemiology. They can reveal truths about what is happening to the health in the population as a whole. They are also helpful in localizing where problems are and who has them, thus enabling resources to be targeted to those with greater need. For example:

- time (are things getting better or worse?);
- place (which locality has the greater health need?);
- person (who has the problem and what are their characteristics?).

Tables 3.7–3.9 illustrate this.

Table 3.6   Clinical work example.

Time	An adult presenting with fever, cough and feeling tired and unwell for 2 days is more likely to have an acute infection like flu or acute chest infection than someone who has had these symptoms for 3 months, who is more likely to have a condition like TB
Place	People who have never been abroad are very unlikely to have malaria. However, this would be a high probability for someone returning home from a holiday in a country where malaria is rife (e.g. Africa), who develops a fever with jaundice. It would be a reason for rapid referral to hospital
Person	
Gender	Men do not get ovarian cancer, so this can be excluded from the differential diagnosis of a lump in the abdomen in a man
Age	It is very unlikely that a lump in the breast in a young woman aged 20 will be cancer, whereas the chances of breast cancer being the cause of a lump in the breast of a woman aged 60 are very high
Ethnicity	A child with anaemia and joint pains of Middle Eastern extraction may well have sickle cell anaemia, but this is unlikely in a child of English parents
Health behaviour	A heavy smoker presenting with weight loss and a cough may well have lung cancer, but the chances of this being the diagnosis in someone who has never smoked are much less

Table 3.7   Mortality rates, 1841–1970, in England and Wales. *Source:* OPCS 2000.

	Time period	
	1841–1950	**1961–1970**
Death rates/1000 population	22.4	11.8

Table 3.8   Cholera death rates in London districts supplied by Southwark and Vauxhall and the Lambeth Water Companies, 8 July to 26 August 1854. *Source:* John Snow (personal communication).

	Water company		
	Southwark and Vaxhaull	**Lambeth**	**Total**
Death	844	18	862
Population served	167654	19133	186787
Death rate/1000 population	5.0	8.9	4.5

Table 3.9   Life expectation (years) in 1841 (Chadwick 1842).

Place	**Professional person**	**Tradesman**	**Labourers, artisans, servants**
Wiltshire	50	48	33
Leeds borough	44	27	22
Bolton	34	23	18

Classical (descriptive) epidemiology uses time, place and person to structure the information you have. Presenting information in this way using simple tables, bar charts, graphs and other types of representation will allow your findings to spring out of the page of any report you may be compiling. This will help enable you to target your resources to the people who need them most.

Conclusion

Public health is about the organised efforts of society to address the issues that stand in the way of people's health. There is a limited amount of resources for doing this and these need to be directed to people who will benefit from them most in a way that is most efficient and effective. Accurately describing the health and absence of health of the population is a prerequisite to being able to do this. This chapter has endeavoured to show how epidemiology can help this to be achieved.

References

Acheson D. (2000) Health inequalities impact assessment. *Bulletin of the WHO* 78 (1), 75–6.

Barker D.J.P., Copper C., Rose G. (1998) *Epidemiology in Medical Practice*, 5th edn. London: Churchill Livingstone.

Bradshaw J. (1972) The concept of social need. *New Society* 30, 640–3.

Centre for Reviews and Dissemination (CRD) (2001) *Undertaking systematic reviews of research on effectiveness: CRD's guidance for those carrying out or commissioning reviews, CRD Report 4*, 2nd edn. http://www.york.ac.uk/inst/crd/pdf/crd4_ph5.pdf

Chadwick E. (1842) *Report on the Sanitary Condition of the Labouring Population of Great Britain*. Edited with an introduction by M.W. Flinn (1965). Edinburgh: Edinburgh University Press.

Chief Medical Officer (2005) *The State of Public Health*. London: HM Stationery Office.

Dahlgren G., Whitehead M. (1991) *Policies and Strategies to Promote Social Equity in Health*. Stockholm: Stockholm Institute of Future Studies.

Department of Works and Pensions (2006) *Households Below the Average Income*. London: HM Stationery Office.

Department of Trade and Industry (2006) *UK Fuel Poverty Strategy*. Fourth Annual Progress Report. London: HM Stationery Office.

DfES (Department for Education and Skills) (2006) *Teenage Pregnancy Next Steps: guidance for Local Authorities and Primary Care Trusts on effective delivery of local strategies*. London: HM Stationery Office.

DH (Department of Health) (2004) Choosing Health: making healthier choices easier. London: Department of Health.

DH (Department of Health) (2006) *Our Health, Our Care, Our Say: a new direction for community services*. London: HM Stationery Office.

Donaldson D. (2005) *The Annual Report of the Chief Medical Officer*. London: Department of Health.

Donaldson L.J., Donaldson R.J. (2003) *Essential Public Health*, 2nd edn. Newbury: Petroc Press.

Farmer R., Miller D., Lawrenson R. (1996) *Epidemiology and Public Health Medicine*, 4th edn. Oxford: Oxford University Press.

Fletcher R.H., Fletcher S.W., Wagner E.H. (1996) *Clinical Epidemiology: the essentials*, 3rd edn. London: Lippincott, Williams & Williams.

Harries A. (1997) *Needs to Know: a guide to needs assessment for primary care*. London: Churchill Livingstone.

Institute of Fiscal Studies (2006) *Poverty and Inequality*. London: Institute of Fiscal Studies.

Johnson M.R.D. (2000) *Black and Minority Ethnic Groups in England: the second Health and Lifestyle Survey*. London: Health Education Authority.

NHS (National Health Service) (2006) *National Health Service Act 2006*. www.opsi.gov.uk/acts/acts2006/20060041.htm.

Office Population Census Surveys (OPCS) (2000) *Annual Abstract of Statistics*. London: HM Stationery Office.

Shaw M., Dorling D., Davey-Smith G. (1999) Poverty, social exclusion and minorities. In: *Social Determinants of Health* (eds Wilkinson R.G., Marmot M.).

Silman A.J., Macfarlane G.J. (2002) *Epidemiological Studies: a practical guide*, 2nd edn. Cambridge: Cambridge University Press.

WHO (World Health Organization) (2004) *International Statistical Classification of Diseases and Related Health Problems. 10th Review*, 2nd edn. Geneva: World Health Organization.

Section 2

Management of Public Health Needs

Section 2 Introduction: Management of Public Health Needs

Key Public Health Skills

- Collaborative working for health and wellbeing
- Working with, and for, communities to improve health and wellbeing

This section offers discussion on how practitioners can stimulate awareness of health needs with individuals, families, groups and communities and in particular with those who are seriously disadvantaged and are socially excluded from society. Evidence provided by the Cabinet Office (2006) in their action plan on social exclusion suggests that social exclusion has a long-term, negative effect on health. Often, immediate survival, or coping with the adverse effects of a hostile environment (where there is crime or racism, for example), prevents people from recognizing their own health needs and acting on them. These groups of people whose needs are unique and complex are particularly difficult to reach. Highly localised and tailored responses are needed to meet the needs of those suffering the effects of social exclusion. Firstly people need to understand what is possible for themselves, their families or community, then they can be supported and empowered to achieve in the way that best suits their needs.

By working closely and in partnership with individuals, families, groups and communities, practitioners can stimulate awareness of what may be possible for them to achieve and develop a plan to manage these needs. This is the first step towards consumer choice, user involvement and empowerment. The skills required here are complex. Practitioners need a positive and proactive attitude towards multiagency and interprofessional collaboration in order to promote and protect the health and social wellbeing of the population, community, families and individuals. The chapters in this section explore the skills required for:

- multiagency and interprofessional team working;
- respecting, understanding and supporting the roles of other public health practitioners involved in health and social care delivery;
- appreciating the changing nature of health and social care roles and boundaries;
- understanding all the public health activities that underpin the delivery of quality client focus services;
- collaboration with a range of public health practitioners;
- involving users and carers in the development, delivery and evaluation of public health activities.

Introduction to Chapter 4

Public Health Skills: collaboration

- Collaboration in community development work: working with communities and others
- Collaborative skills of practitioners: consciousness raising, community action and participation

This chapter looks at collaborative working between service providers and communities. It explores the organizational structures and cultures needed to develop effective collaboration between organizations and the communities they work with. To highlight these issues, the findings of an action research study conducted within a community health programme in a regeneration area are drawn upon. The final section pulls out broader lessons learnt from the study that may be of use to practitioners in establishing a community health programme that can collaborate effectively with its constituent communities, including:

- the problem of community participation;
- design of the action research study;
- study findings;
- constraining and enabling factors in building a participatory programme;
- lessons learnt: organizational changes for collaboration with communities.

Introduction to Chapter 5

Public Health Skills: partnership and user involvement

- Skills of partnership working: what it means to work in partnership, issues of power in partnerships, values to support effective partnerships, trust in partnership working, empathy, enablement, acceptance, genuineness and empowerment
- Dialogue and learning together: engaging with service users, statutory and voluntary agencies, negotiating and action planning
- Facilitation skills: managing conflict, advocacy and leadership

Chapter 5 is the first of two chapters on partnership and is about partnerships for public health and, in particular, user involvement to improve health and wellbeing. The chapter examines the knowledge and skills required for establishing and maintaining effective partnerships by guiding the reader through strategies for developing awareness of their own professional and personal value base, through gaining knowledge about the actions that communities, groups, families and individuals can take to improve their health and wellbeing. It takes the perspective that for public health practitioners to work effectively, they need a deeper understanding of the diversity of people, their motivations and the consequent dynamics of partnership work. Through this understanding the practitioner can assist in developing the capacity and confidence of communities, groups, families and individuals to influence and use available services and information and build skills to enhance choice leading to health improvements.

Introduction to Chapter 6

Public Health Skills: partnership and professional involvement

- Developing partnerships: managing, implementing, evaluating and the facilitation of health-enhancing activities
- Examination of prerequisites for partnership working

- Skills for working in partnership with families and individuals in the identification of health need
- Facilitation skills for working in partnership with families and individuals to promote health-enhancing activities
- Skills in offering support and encouragement with development of life skills
- Constraints and barriers to working in partnership

Chapter 6 is the second chapter on working in partnership and explores a range of varied discourses to determine how partnership has reached prominence in the health care literature. It examines what partnership working is and focuses particularly on considering the type of skills that public health practitioners need to work in this way. It also seeks to examine what factors might mitigate against working in partnership and what factors may promote it. The health gains from partnership working are considered and presented.

Introduction to Chapter 7

Public Health Skills: communication

- Effective communication: perspective, beliefs and values, environment, rapport, pacing, listening and hearing, language and goal setting
- Communication feedback: conflict, emotion, trance and endings

Chapter 7 is a very practical one and offers you, the reader, the opportunity to examine the field of communication and its relationship and meaning for you as a public health practitioner. It challenges you to examine yourself, your presuppositions, prejudices, perspective, beliefs and responses to the communication process. The aim of the chapter is to understand how you can use communication skills to influence effective communication and appreciate how your perspective, reactions and responses can affect the desired communication outcome.

Reference

Cabinet Office (2006) *Reaching Out: an action plan on social exclusion*. www.cabinetoffice.gov.uk.

CHAPTER 4

Collaborative Working: Organizational Development for Community Participation

Helen Elsey

Public Health Skill: Collaboration

- Collaboration in community development work: working with communities and others
- Collaborative skills of practitioners: consciousness raising, community action and participation

Introduction

This chapter looks at collaborative working between service providers and communities. In particular it explores the organizational structures and cultures needed to develop effective collaboration between organizations and the communities they work with. To highlight these issues, the findings of an action research study conducted within a community health programme in a regeneration area will be drawn on. The final section pulls out broader lessons learnt from the study that may be of use to others in establishing a community health programme that can collaborate effectively with its constituent communities.

Increasingly, public health programmes are developed and implemented through collaboration between NHS organizations, local authorities and other statutory bodies, the voluntary sector and communities. The mandate for, and value of, collaborative working has been evident in both Department of Health (DH 1998, 2000, 2003) and regeneration policies (Social Exclusion Unit 2001; Neighbourhood Renewal Unit 2004) for several years. This has led to a great variety of collaborative ventures, including local strategic partnerships and regeneration schemes such as 'New deal for communities' (NDC), which pull together the public, private and voluntary sectors to work with communities.

The study used in this chapter is set within an NDC area, so it is worth explaining the background to the scheme. The NDC is funded by central government through the Office of the Deputy Prime Minister and works in 39 of the most deprived communities in England. NDC draws together statutory and voluntary organizations to work on programmes under the theme areas of health, education, the environment, crime and employment. The overarching focus that underpins all these themes is community participation and ownership.

4.1 The Problem of Community Participation

However, while these initiatives have burgeoned across the UK, research has highlighted the problematic nature of involving communities in these partnerships. For example, Burton *et al.* (2004) conducted a systematic review of 26 studies of regeneration areas in the UK and found that while there had been an increase in community involvement in policy, this was not reflected in practice. They found the most common participation modes were consultation to solicit community views and representation of community members on organizational bodies. While consultation is an important aspect of community health programmes, it can also be seen as a fairly limited form of participation. The dominance of consultation as a means of participation is also a consistent theme in the literature (Jordan *et al.* 1998; Anderson & Florin 2000; Fitzpatrick *et al.* 2000; Wood 2002; Farrell 2004), with many studies identifying a lack of structured mechanisms for ensuring that the results of consultation exercises are successfully fed into the organizational decision-making processes.

Burton *et al.*'s (2004) study also identified a number of difficulties in relation to community representatives, particularly the high expectations placed on them, the limited extent to which they can be said to 'represent' the diversity of their communities, and the inadequate organizational structures for ensuring they can influence decisions taken. Burton *et al.* (2004) further recognised a general lack of evaluation of participation strategies within programmes. Burton *et al.*'s (2004) findings of the tensions within the concept of the community representatives and their ability to not only 'represent' their communities but also influence the health or regeneration agenda are a constant theme within the literature on participation in the UK and beyond (Jewkes & Murcott 1998; Foley & Martin 2000, McInroy 2000; Purdue *et al.* 2000; Pickard & Smith 2001; Perrons & Skyers 2003; Dinham 2005).

An extensive national evaluation of NDC schemes is currently being conducted by the Centre for Regional Economic and Social Research at Sheffield Hallam University. While it is too early to assess any conclusive findings, the evaluation team produced a 2003/4 annual report. The report draws on a variety of survey and qualitative interviews to assess the views of NDC boards (staff and residents), programme teams and agencies to conclude that the community has become more involved in a range of partnership tasks. However, their findings also indicate that while a few community members may be heavily involved, participation does not extend to the wider community and that there are still a whole range of partnership tasks that do not have much involvement – particularly monitoring and evaluation, project design, development and management (CRESR 2004).

Clearly, collaborating with communities is a great challenge and lack of meaningful participation would appear to be a widespread problem. This leads us to ask why is collaborating with communities so challenging for statutory and partnership organizations? In order to help answer this question, the findings of an action research study conducted in a NDC regeneration area are presented here.

4.2   Action Research Study: Community Participation in a Collaborative Health Programme

As described above, NDC is the national regeneration scheme in which this action research study was situated. More specifically, the study was located within one of the community health programmes whose aim was to support families with children aged from 0 to 17 years. The programme brought together health visiting and midwifery services and introduced a new locality family worker service. The role of the locality family workers was to support the work of the health visitors and midwives by providing practical support to families in the area. The family workers often live in or near the area and are very familiar with the challenges facing local families. The aim is that their support may prevent families reaching crisis point.

In the research cited above, the problem of increasing levels of participation among anything more than a small group of committed community activists was also identified by both staff and residents involved in the NDC regeneration area. It was the recognition of these challenges that led to the development of the action research study. Both programme staff and residents were keen to try out new approaches to encouraging participation and action research provided the ideal methodology to not only develop participation within the programme but also to document and analyse the experiences of staff and community members in trying to establish a participatory programme.

4.2.1   Design of the action research study

In light of this, the study used an action research methodology. While there are many different types of action research, Kemmis and McTaggart's (1982) definition helps to clarify the fundamentals of the approach. They describe action research as:

> A form of collective self-reflective enquiry undertaken by participants in social situations in order to improve the rationality and justice of their own social or educational practices, as well as their understanding of these practices and the situations in which these practices are carried out.

In essence, action research involves a series of cycles of planning, acting, observing and reflecting and is normally conducted by a group of co-researchers. The observation stages often draw on a variety of quantitative and qualitative methods resulting in the action research cycle (Figure 4.1).

The aim of this study was to identify what helped and hindered the development of a participatory programme. More specifically the objectives of the study were:

1. To understand the meanings and motivations for participation from the perspectives of agency staff and community members.
2. To assess the effectiveness of various action strategies in improving the extent and quality of participation from the perspectives of community members and programme staff.
3. To explore the value and effectiveness of techniques to measure participation.
4. To analyse the experiences of a team of co-researchers in their efforts to encourage participation.

At the heart of the study was a core group of seven co-researchers, all of whom volunteered to participate. The co-researcher group consisted of three locality family workers, a health visitor, a resident, the programme co-ordinator and the facilitator/researcher. The group met roughly every 4 weeks over an 18-month period. Initially, a reconnaissance phase, as recommended by Titchen and Binnie (1994), was conducted. This involved seven semi-structured interviews with staff, 15 questionnaire-based interviews with community members, and group exercises with residents, health and regeneration staff and other stakeholders to explore what helped and hindered participation.

The findings of this first phase provided the group with the information needed to try out different strategies for encouraging participation within the action research cycles of planning, acting, observing and reflecting. The observation stages of the action research cycles drew on a variety of quantitative and qualitative methods including observation, interviews with residents and staff, and a survey of the programme's clients.

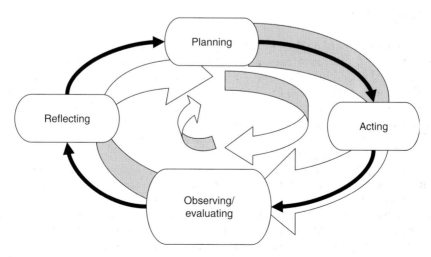

Figure 4.1   The action research cycle.

Throughout the study, where possible, all the co-researchers were involved in the analysis process to some extent. However, given the time pressures on frontline health workers, often the co-researchers could only get involved in the final stages of the analysis. Hence, with the qualitative data, the facilitator/researcher used the 'framework approach' as developed by Ritchie and Spencer (1994). The advantage of this structured approach was that a thematic framework could be developed to be closely based on the research objectives but also to allow for other themes to emerge from the data. One of the final stages of the approach was to map the key themes that emerged from the data; these maps provided a clear visual representation that the co-researchers could use as a basis for discussion of the validity of the themes chosen and their meanings. For the quantitative data, the co-researchers played a valuable role in identifying variables to be compared. Analysing the quantitative and qualitative data in this way led to thoughtful, reflective discussions among the co-researchers which then led naturally into the next cycle of planning and action.

In addition to this, the facilitator/researcher also analysed the overall process and experience of the co-researchers over the 18-month period. The aim here was to solicit deeper insights into the factors that constrained and enabled the co-researchers in developing a participatory programme. In order to do this, the transcripts of all the action research sessions and individual interviews with the co-researchers throughout the study period were analysed.

4.2.2   What the study found

Throughout the 18-month study period the co-researchers became increasingly aware that in order to develop a participatory programme they needed to address many different aspects of their relationships with communities and the functioning of their organizations. They started to appreciate that participation should be seen as a coherent system within the organization. The co-researchers felt strongly that this system must include:

- the means to effectively communicate with all the community, so community members are aware that the organization is actively seeking their participation;
- many different ways for clients and the wider community to participate;
- a mechanism for this participation to influence decisions made about the design and development of the programme;
- effective ways of communicating the impact of their participation back to clients and the wider community, explaining what changes have been made in light of their participation and, if no changes can be made, why not.

The findings from the action research cycles show which strategies proved most effective in developing the different components of this participation system identified by the co-researchers. In terms of communicating with clients and soliciting their feedback, a simple survey, developed with user involvement, proved to have the highest response rate of all the feedback methods tried, with 53 per cent of questionnaires returned. However, it must also be noted that those responding to the survey were invariably the most articulate and literate in the community. The other participation methods tried – such as drop-in sessions and group discussions, where clients or the wider community could talk through their concerns about family support services more informally – generated much more in-depth and valuable information to help improve the service. A texting service was also established so that community members could feed in their comments quickly and, if desired, anonymously. This proved popular with younger parents, but was used predominantly after key events rather than for giving feedback on regular health visiting, midwifery or other family support services.

The overriding finding, however, was that the most successful method for encouraging participation, particularly from the more isolated in the community, was through the direct one to one support offered by the locality family workers. Through these interactions the family workers were able to communicate what participation pathways were available, hear feedback about the services and, importantly, provide the support and encouragement for their clients to begin attending groups or get involved in decision making within the programme. This individual communication, support and encouragement proved far more effective than relying on the written word – such as flyers, adverts and newsletter articles – in encouraging community members to participate either on a passive or more active level.

4.2.3   Constraining and enabling factors in building a participatory programme

While the co-researchers did make some progress through these strategies in developing the participation system, overall progress was slow and by the end of the action research study, participation within the programme went no further than improved feedback on some parts of the service and a gradual increase in the number of community members attending toddler groups and play sessions. The findings from the overall analysis of the co-researchers' experience of attempting to develop a participatory programme identify five key themes. Firstly; the characteristics of the area and its community with its history of suspicion of statutory agencies, complex family lives and a transient population made developing a participatory programme challenging. However, it could be said that any area has its challenges and certainly the other themes point to some fundamental organizational constraints to developing a participatory programme. In particular, the other themes were: the level of organizational commitment to participation, the extent of empowerment among frontline staff, the traditional health professional approach, and levels of empathy shown towards the local community.

The findings clearly show that while the policies of all the statutory agencies working in partnership in the area were very favourable towards community engagement, often specifying it as one of their main aims, in practice there were many organizational constraints to achieving participation. Many of those interviewed both from the statutory agencies and the community identified the formal structures and processes, with their emphasis on paperwork, long meetings and the use of jargon, as a constraint to participation.

> I think the structures don't empower people. Too often they are geared up to the way the agencies work. Yeah and even say, sometimes we set up a project and the question they ask is how to involve the community and they pull an answer off the peg – oh we'll set up a steering group. (Individual interview with an agency representative, regeneration scheme)

During the action research sessions, the co-researchers often expressed frustration that the idea of community participation seemed alien to many within statutory agencies.

> They were talking about vandalism and I said, surely there are things that could be done with the community and they all looked at me askance. I said, well actually we have got some youth projects working on the estate and surely when we get to that point, the young people should be involved in the design and the planting. … All these great wonderful architect people there and the PCT planning team and they all looked at me askance. (Co-researcher, action research session 10)

This limited practical drive for participation presented itself in many ways, for example, given that the programme provided family support services, one crucial organizational limitation was the lack of resources available to pay for childcare during meetings or other events where community members were encouraged to participate. This issue shed light on another organizational constraint to participation, namely that frontline staff who were actively wishing to promote participation from the community had no access to resources to support such engagement. The dialogue below between the co-researchers (CR1 to CR3) illustrates just how those keen to encourage participation were often left to use their own ingenuity to find resources to cover childcare or other costs to facilitate the participation of their clients and members of the wider community:

> *CR1:* Yes, we'll have to think carefully about how they [the parents' group sessions] work.
>
> *CR2:* We should definitely provide childcare.
>
> *CR3:* But how do I pay for it?"
>
> *CR1:* Didn't you say you could maybe get £50 or so to pay for it?
>
> *CR3:* Maybe as a one-off, but not on a regular basis.
>
> (Discussion among co-researchers, action research session 9)

This lack of direct decision-making power over resources was further exacerbated by the hierarchical system within the NHS Trusts. Those involved in the programme were required to work their way up a decision-making hierarchy before being able to change elements of their practice in response to client and community feedback or to facilitate participation. Furthermore, access to decision making was hampered by the processes of constant change and restructuring within the Trusts.

> 'A' has looked at it as my line-manager, she said I have to show it to 'B' [next level of management], who then passed it on to 'C' [next layer of management] so I'm waiting for her to come round! (Co-researcher, action research session 8)

This reliance on traditional structures and processes, lack of resources targeted to stimulate and facilitate participation along with a lack of devolved decision-making authority to frontline staff all played their part in restraining the co-researchers' attempts at developing a participatory programme. However, the findings also show the importance of the attitudes of those working with communities in their attempts to encourage participation. The differences in attitudes among the co-researchers, particularly between those residing in the area and those from outside, were striking throughout the study.

Those living within the area frequently displayed more empathetic attitudes towards the community than frontline health staff not resident in the area. The two quotations below typify the attitudes often displayed by non-resident (the first quotation) and resident (the second quotation) co-researchers:

> There are also the people who don't do it because they've got nothing else to do, they just can't be bothered. It's fair enough if you've got something to replace it, but for lots of people round here they just can't be bothered. (Non-resident co-researcher, action research session 7)

> Because I think lots of the parents just lack confidence don't they. I mean we find that all the time, that they lack self-esteem and confidence. They have got the skills, and they want to learn but they've just not had that praise, you know, 'you could do it'. (Resident co-researcher, action research session 16)

There was constant tension among the co-researchers as some explained non-participation as the result of high levels of apathy within the community, while others felt participation was constrained by community members' limited confidence to participate. Further analysis identified that resident staff with more empathetic attitudes were more likely to acknowledge that organizational policies and practices were often responsible for restricting participation, a point they found frustrating as they believed strongly that participation was of benefit to both the individual and for the development of the community. For non-resident professionals with lower levels of empathy there was a tendency to see limited value in participation, often fuelled by a sense of disillusionment with the possibility for change within their organizations. Furthermore, there was a tendency among the least empathetic to put the needs of staff on an equal level with, or even above, the needs of the community. The full report of the research study can be found in Elsey (2006).

4.3   Lessons Learnt: Organizational Changes for Collaboration with Communities

The study highlights some important lessons for statutory and partnership organizations keen to encourage participation and collaborative working with their communities. There is much emphasis in guidelines and toolkits on the kinds of techniques that can be used to encourage community participation; in fact it often seems that a new technique is always appearing which those working with communities are keen to learn and try out. The study shows that while these techniques are important – particularly having an assortment of techniques that meet the varied needs of all in the community and having one to one support from community health workers to help build confidence for participation – they are only part of the picture. In addition the organization needs to develop a coherent system that ensures effective communication with communities and, importantly, mechanisms for ensuring that community views directly influence decisions made about their services. The components of the participation system identified by the co-researchers in the study are presented in Figure 4.2.

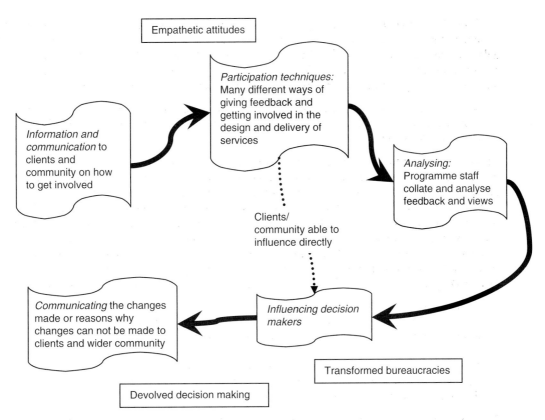

Figure 4.2 The Participation System.

The study shows how important it is for an organization to develop an effective participation system; however there is a need to look beyond organizational systems alone. The attitudes of those at the frontline, working with communities, are of vital importance. The more empathetic staff can be towards the community and the greater understanding they can have of the community's needs, the more likely they are to be able to encourage participation and to establish equal and effective collaborations. In the study, the fact that some of the frontline health workers – the locality family workers – were resident in the community seems to have given them a natural empathy with the community.

This is not to say that health workers who may not be resident in the community can not also be empathetic. However, it does highlight the importance of paying attention to the values and attitudes of staff. One way of building empathy is to develop an in-depth understanding of the issues facing all the various groups within the community. Where staff are able to 'put themselves in the shoes' of community members and understand their perspective they are much more likely to be able to work in an open and responsive way. Valuing time to talk to a wide range of people in the community and even undertaking small pieces of research – or even action research – projects can help in building up this understanding.

The study highlights how extensive organizational changes must be in order to encourage community participation effectively. In fact, the study shows that for this particular Health Trust a transformation of traditional hierarchical ways of working is required. Frontline staff can not be responsive to the needs of the community and the results of participation exercises if they do not have the power to take decisions and back them up with speedy access to resources.

Conclusion

While the study is based on only one Trust and its regeneration partners, the literature discussed earlier in the chapter indicates that the problems faced in this study are common elsewhere too. There would seem to be a great need for statutory and complex partnership organizations to transform the way they work, both by establishing systems to ensure participation and by devolving decision-making power to frontline staff who themselves are encouraged to be empathetic towards the communities they work with.

References

Anderson W., Florin D. (2000) *Involving the Public – One of Many Priorities: a survey of public involvement in London's Primary Care Groups*. London: Kings Fund.

Burton P., Croft J., Hastings A., Slater T., Goodlad R., Abbott J., Macdonald G. (2004) *What Works in Community Involvement in Area-based Initiatives? A systematic review of the literature*. Home Office Report No. 53/04. London: Home Office.

CRESR (Centre for Regional Economic and Social Research) (2004) *New Deal for Communities: the National Evaluation the Programme Wide Annual Report 2003/2004*. Sheffield: Sheffield Hallam University.

DH (Department of Health) (1998) *Our Healthier Nation – a contract for health*. London: HM Stationery Office.

DH (Department of Health) (2000) The *NHS Plan: a plan for investment, a plan for reform*. London: HM Stationery Office.

DH (Department of Health) (2003) *Tackling Health Inequalities: a programme for action*. London: HM Stationery Office.

Dinham A. (2005) Empowered or over-powered? The real experiences of local participation in the UK's New Deal for Communities. *Community Development Journal* 40 (3), 301–12.

Elsey H. (2006*) Encouraging participation in a community health programme*. Unpublished PhD thesis, University of Southampton.

Farrell C. (2004) *Patient and Public Involvement in Health: the evidence for policy implementation*. Department of Health: London: HM Stationary Office.

Fitzpatrick S., Hastings A., Kintrea K. (2000) Youth involvement in urban regeneration: hard lessons, future directions. *Policy and Politics* 28 (4), 493–509.

Foley P., Martin S. (2000) A New Deal for the Community? Public participation in regeneration and local service delivery. *Policy and Politics* 28 (4), 479–91.

Jewkes R., Murcott A. (1998) Community representatives: representing the community? *Social Science and Medicine* 46 (7), 843–58.

Jordan J., Dowswell T., Harrison S., Lilford R., Mort M. (1998) Health needs assessment: whose priorities? Listening to users and the public. *British Medical Journal* 316, 1668–70.

Kemmis S., McTaggart R. (1982) *The Action Research Planner*. Deakin: Australia: Deakin University.

McInroy N. (2000) Urban regeneration and public space: the story of an urban park. *Space and Polity* 4 (1), 23–40.

Neighbourhood Renewal Unit (2004) *New Deal for Communities*. Presentation from NDC Stakeholders Conference 12 May 2004. http://www.neighbourhood.odpm.gov.uk/ndcomms.asp.

Perrons D., Skyers S. (2003) Empowerment through participation? Conceptual explorations and a case study. *International Journal of Urban and Regional Research* 27 (2), 265–85.

Pickard S., Smith K. (2001) A 'third way' for lay involvement: what evidence so far? *Health Expectations* 4, 170–9.

Purdue D., Razzaque K., Hambleton R., Stewart M. (2000) *Strengthening Community Leaders in Area Regeneration*. York: Joseph Rowntree Foundation.

Ritchie J., Spencer L. (1994) Qualitative data analysis for applied policy research. In: *Analyzing Qualitative Data* (eds Bryman A., Burgess R.), Chapter 9. London: Routledge.

Social Exclusion Unit (2001) *A New Commitment to Neighbourhood Renewal: National Strategy Action Plan*. London: HM Stationery Office.

Titchen A., Binnie A. (1994) Action research: a strategy for theory generation and testing. *International Journal of Nursing Studies* 13 (1), 1–12.

Wood M. (2002) Resi*dent Participation in Urban and Community Renewal*. Australian Housing and Urban Research Institute, Queensland Research Centre.

CHAPTER 5

Partnerships for Public Health: User Involvement to Improve Health and Wellbeing

Steve Tee

Public Health Skills: Partnership and user involvement

- Skills of partnership working: what it means to work in partnership, issues of power in partnerships, values to support effective partnerships, trust in partnership working, empathy, enablement, acceptance, genuineness and empowerment
- Dialogue and learning together: engaging with service users, statutory and voluntary agencies, negotiating and action planning
- Facilitation skills: managing conflict, advocacy and leadership

Introduction

Public health nursing is, according to McMurray and Cheater (2003), a complex endeavour requiring a sophisticated range of skills enabling practitioners to work flexibly and in new ways. The new ways of working are those that transcend traditional boundaries and engage individuals, groups and communities in partnerships focused on improving health and wellbeing. Social, cultural and political factors interact to create a practice environment that demands a workforce which can embrace and adapt to change. Therefore, to be effective, practitioners require a deep appreciation of factors that enable the building of effective partnerships with service users at an individual, family, community and population level. As Cornwall *et al.* (2003, p. 30) point out:

> Bridging the gap between professionals and communities and establishing new forms of partnership is essential if service provision is to be made more responsive and accountable.

This chapter examines the knowledge and skills required for establishing and maintaining effective partnerships by guiding the reader through strategies for developing awareness of their own professional and personal value base, through gaining knowledge about the actions families, groups and individuals can take to improve their health and wellbeing. It takes the perspective that for public health practitioners to work effectively, they need a deep understanding of the diversity of people, their motivations and the consequent dynamics of partnership work. Through this understanding the public health practitioner can assist in developing the capacity and confidence of individuals, families and communities to influence and use available services and information and to build skills to enhance choice leading to health improvements.

The chapter includes a case study example presenting a dynamic, multiagency approach to the health, education and social care needs of a population of vulnerable children, their families and the wider community. The case study example is used as a vehicle for illustrating the skills that can lead to tangible benefits for all involved.

5.1   The Skills of Partnership Working

5.1.1   Why public health partnerships?

Modern public health nursing approaches seek to improve the health of whole populations through working in partnerships with groups and individuals to systematically address health needs within a community. Sir Donald Acheson (1998) defined public health as:

> The science and art of preventing disease, prolonging life and promoting health through the organised efforts of society.

Acheson's definition emphasises harnessing the power of individuals and communities towards improved health outcomes. Policy initiatives which are driving the partnership agenda highlight the professional responsibility for working in new ways (DH 2004). Stages of the process include monitoring the community health status, identifying the needs of that community and then planning systematic programmes, in partnership, which reduce health risks. Within such partnerships the practitioner collaborates to both develop policies that promote healthy behaviours and evaluate the care provided.

Similar developments are taking place in other parts of the world. In the United States, the Quad Council of Public Health Nursing Organizations (1999) have identified some principles of population-based practice. As well as a focus on entire populations possessing similar health issues, they include the creation of healthy environmental, social and economic conditions in which people can thrive and the requirement to 'reach out' to collaborate with other organizations, agencies and professionals. The Quad Council stresses the need for nurses to consider all levels of practice, including individual/family, community and systems.

This emphasis represents a broadening of practice from approaches primarily targeted at the needs of individuals and families, toward approaches that also embrace communities and populations (Caraher & McNab 1997; Smith 2004). To illustrate the dimensions of the role, Carr (2005) identified five potential levels of practice that help to demonstrate the full scope of the public health nurse's role. The adapted version of Carr's model is shown in Figure 5.1.

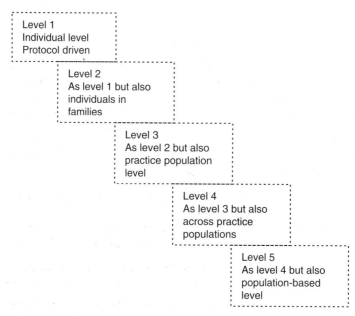

Figure 5.1   Levels of practice with a primary care public health continuum. *Source*: Adapted from Carr (2005).

This model is useful in that it provides a reflective tool to determine the focus of the intervention according to need and context. As Carr (2005) points out, the levels of practice are bounded by a broken line to indicate permeability and to acknowledge the functions shared between levels. Importantly, from the perspective of partnerships, the model also illustrates that moving through the levels require practitioners to work in collaboration with service users, workers and agencies from different health and social care sectors in order to achieve the desired health benefits.

The emphasis on partnerships in this model highlights three significant challenges to traditional approaches to public health practice in the UK:

1. Health and social care providers have been located in silos derived from functional, departmental and professional legacies preventing effective collaboration between organizations (Flynn 2002).
2. Health providers have tended to adopt paternalistic approaches to decisions about care, treatment and service provision with service users and their families being passive in the decision-making process (Tee 2002a).
3. Health services have been provided following little, if any, consultation with the public or service users and a 'one-size fits all' mentality (Rook 1998; Barker *et al.* 1999).

Today, higher public expectations, an increase in well-informed, assertive consumers and the need to provide greater choice and diversity have been at the forefront of policy and have changed the culture of practice. McKenna and Keeney (2004) highlight the key challenges that face providers of modern health and social care provision:

- expectation of choice;
- an increase in well-informed assertive consumers;
- an increase in perceptive questions;
- an increase in individual access to health information;
- the challenge of professional autonomy and increased empowerment of consumers;
- an increased access to best evidence through the internet and other media.

It is clear that working effectively within this context requires practitioners who can not only appreciate the best evidence for health intervention but who have the skills to work alongside the public, service users, their families and the wider community. In other words, the practitioner needs to work flexibly, creatively, innovatively and in ways that address health needs holistically in order to acknowledge the factors identified by McKenna and Keeney (2004) and to lead to meaningful outcomes valued by all concerned.

5.1.2 What does it mean to work in partnership?

The characteristics of a partnership are derived from relationships formed through mutual participation and contracts (Towle & Godolphin 1999). Partnership can therefore include relationships between individuals or groups characterised by mutual cooperation and responsibility or can be legal contracts entered into by two or more persons. Within a public health context, partnerships are essentially relationships established within the social, political, cultural and familial context of people's lives. Informal partnerships may be formed where there is an understanding between people, and informal agreements may precede more formal arrangements. Whatever their status, Towle and Godolphin (1999) suggest partnerships imply:

- shared responsibility with all parties involved having something to gain and contribute;
- focused discussion about the nature of the relationship;
- a dynamic and evolving process that accommodates changed circumstances;
- something that can be initiated anytime but which will need time to develop.

These factors are important considerations for nurses attempting to develop partnerships with service users, organizations or other health and social care workers as they indicate that the nurse will require:

- an understanding of their own and others' motivations for establishing the partnership;
- time and commitment to develop and maintain the partnership.

To help contextualise the focus of partnership working, Scragg (2001) suggests there can be three levels of partnership:

1. *Strategic*: a shared vision, with joint planning and commissioning.
2. *Operational*: co-located teams, interdisciplinary groupings and virtual teams.
3. *Service delivery*: mutually agreed plans of action based on individual or community need.

It is, of course, conceivable that the public health nurse is simultaneously engaged in partnership working at all three levels. They may, for example, be working with a number of statutory and third sector organizations to facilitate a shared vision of how to tackle a particular health issue within a community. At an operational level, to support interagency collaboration, they may be co-located with a number of agencies to support the development of a particular project. Similarly they may be working at an individual or family level to enable community participation.

5.1.3   Issues of power in partnerships

Developing public health partnerships requires an understanding of how power relations between individuals and groups or the wider community can impact on the relationship. In professional relationships there is often an imbalance in power. The source of the imbalance can be manifold. As Handy (1990, p. 359) points out relations between individuals and group may be subject to:

> systematic distortions by dominant power holders whose structural position in society gives them an enhanced ability to make their own sectional interests appear to others as a universal one.

The structural position of dominance may, for example, arise from access to knowledge, information and channels of communication, control of budgets and resources or professional domination of decision making. Discussion of the required systemic and structural changes, characteristic of anti-oppressive practice in social work (Preston-Shoot 1995; Garcia & Melendez 1997), is beyond the scope of this chapter. However, at the level of day to day practice, effective partnership working requires practitioners to anticipate, understand and begin to manage power differentials in order to avoid actions which may lead to further disempowerment.

These issues were illustrated in work undertaken by Sherry Arnstein in the 1960s, who outlined a ladder of participation toward greater citizenship (Figure 5.2). The items identified down the left are

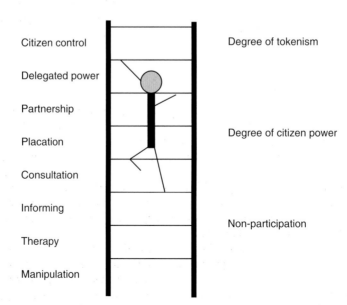

Figure 5.2 The ladder of participation. *Source*: Adapted from Arnstein (1969). Reproduced with permission of *The Journal of the American Planning Association*.

> **BOX 5.1**
>
> **Openness towards partnership.**
>
> - Health and social care is affected by social, political and personal circumstances
> - People experience discrimination as a consequence of their ethnic origin, age, gender, sexuality and disability
> - Service users' needs and preferences should be at the centre of service delivery
> - Uphold the right of the individual to make informed choices that enable them to participate in life opportunities
> - Be sensitive to and embrace difference
> - The safety, health and wellbeing of service users and their carers is paramount
> - People should be treated with respect and dignity, observing their right to privacy and confidentiality

activities that may be undertaken or provided by an individual practitioner or an organization in order to engage the individual citizen, group or community within the decision-making process. The outcomes listed on the right of the ladder are the degree of actual participation experienced by the citizen(s).

The ladder can be used to analyse activity at both an individual level, through the process of negotiating care, and at a community level when developing a population-based intervention. The ladder makes it clear that certain behaviour, such as the giving of information to clients or consulting clients through a questionnaire, whilst useful, involves minimal active participation and tends to be a one-way process with all the power over decisions remaining with the professional service provider. As one goes further up the ladder, power becomes increasingly shared and devolved to the point where the individual or community has complete control and can make decisions independently.

It is evident from Arnstein's (1969) work that there may be considerable activity that purports to be partnership working but which may be experienced as manipulative and tokenistic by individuals or communities where the decisional power does not get shared. An example of this would be where families are asked by survey to comment on the development of a new service when in fact, behind the scenes, professionals have been meeting and have already determined the scope of the service and are just seeking to validate their plans. Such practice is not only ethically questionable but, importantly, maligns participation and involvement, making it more difficult to engage people in future projects. Of course it is unlikely with any new public health initiative or service development that there will be unlimited resources to develop services or scope to give the public complete control over funding, but it needs to be stated from the outset the limits of their influence so that they can make an informed choice about participation.

5.1.4   Values to support effective partnerships

An awareness of differentials in power relations in order to overcome or avoid the types of manipulation and coercion identified in Arnstein's model requires an understanding of how one's own beliefs, values and assumptions affect decisions. The personal and professional values held by individual practitioners can both enhance and hinder effective partnership working. Values are deeply held convictions that influence individual behaviour and action. They are of crucial importance when it comes to taking decisions about service delivery, priorities and needs. Public health practitioners need to become aware of their values and beliefs about other people so that they do not bias or cause adverse influence on decisions. Examples of the type of values that might suggest openness toward partnership working in public health are identified in Box 5.1.

Whilst this is not an exhaustive list, the points do illustrate an important attitudinal shift from services based on the values of professionals toward those based on the values of service users. Awareness of personal values and beliefs can be developed through reflection in practice as well as through supervision. To explain how beliefs evolve and are maintained, Argyris (1990) constructed a progressive model that illustrates the relationship between individual values and beliefs and the attachment of meaning to experience (Figure 5.3).

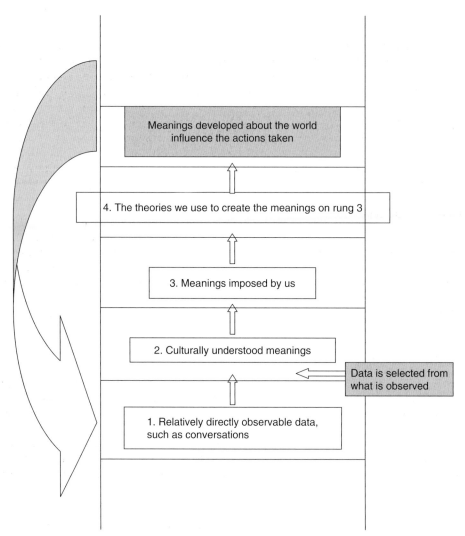

Figure 5.3   Ladder of inference. *Source:* Adapted from Argyris (1990, p. 88). Reproduced by permission of Pearson Education, Inc., Upper Saddle River, NJ.

5.1.5   Trust in partnership working

Awareness of our own values and beliefs helps us avoid making premature assumptions which may lead to prejudicial behaviour and impede the development of trust in a partnership. A high degree of trust is essential for partnership working. Trust takes time to build and is easily broken, so sensitivity and competent communication skills are important tools in the practitioner's toolbox. Active listening, conveying empathy and the ability to promote meaningful dialogue between participants are essential for building trust. These can be used to facilitate two-way communication in order to develop insight and understanding into each other's perspectives. Where people can get to a place of mutual respect and understanding there is a much higher likelihood of participants moving toward a successful outcome. However, where individuals sense that they are being misunderstood, coerced or manipulated, trust will break down and efforts to bring about change will quickly falter. To avoid such an outcome the practitioner needs to be sensitive to how people behave in groups and the cultures and values which influence the ways other people work. Carl Roger's (1970) work on encounter groups indicates that the three core conditions of *empathy*, *acceptance* and *genuineness* need to be present if any helping activity is to be effective.

5.1.6   Empathy

Empathy is the ability to be able to appreciate the perspective (thoughts and feelings) of another person and to express this back in a way that the person can hear. Achieving empathy for another's predicament requires the skills of reflecting back, paraphrasing and active listening. It is about getting in touch with the person's world and expressing an appreciation of what the person faces. However, it is not sentimental. There is a commonly used comparison of the differences between being sympathetic, being unsympathetic and being empathic toward a person who falls in a ditch. The sympathetic helper goes in and lies in the ditch and bewails the situation with him. The unsympathetic helper stands on the bank and shouts to the victim 'get yourself out' and the empathic helper climbs down, keeping one foot on the bank thus being able to help the victim out of trouble and on to firm ground again (Tschudin 1995).

5.1.7   Empathy and enablement

Empathy is also a core component in enablement. Enablement is the effect of a helping encounter on an individual's ability to understand, cope with and manage their difficulties. One study by Mercer *et al.* (2001) measured empathy and enablement in outpatient attendees. They found that no patient reported a high enablement score with a low empathy score, suggesting practitioners need the time and skill to develop empathic approaches in order to facilitate enablement. Similarly, in general practice, Howie *et al.* (1999) found that enablement was strengthened by lengthier consultations and continuity of care.

5.1.8   Acceptance and genuineness

Fostering a relationship of trust demands an atmosphere of acceptance in which people can feel free to explore their difficulties/problems and where they do not feel judged. Sometimes known as unconditional positive regard, it is about acknowledging the worth of people regardless of what that person may have done. However, seeing someone as worthy does not require the nurse to approve of another's behaviour or admire them, it is simply seeing them as a human being of equal value. Genuineness is about being honest and true to yourself without front or façade. It is about avoiding adopting the role of 'expert' but being what Rogers (1970) suggested was 'transparently real'.

5.1.9   Empowerment

Empowerment refers to a process that enables choice and the achievement of individual consumer rights. It can be seen as a tool for challenging oppression (Ward & Mullender 1991) and, as Solomon (1976) suggests, should promote the individual's potential for managing their own problems. However, some within the disability movement express concern about a model where professionals have the responsibility for empowering the client (Barnes *et al.* 1999). They suggest such notions of 'powerful professionals', however well intentioned, can maintain the power imbalance and lead to disempowerment. Therefore, as Fazil *et al.* (2004) point out, trust and partnership are central to any empowerment approach with professionals, as previously discussed, requiring strategies for dealing with potential power differentials. It is only when these core conditions have been addressed that it will be safe for the process to move on toward open and creative dialogue.

5.1.10   Dialogue

Senge (2006) suggests that learning happens through networks and a climate of openly talking about problems and challenging thinking – it is dialogue rather than discussion. Dialogue is an open conversation, without retreating to polarised views caused by what Isaacs (1999) called the limitations created by our inability to think beyond our vested interests. Dialogue is therefore a conversation with a focus but which does not take sides, a living experience of inquiry within and between people. Senge (2006) adds that dialogue is the ability of the group to explore complex issues from many viewpoints, suspending their assumptions but communicating assumptions freely. Thus each contributes to the pool of co-created meaning which is open to constant development and learning.

Section 2

However, to do this one needs an understanding of how beliefs about health can affect health-seeking behaviour. As Halligan (2006) points out, beliefs provide the mental structures for making sense of who and what we are and for managing our world. They also influence how individuals deal with their health, interpret symptoms of illness and cope with their condition. Therefore, knowing what individuals, families and communities believe about health will be relevant to the process of negotiation and, whether working individually or with a group, to the process of setting mutually agreed, realistic targets and objectives.

Drawing on the creative energies of all partners and valuing all contributions will facilitate support of any endeavour. It is here that the nurse will be able to introduce their knowledge of health issues and local services to any discussions, but also to be actively listening to others so that they do not dominate the agenda and can respond sensitively. Of course the actions that individuals, families and groups can take will vary according to the type of public health issue being addressed. One example might be to involve young people in discussions about reducing vandalism in the community, thus improving the local environment. A high handed, prescriptive approach is sure to fail, but working with community and youth leaders, seeking local solutions from the young people themselves, may have a greater chance of success.

5.1.11   Learning together

Building the empathy that reflects the perspectives of individuals, families and communities requires strategies which enable practitioners and clients to work closely together on shared problems. However, Parker (1997) makes the point that professional practice, particularly in health care, has created divisions between 'expert' practitioners and those that use or require services. As a consequence practitioners wanting to adopt emancipatory approaches toward partnerships between practitioners and service users and service user groups, must develop new strategies. Parker (1997, p. 43) further suggests that more equitable relationships can be achieved by constructing situations in which professionals and individuals, families and groups come together within a 'framework of participatory democracy'.

Such a framework implies a model enabling those involved having regular contact with active involvement of all parties and power sharing within an equal partnership. However, it is important to consider more fully the nature of the 'contact', particularly if public health practitioners are to promote participation as a technique for overcoming oppression and responding to the aspirations of service users. Contact theory postulates that if contact between groups of people increases then this leads to more positive attitudes toward each other. Originating in Allport's (1954) classic text on prejudice, contact theory indicates that more 'intimate' acquaintance leads to increased tolerance. Intimate in this context refers to informal, friendly and less professionalised contact. Lewin and Grabbe (1945) also proposed that a psychological linkage is needed between an individual and the person or group in order to impact on stereotyped attitudes.

Further work on contact theory (Ford 1973; Barnard & Benne 1988; Carpenter 1995) has identified up to six factors that should be present in any experience in order to have a positive impact on attitudes:

- equality of status between the groups;
- group members working toward common goals;
- cooperation during the contact;
- positive expectations by participants;
- successful experience of joint working;
- a focus on understanding differences as well as similarities.

Such conditions are important considerations in the development of an individual or community-focused public health initiative. Cornwall *et al.* (2003) put key concepts about participation and partnership into practice within a 5-year project on a south London housing estate which aimed to bring about change in community wellbeing through alliances with local people. The emphasis was on engaging with local knowledge and on 'strategies to democratise otherwise hierarchical interactions and encounters'.

Box 5.2 highlights the skills required for partnership working.

> **BOX 5.2**
>
> **Skills required for partnership working.**
>
> - High level of self-awareness
> - Trust building skills
> - Empathic approaches
> - Acceptance
> - Genuineness
> - Dialogue
> - Learning together
> - Contact

5.1.12   Engaging with service users and statutory and voluntary agencies

Undertaking participatory approaches with individuals and organizations across sectors, whilst a keystone of good public health practice, clearly does not happen by chance. It requires considerable effort, openness and emersion within the communities who are the focus of the intervention. Cornwall *et al.* (2003) in their work with a deprived south London housing estate suggested it was the networks established between professional health and social care workers, local institutions and residents that broadened involvement. They add that if they had relied on the usual consultative processes with community representatives, they would have missed many potential participants who did not feel part of local institutions.

Therefore a key skill for the public health worker is to be able to reach out to the community by undertaking activities that will engage a wider spectrum of people. In other words, rolling up their sleeves and being prepared to, metaphorically speaking, get their hands dirty. This can be achieved by working with schools, health clinics, retirement clubs and youth organizations, and by running activities within areas frequented by local residents, such as libraries, community centres and shopping areas. Adapting an approach known as participatory rural appraisal (PRA), Cornwall *et al.* (2003) used a range of methods such as a 'problem wall', used to develop a list of perceived problems, and a 'solution tree', which focused on encouraging participants to generate potential solutions. The methods that can be employed are endless, such as pictures, diagrams, flowcharts, videos, film, etc. and are really only limited by the creativity of those leading the initiative. Whatever method is chosen, to gauge opinion or seek views, it is important that they are relevant, accessible and understandable to the target audience.

A further example of public health nursing engagement has been reported by Westbrook and Schultz (2000). They adopted an approach which Kulbok *et al.* (1999, p. 1191), described as a 'strengthening agency within groups and communities to co-create health through partnership'. The approach started with individual home visits to Iraqi mothers to provide maternal–child services but, realizing they were experiencing common problems of isolation, discrimination and harassment, connections between the mothers began to be facilitated. This resulted in the sharing of problems, mutual support and shared solutions.

Importantly, from a partnership perspective, studies have found that involving service users in decisions increased self-esteem (Mowbray *et al.* 1996) and facilitated the development of new skills (Mowbray *et al.* 1998). One significant area of work in mental health by Simpson *et al.* (2002) views involvement in terms of a 'health technology' approach. They propose that user involvement can be considered by organizations as a 'health technology' in the same way as any other health service intervention. The 'technology' is the method by which users are involved and, they argue, by viewing involvement in these terms ensures more rigorous and active participation in the planning, delivery and evaluation of services. In producing a guide for service providers, it includes a useful series of checklists to help shape the work and provides insights for developing a reflective culture of participation within organizations.

5.1.13   Negotiating and action planning

Whether working at an individual or community level, achieving a mutually agreed action plan will be an important determinant of success. Many initiatives arguably falter because, despite considerable effort to understand participants' perceptions of and potential solutions to health problems, concerns become lost in bureaucratic processes. Service users engaged in community consultations share their frustrations at being asked their views but not seeing any tangible outcomes (Tee 2002b). Partnerships therefore need to be nurtured in order to maintain an action-oriented focus toward mutually identifying potential solutions.

This is important because, as Cornwall *et al.* (2003) point out, one of the underpinning assumptions of community approaches is that communities should do as much for themselves as possible. Consequently this may demand a shift in mindset amongst communities who may not see themselves as having responsibility for problems in their environment. Bringing about change, in what is termed the 'locus of control', can be achieved by community members and professionals working together to identify and plan the implementation of solutions. Cornwall *et al.* (2003) describe an excellent example of this involving a day-long session where participants could view solution cards that had been pinned to the walls of a community centre. A process of voting was facilitated which achieved consensus on a list of initial priorities.

This process of sharing problems and solutions is an important leveller as it brings professionals, who may be seen as distant and out of touch, into direct contact with the community they are serving. It is at this point that the public health nurse can share their experience and evidence for ways of dealing with health problems. The difference is that interventions can be contextualised according to the expressed needs of the community and, perhaps more importantly, the process of partnership will have provided a mandate for change which can be used to bring pressure to bear on an authority's priorities.

It is interesting to note from the south London experience (Cornwall *et al.* 2003) that change was acted upon and resulted in new styles of partnership away from paternalistic approaches. The action taken was proof to the residents that their concerns were being taken seriously.

5.1.14   Facilitation skills and managing conflict

Getting to the point at which priorities are agreed may not be a straightforward journey as there will inevitably be disagreement with passions probably running high. Any participatory approach that involves people coming together requires an understanding of how people behave and interact in groups. Tuckman's (1965) framework, which has been used to determine the progress of team development, suggests that teams, or partnerships, work through discrete development stages namely: forming, storming, norming and performing. Awareness of these stages can alert the facilitator of a group to expected behaviours that may demand skilled facilitation techniques.

When a group of people first come together there is a tendency to be overly polite, with guarded communication patterns creating a rather impersonal atmosphere. This was certainly something observed in a cooperative inquiry involving mental health service users and student nurses coming together in a process of mutual learning (Tee 2005). As the participants become more familiar with each other, storming behaviour may be exhibited where group members may feel uncertain, challenge each other and want to withdraw. However, as the chaos disperses and the stage is successfully negotiated, positive norms emerge enabling a more honest, open atmosphere which allows conflicts to be managed effectively. This finally allows for the group or partnership to perform and collaborate effectively within an atmosphere of authentic participation.

The skills of group facilitation require an acute sensitivity to the atmosphere of the group at a particular point, as well as the ability to contribute to an atmosphere of trust, hope, safety, appreciation and respect. The communication skills required will be those of reflection, summarizing and paraphrasing in order to acknowledge and value contributions as well as demonstrating understanding and accuracy of recording. A key outcome is to be able to facilitate the decision-making process toward consensus rather than domination by one particular group, individual or special interest. Within such a process there may often be a need to advocate on behalf of an individual or group.

5.1.15   Advocacy

Advocacy in the UK is a broad concept, closely linked to empowerment, encapsulating the promotion of the interests of service users considered incapable of representing themselves. It is defined as:

BOX 5.3

Forms of advocacy.

- Legal advocacy
- Citizen advocacy
- Formal advocacy
- Peer advocacy
- Self-advocacy

Either an individual or group with disabilities or their representative, pressing their case with influential others, about situations which either affect them directly or, and more usually, trying to prevent proposed changes which will leave them worse off. (Brandon *et al.* 1995, p. 1)

The aim of any public health initiative should be to promote autonomy and self-management that recognises the expertise and capability of the individual, family or community to develop strategies for managing their difficulties. However, this does not imply that help is not required, for it is sometimes necessary to advocate on behalf of individuals or groups of people to ensure their rights and interests are safeguarded. Advocacy is best described as a process for ensuring that the individual or group voice is heard, valued and defended.

In many ways advocacy can be seen as an element of anti-oppressive practice that underpins the preparation of social workers. Anti-oppressive practice adopts a set of principles/values drawn from critical, feminist, post-structural and post-modern theories (Payne 1997) that focus on structures of power and oppression within marginalised groups and service provision (Preston-Shoot 1995; Garcia & Melendez 1997). It is concerned with the practice of challenging structural inequalities. It therefore focuses on empowering individuals to understand their rights and to progress toward effective citizenship.

Whilst there are several forms of advocacy (Box 5.3), wherever possible each should be independent of the provider organization and have the common aim of working toward self-advocacy. As Onyett (2003) points out, practitioners often do not have the required level of independence from service provision required for true advocacy to be achieved. However, they do have an important role in helping individuals or groups to identify advocates to represent them or in articulating the needs of a community in order to argue for more resources. It is clearly important for the practitioner to be aware of the power they have in this situation and to recognise when they are working towards the needs of the community or their own professional self-interest.

To expand on these ideas a little further, citizen advocacy, which is also known in some areas as independent advocacy, involves an individual service user developing a partnership with an advocate. The partner advocate then behaves as if the user's interests are their own (Monarch & Spriggs 1994). As with any partnership, achieving such a relationship requires an open and trusting dialogue in order to fully appreciate the user's situation and then be able to advocate on their behalf. Self-advocacy, according to Croft and Beresford (1990), moves the emphasis of the role of partner to that of coach, supporting the user to develop skills and build relationships and alliances with other users who have similar issues of concern. The underpinning philosophy of self-advocacy emphasises self-determination and control.

5.1.16 Leadership

In many ways, working in partnership across organization boundaries and with diverse communities requires a clear sense of purpose and vision. The qualities required could be said to be characteristic of the transformational leader. Transformational clinical leaders will often motivate followers by appealing to higher ideals and moral values and articulate a clear vision of where the service is going (Mullins 2002). They will recognise and embrace change and quickly institutionalise systems so that new working patterns and relationships emerge and become embedded. However, they will also recognise the interpersonal impact of change and seek to provide individualised support to those involved.

BOX 5.4

Methods to support partnership working.

- Networking
- Hearing strategies
- Talk-back panels
- Negotiating and action planning
- Facilitating groups and conflict resolution
- Advocacy
- Leadership

Leading change also requires support at a senior level of health and social care organizations. At a national level, strategic partnerships are being facilitated through strategic agreements between the Department of Health, the NHS and the voluntary and community sector (VCS) (DH 2004). These agreements are seen as the realization of a trend toward greater joint working and are a framework for promoting greater VCS participation in the planning and delivery of services. At a local level, Local Strategic Partnerships bring together many agencies, co-terminus with local authority boundaries, from the public, private, voluntary and community sectors. They have responsibility for the delivery of a community strategy and advising Primary Care Trusts about local delivery plans creating healthier communities. The outcomes of this important work can be viewed at www.the compact. org.uk. A good practice guide has also been produced that emphasises the importance of strong relationships built on 'openness and integrity' (Compact 1998, p. 1). These are important considerations for public health practitioners leading initiatives, as they create strategic frameworks in which practitioners can begin to develop more effective and sustained partnerships and use the skills of partnership development to best effect.

Box 5.4 Highlights methods used to support partnership working.

5.2   Case Study Example: The Family and School Support Team (FASST)

The following case study example provides a working illustration of the skills outlined in Section 5.1. This case study example has been developed from interviews with the originator of the project, Penny Corsar, and describes a multiagency and multidisciplinary approach to working with disadvantaged and socially excluded groups of people. It draws on the experience of health, social care, education and other agencies and illustrates the skills that those working with the public health agenda would find useful in harnessing the resources of the community and achieving positive change.

5.2.1   Making an assessment of the problem

The project known as FASST was established following 2 years of initial work undertaken by an inclusion social worker in Leigh Park in Hampshire, UK. This initial mapping work revealed a complex array of challenges within a community that could not be addressed by a single agency alone (Box 5.5). Problems such as domestic violence, deprivation of all kinds, a multitude of general and mental health issues and unsupported learning difficulties were identified. Leigh Park is a large social housing estate with high levels of deprivation and consequent health and social care challenges characteristic of such areas. The area was subsequently designated an Education Action Zone.

Families, and the young people within the area, often had a complex array of difficulties with the children being at risk of exclusion due to behavioural problems. Despite the school's best efforts, school staff felt overwhelmed by the complexity of the difficulties, which were made more complex by communication problems between the family, the school and the many agencies that may be involved. Consultation by Corsar and her team, with key stakeholders, identified the need for support for children, families and school staff as well as more effective and open communication system indicating what was being provided for a particular family (Osgood 2006).

BOX 5.5

Problems identified by a family and school support team in Hampshire, UK.

- Domestic violence
- Deprivation
- Mental health issues
- Poor school performance
- Lack of available eye tests
- Hearing tests not being accessed
- Obesity
- Sexual health issues
- Dyslexia
- Speech and language problems

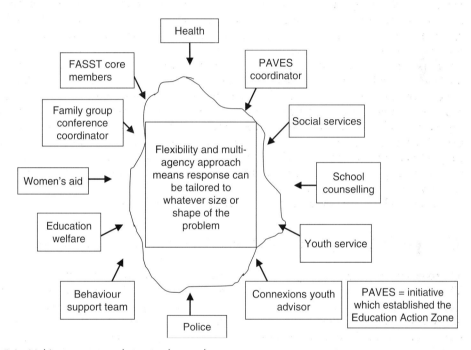

Figure 5.4 Multiagency approach to complex needs.

5.2.2   How the service works

As is the case with many such initiatives, there was no additional pump-priming funding made available so FASST had to be resourced through existing budgets. It was important for this to be achievable if such a project was to be replicated in other areas. FASST is essentially a multiagency approach which is needs-led. Some of the many agencies involved are identified in Figure 5.4 and have developed strong relationships and communication. An open referral system now operates that enables any member of school staff within the Education Action Zone to refer. The referral form used facilitates a process of open communication and sharing of information. The team meets weekly and the speed of support is crucial to the success of the project.

5.2.3   Evidence of effectiveness

Established in 2003, the project has worked with many children and families across 14 primary and secondary schools whose needs could not be met by one agency alone. Fourteen professionals are involved with representatives drawn from the police, behaviour support, youth services, public health nursing, mental health services, education, home–school link worker service, psychotherapy and psychology fields. The most tangible evidence that the service is successful has been the sheer volume of families accessing the service. In the 3.5 years of operation, many of the 530 families who have received support from FASST have given very positive feedback.

Benefits previously reported (Osgood 2006) include a reduction in permanent exclusions, reduced referrals to social service departments and improved learning experiences within school. Importantly, the children and their parents feel supported and their needs acknowledged. Teachers in schools have data demonstrating improvements in the behaviour of children, attendance and cooperation. Improved self-esteem of both the children and parents has been reported, as well as a reduction in referrals to social services and a fall in the number of school exclusions (Osgood 2006). The FASST project has also received considerable media attention due to the pioneering nature of the approach (Burt 2004; Jackson 2005; Osgood 2006).

5.3   What are the Key Learning Points from the FASST Project for the Public Health Nurse?

5.3.1   A shared vision

The underpinning rationale for FASST was that the team would work jointly to provide intervention and prevention at a whole community, school, group, individual and family level. This has meant working strategically, to develop a vision for the service, and operationally, to ensure the many agencies come together and contribute to integrated processes, and at the level of service delivery, to ensure support is inclusive and appropriately targeted at those in need.

5.3.2   Managing issues of power

Conceived as a multiagency approach with the aim of providing support to families, pupils and schools, FASST was focused on changing cultures and behaviour amongst agencies in order to focus on the collective needs of the community. Therefore the choice of name was an important consideration as feedback from potential service users suggested a poorly titled service could doom it from the start. Names can be stigmatizing and cause potential users to make assumptions about the service being delivered. It was determined that the word 'behaviour' would be avoided as the term implies the problem lies solely with the child.

The title eventually chosen reflected the essential partnership between the family and the school. It also emphasised 'support', and a model of working alongside families, rather than any physical or psychological treatment approach. This had the effect of putting decisional power in the hands of service users rather than 'experts' who purport to be able to diagnose and treat a problem. The intended message was to be 'we are in this together'. The overall vision of the project was for the school to be seen as part of the process and part of the solution.

5.3.3   Working with others to develop a shared set of values

It was clear from the outset that different agencies had evolved their own ways of working based on their own ideas of what is a successful outcome. Powerful socialization processes imbue individuals with the cultural norms, values and expectations of the way things should be done in that service. Sometimes this can create barriers to collaboration through defensive or avoidant behaviours.

What was apparent in the FASST study was that through bringing stakeholders together, including the families themselves, a shared set of values was agreed around which the team could move toward a shared set of outcomes. Strong relationship building, mutual support and effective communication were the tools used to encourage agencies to work in different ways. This was considered to be a significant step forward and reflective of a high degree of commitment to collaborative working across boundaries.

The 'values' or working agreement of the team can be summed up as a series of simple action-orientated statements that put the service user at the heart of the service.

5.3.4 Empathy and trust building

The skills most immediately apparent were those of engagement with parents and children who were, by and large, suspicious of such help. The approach involved working collaboratively, alongside and in partnership to ensure decisions were shared and communication was open. It was important that agency workers were aware of the wider community cultures in which they were working. This, arguably, can only be achieved through emersion in the locality in order to appreciate the difficulties the families face. The originator of the FASST project, Penny Corsar, talked of being in an advantageous position having grown up in the area and having 'insider knowledge' into the day to day challenges of living in that environment. Through this process Corsar was able to display qualities of acceptance and genuineness and to purposively tune into the needs and aspirations of the community. Whilst this degree of emersion may be unrealistic for many working in similar public health environments, this does not preclude the need for workers to employ strategies, including regular contact, that will achieve insight into need at both an individual and population level.

5.3.5 Acceptance and genuineness

Sensitivity to the individual has been the cornerstone of the project through respect for where people are at in terms of their perspective on the world, their values and beliefs. Many of the families had previously experienced adversarial relationships with professionals and agencies, which often antagonised situations rather than leading to constructive solutions. It has been reported that health care professionals, in particular, can be discourteous and insensitive, have poor communication patterns and may neglect human aspects of the relationship with service users (Office for Public Management 2000; Mind 2005). Parents involved in FASST had reported this through statements such as 'no-one listens'. Working with diverse groups and communities of service users demands particular interpersonal skills to ensure that issues are handled with sensitivity and dignity. FASST workers are acutely aware of how language is used and avoid confrontation that would embarrass or belittle an individual or contribute to an atmosphere of blame.

5.3.6 Dialogue, engagement and learning together

The FASST project would not be as effective without open communication and dialogue. The byword is cooperation and a 'can do' attitude that can challenge the functional integrity of some agencies. However, this is essential to achieve the sharing of information and avoiding the duplication which so often characterises service users' experiences of multiagency initiatives. FASST functions in such a way as to avoid multiple assessments.

Learning together required a process of listening to the complexities of what was going on in practice. There was a need to understand the perspective of the teachers and the challenges they face in operating an effective school system, as well those of health professionals, the police and social services. But ultimately the success of FASST has been about learning from the people who are living in the community.

5.3.7 Negotiation and action planning

A key worker in the whole process is the home–school link worker who makes a home visit to negotiate an action plan. They discuss the situation with the parents and the child before arranging a meeting in the school. The issues identified may involve health, education or social care and these will be discussed at the multiagency team meeting. According to Osgood (2006), this process ensures that there is constant availability of someone who is both accessible and knowledgeable about the circumstances of the case and the local community.

5.3.8   Facilitation skills, managing conflict and advocacy

Agreeing a group of shared values is one thing, operating and maintaining the 'contract' between agencies is another, but remains essential to the integrity of the whole operation. Therefore a further skill has been that of being vigilant of any apparent deviation from these shared values and creating opportunities where these can be debated, refined and agreed by all stakeholders.

When many agencies are brought together there are invariably unhelpful dynamics, resulting potentially in professional dominance of the agenda, which have the potential to derail progress. Facilitating the multiagency FASST meetings are no exception and require the skills of attentive listening, assertive management of group dynamics and efforts to ensure the centrality of the family's concerns. On occasions there is a need for individuals to advocate on behalf of service users when it appears their perspective is not being heard or their interests are being misrepresented.

5.3.9   Leadership

Effective leaders are those that listen and shape their ideas accordingly. Listening to what is being said and how it is being said, observing the culture and being open to ideas enabled the FASST team to build up a picture of what might work in practice and to see the gaps or shortfalls in the current system. An essential skill in bringing about the required cultural and behavioural change was that of leadership. This involved facilitating a process toward visioning a service that would engage with service users differently through the use of delegated power and partnership working, as illustrated in Arnstein's ladder of participation. Described as a 'can do' mindset, and a service that was there for everyone, it was necessary to paint a clear picture of how such a service might work. In the case of FASST, there were two key people – the school inclusion social worker and the home–school liaison worker – who combined to ensure the vision could be translated into practice.

It was clear that the transformational leadership skills of the project enabled the service to develop whilst ensuring that the many stakeholders were on board and felt supported. From a policy perspective the project has been able to take advantage of its Education Action Zone status and use the impetus to bring about the desired cultural change, again reflecting a key leadership skill of having a keen awareness of the political context of a change initiative and taking advantage of opportunities that may present themselves.

Conclusion

Working in partnership is as much about an attitude of mind as it is about the skills used to facilitate partnership. A prerequisite for effective public health practice is a determination to ensure the minority voices of the vulnerable and socially excluded are not only heard and valued but contribute to meaningful outcomes. Developing an appreciation of the public health issues facing individuals and communities cannot be achieved at a distance, but require contact and emersion to develop an accurate picture of the issues so that interventions can be appropriately contextualised. It is also clear that to be effective, a public health nurse requires an understanding of organizational systems and dynamics to help bring about greater integration between agencies focused on public health needs at an individual and community level.

The FASST project was established following the realization that the problems were so complex that no single agency could provide the holistic approach demanded. However, it relied on the energy, vision and determination of a single individual to work flexibly and across traditional boundaries in order to realise the outcomes that were valued by the community being served.

References

Acheson D. (1998) Public Health in England: report of the committee of inquiry into the future development of the public health function. London: Department of Health.

Allport G. (1954) *The Nature of Prejudice*. Cambridge, MA: Addison-Wesley.

Argyris C. (1990) *Overcoming Organisational Defences: facilitating organisational learning*. Needham, MA: Allyn & Bacon.

Arnstein S. (1969) A ladder of participation. *Journal of the American Institute of Planners* 35 (4), 216–24.

Barker J., Bullen M., De Ville J. (1999) *Reference Manual for Public Involvement*. London: South Bank University.

Barnard W.A., Benne M.S. (1988) Belief congruence and prejudice reduction in an interracial setting. *Journal of Social Psychology* Feb, 125–34.

Barnes C., Mercer G., Shakespeare T. (1999) *Exploring Disability: a sociological introduction*. Cambridge: Polity Press.

Brandon D., Brandon A., Brandon T. (1995) *Advocacy: power to people with disabilities*. Birmingham: Venture Press.

Burt C. (2004) My nine-year-old son wanted to plunge a knife into his heart. *BBC News* 14 Dec.

Caraher M., McNab M. (1997) Public health nursing: an alternative viewpoint. *Health Visitor* 70, 380–4.

Carpenter J. (1995) Doctors and nurses: stereotype and stereotype in inter-professional education. *Journal of Interprofessional Care* 19, 151–62.

Carr S.M. (2005) Refocusing health visiting – sharpening the vision and facilitating the process. *Journal of Nursing Management* 13, 249–56.

Compact (1998) *Code of Good Practice*. www.thecompact.org.uk.

Cornwall A., Lall P., Kennedy K., Owen F. (2003) Putting partnership into practice: participatory wellbeing assessment on a south London housing estate. *Health Expectations* 6 (1), 30–43.

Croft S., Beresford P. (1990) *From Paternalism to Participation: involving people in social services*. London: Open Services Project.

DH (Department of Health) (2004) *Making Partnerships Work for Patients, Carers and Service Users: a strategic agreement between the Department of Health, the NHS and the voluntary and community sectors*. London: Department of Health.

Fazil Q., Wallace L.M., Singh G., Ali Z., Bywaters P. (2004) Empowerment and advocacy: reflections on action research with Bangladeshi and Pakistani families who have children with severe disabilities. *Health and Social Care in the Community* 12 (5), 389–97.

Flynn N. (2002) *Public Sector Management*. Harlow: Pearson Education.

Ford S.W. (1973) Interracial public housing in a border city: another look at the contact hypothesis. *American Journal of Sociology* 78, 1426–47.

Garcia B., Melendez M.P. (1997) Concepts and methods in teaching oppression courses. *Journal of Progressive Human Services* 8 (1), 23–40.

Halligan P.W. (2006) *The Relevance of Belief for Understanding and Managing Illness Behaviour. Chapter 1 In: The Power of Belief: Psychological influence on illness, disability and medicine* (eds Halligan P.W., Aylward M.). Oxford: Oxford University Press.

Handy J. (1990) *Occupational Health in a Caring Profession*. Aldershot: Avebury.

Howie J.G.R, Heaney D.J., Maxwell M., Walker J.J., Freeman G.K., Rai H. (1999) Quality at general practice consultations: cross sectional survey. *British Medical Journal* 319, 738–43.

Isaacs W. (1999) *Dialogue and the Art of Thinking Together: a pioneering approach to communicating in business and life*. New York: Doubleday.

Jackson L. (2005) Region rises to the challenge. *The Guardian* 16 Feb.

Kulbok P.M., Gates M.F., Vicenzi A.E., Schultz P.R. (1999) Focus on community: directions for nursing knowledge development. *Journal of Advanced Nursing* 29 (5), 1188–96.

Lewin K., Grabbe P. (1945) Conduct, knowledge and the acceptance of new values. *Journal of Social Issues* 3, 53–64.

McKenna H., Keeney S. (2004) Community nursing: health professional and public perceptions. *Journal of Advanced Nursing* 48 (1), 17–25.

McMurray R., Cheater F. (2003) Partnerships for health: expanding the public health nursing role within PCTs. *Primary Health Care Research and Development* 4 (1), 57–68.

Mercer S.W., Watt G.C.M., Reilly D. (2001) Empathy is important for enablement. *British Medical Journal* 322, 865.

Miller N. (2002) Personalisation and the promise of contact theory. *Journal of Social Issues* 58 (2), 387–410.

Mind (2005) *Ward Watch Campaign*. London: Mind.

Monarch J., Spriggs L. (1994) The consumer role. In: *Implementing Community Care* (ed. Malin N.), pp. 138–53. Buckingham: Open University Press.

Mowbray C.T., Moxley D.P., Collins M.E. (1996) Consumers as community support providers: issues created by role innovation. *Community Mental Health Journal* 32 (1), 47–67.

Mowbray C.T., Moxley D.P., Collins M.E. (1998) Consumers as mental health providers: first-person accounts of benefits and limitations. *Journal of Behavioural Services and Research* 25 (4), 397–411.

Mullins L.J. (2002) *Management and Organisational Behaviour*. London: Pitman.

Office for Public Management (2000) *Shifting Gears Towards a 21st Century NHS*. London: Office for Public Management.

Onyett S. (2003) *Team Working in Mental Health*. Basingstoke: Palgrave.

Osgood W. (2006) Integrated services should now lead to FASST improvement. *Early Years Education (EYE)* 7 (10).

Parker S. (1997) *Reflective Teaching in the Post Modern World*. Buckingham: Open University.

Payne M. (1997) *Modern Social Work Theory*, 2nd edn. Chicago: Lyceum Books.

Preston-Shoot M. (1995) Assessing anti-oppressive practice. *Social Work Education* 14 (2), 11–29.

Section 2

Quad Council of Public Health Nursing Organisations (1999) *Scope and Standards of Public Health Nursing Practice.* Washington, DC: American Nurses Association.

Rogers C. (1970) *Encounter Groups.* London: Penguin.

Rook S. (1998) *Public Engagement Toolkit.* Durham: NHS Executive N&Y Regional Office.

Scragg T. (2001) *Managing at the Front Line: a handbook for managers in social care agencies.* Brighton: Pavilion Publishing.

Senge P. (2006) *The Fifth Discipline*, 2nd edn. Oxford: Oxford University Press.

Simpson E.L., House A.O., Barkham M. (2002) *A Guide to Involving Users, Ex-users and Carers in Mental Health Service Planning, Delivery or Research: a health technology approach.* Leeds: University of Leeds, Academic Unit of Psychiatry and Behavioural Sciences.

Smith M.A. (2004) Health visiting: the public health role. *Journal of Advanced Nursing* 45 (1), 17–25.

Soloman B. (1976) *Black Empowerment.* New York: Columbia University Press.

Tee S. (2002a) Promoting patient and public involvement in primary health care. Part 1 Literature review. *MCC Building Knowledge for Integrated Care* 10 (3), 39–45.

Tee S. (2002b) Promoting patient and public involvement in primary health care. Part 1 Literature review. *MCC Building Knowledge for Integrated Care* 10 (4), 41–8.

Tee S. (2005) *A co-operative inquiry: participation of mental health service users in the clinical practice decisions of mental health student nurses.* DClinP thesis, University of Southampton.

Towle A., Godolphin W. (1999) Framework for teaching and learning informed shared decision making. *British Medical Journal* 319, 766–71.

Tschudin V. (1995) *Counselling Skills for Nurses*, 4th edn. London: Bailliere Tindall.

Tuckman B.W. (1965) Development sequence in small groups. *Psychol Bulletin* 63 (6), 384–99.

Ward D., Mullender A. (1991) Empowerment and oppression: an indissoluble pairing for contemporary social work. *Critical Social Policy* 11 (2), 21–30.

Westbrook L.O., Schultz P.R. (2000) From theory to practice: community health nursing in a public health neighbourhood team. *Advances in Nursing Science* 23 (2), 50–61.

CHAPTER 6

Partnerships for Public Health: Professional Involvement to Improve Health and Wellbeing

Palo Almond and Sarah Cowley

Public Health Skills: Partnership working and professional involvement

- Developing partnerships: managing, implementing, evaluating and the facilitation of health-enhancing activities
- Examination of prerequisites for partnership working
- Skills for working in partnership with families and individuals in the identification of health need
- Facilitation skills for working in partnership with families and individuals to promote health-enhancing activities
- Skills in offering support and encouragement with development of life skills
- Constraints and barriers to working in partnership

Introduction

Partnership working with health service users, that is clients, patients or families, has been described in various ways, ranging from an impossible ideal (Watson 1999), or a fashionable buzzword (Kirkham 2000), to a way of working that promotes health and wellbeing (Cowley & Almond 2001).

This chapter aims to explore a range of varied discourses to determine how partnership has reached prominence in the health care literature. It examines what partnership working is and focuses particularly on considering the type of skills that public health practitioners need to work in this way. It also seeks to examine what factors might mitigate against working in partnership and what factors may promote it. The health gains from partnership working are considered and presented.

Whilst it is accepted that partnerships can involve several partners, for simplicity the discussion centres on partnerships involving two people, the health professional and the service user. A case study amalgamated from two empirical studies – *Health Visiting in Partnership Project* (Cowley & Almond 2001) and *A case study of equity in health visiting postnatal depression policy, services and practice* (Almond 2007) – is provided to illustrate some of the elements of partnership working in a health visiting context.

6.1 Tracing the Impetus for Partnership Working

Partnership working appears to have come about from a number of key sociopolitical factors and changes in illness patterns occurring over several decades. The principles that are embedded in partnership are those espoused by the United Nations: equity, and a free and just society. Such principles and ideologies underpin moral and ethical practices that do not seek to conquer or dominate but which instead are informed by a sense of equality and democracy (Almond 2001a). Such views informed the 1978 declaration by the World Health Organization (WHO) that primary care should be founded on justice and equity. These instigated a change in attitude as to how health care should be provided, and led to service users being seen as consumers, rather than witless and passive recipients (Almond 2001b).

These principles may not on their own actually influence or pervade the mindset of health care providers; other sociopolitical factors have contributed to these attitudinal changes. Health care services were initially focused on acute illness management and such systems promulgated paternalistic attitudes and created patient dependency on the seemingly more knowledgeable health care practitioner (Holman & Lorig 2000). Epidemiological and social studies served to increase knowledge about the links between lifestyle and disease. The preventability of some diseases resulted in a policy shift to bring about radical changes in how health care was delivered (Lalonde 1974). In 2002 the WHO stated that chronic medical conditions such as diabetes, heart failure and mental illness were the new major challenges for health care systems worldwide.

These changes in illness patterns, such as the decline in acute illness and increase in chronic ill health, have stimulated changes in policy and services (DH 2004a). If health care providers were to combat lifestyle factors, new methods of disease management would need to be found as autocratic and paternalistic practice will not win patient's cooperation to change their lifestyle behaviours. At about the same time as this political enlightenment, and philosophical shift in health care policy and practice, the general public began to demand more education and information about disease and health and expected more involvement in decision making and care. Political transformations also saw the rise in patients being seen as consumers with legal rights (Almond 2001b). These changes brought about a re-allocation of power with more power transferring to service users. Services users were no longer passive recipients but were becoming more active players in medical and health care encounters.

6.2   Theoretical Interpretations of Partnership

One of the earliest models that relates to partnership is that proposed by Arnstein (1969) (see Chapter 5). This model describes the different levels of participation (partnership is rung 6 on the ladder). The rungs are:

1. Manipulation
2. Therapy
3. Informing
4. Consultation
5. Placation
6. Partnership
7. Delegated power
8. Citizen control

This model can be used to plot health practitioner activities to determine the levels of partnership these may involve. As can be seen, many clinical interactions are on the lower rungs of the ladder; however, if these interactions are conducted using the philosophy and skills of partnership as described later in this chapter, clinical interactions may move higher up the ladder.

Although the philosophical movement towards egalitarian health care started several decades ago, partnership working as an academic interest and a clinical priority only began to emerge in the last two decades. Two medical articles on partnership (Coulter 1999; Bleker 2000) generated a flurry of 19 letters in the *British Medical Journal*. Partnerships with patients were largely concerned with decision making around treatments. Decision making is indeed a complex and important clinical process (Almond 2001c) but the primacy for efficiency and effectiveness of interventions and a need for patient compliance seemed to be the main triggers for an adjustment in medical attitudes from paternalism to partnership (Holman & Lorig 2000).

Charles *et al.* (1999) suggest three types of medical relationships with patients:

1. The *paternalistic* model (the doctor is the expert and the patient is passively acquiescent).
2. The *informed* model (there is information transfer between the doctor and patient but the relationship is still largely dominated by the doctor).
3. The *shared* model (a two-way exchange of information and decisions are negotiated and agreed by both the doctor and patient).

They suggest that in reality a 'hybrid' model (a blend of two or more of the approaches) is most likely to be utilised. The hybrid model may well be suited to the complex world of human interaction and variations in human nature. It would seem unethical to apply a shared model if the patient were unwilling to engage in decision making. Waterworth and Luker's (1990) study found some patients were indeed reluctant and unwilling to be involved in making decisions about care.

The community nursing press has largely reported conceptual papers on partnership working (McIntosh & McCormack 2001; Gallant *et al.* 2002; Bidmead *et al.* 2002; Bidmead & Cowley 2005). Nursing has sought to explore the meaning and application of partnership (Casey 1995; Kawik 1996). Examples are also found in the midwifery literature (Fleming 1998). The literature reveals the concept of partnership to be a multidimensional term. This might explain why much of the literature is not specifically focused on partnership working, but discussions include collaboration, negotiation, participation and involving patients in care. Gallant *et al.*'s (2002) conceptual analysis concluded that the concept was still immature. This means that there is little consistency in how the term is used and applied (Morse *et al.* 1996).

Partnership working has attracted theoretical attention but little empirical interest within the public health field. Cowley and Almond's (2001) qualitative study explored partnership in health visiting. Health visitors are nurses who have undertaken further education and training to work with populations to improve health, prevent illness and encourage behaviours to protect health. Box 6.1 briefly outlines the study.

The primary home visit to mothers generally took place between the 10th and 14th postnatal day and was normally preceded by a phone call from the health visitor to arrange a suitable time for the home visit. These primary visits were dominated by the health visitors. This was clearly evident from the research transcripts of the interactions as well as the observations. In some instances the number of lines of health visitor speech numbered 20 compared to four lines of the mother's speech, and this pattern of conversation persisted virtually throughout the visit. The reasons for this offered by the health visitors were that the first visit required them to impart a lot of information (for example the health visiting service, immunizations, clinics, infant feeding, sleeping, prevention of cot death, etc.). Partnership did not exist at these visits although it was claimed that it was being established. The health visitors perceived their role to be one of imparting information rather than collecting information from the mother. The mothers felt themselves to be the recipient, and at most times a grateful recipient.

BOX 6.1

Health visiting in partnership study. *Source*: **Cowley and Almond (2001).**

The research took place within in a South London Primary Care Trust (PCT) that serves a population with high levels of social and economic deprivation. The PCT has a policy whereby health visitors are allowed to conduct more than one home visit if the client's health and situation meet the criteria for more health visiting. It also states explicitly that health visitors work in partnership with clients requiring extra health visiting.

Ethical approval was gained to conduct interviews and observations of home visits by health visitors to postnatal women to explore partnership working.

Twenty-six observations of health visitor home visits to mothers during their first postnatal year were carried out. These observations were preceded by interviews with six health visitors (HV1–HV6). Twenty-six post-observation interviews were conducted with 26 mothers (Client 1–Client 26) and 26 interviews with the six health visitors.

The sample was a mix of white, Indian and African women. All but one of the health visitors was white and one was African. Data analysis drew on the principles of grounded theory.

Partnerships cannot exist when there is no conversation and when it is one-sided. This is akin to Charles *et al.*'s (1999) paternalistic and informed models. The health visitors said the first visit was the most crucial as it was the one where they established a relationship with the client and it was the quality of this relationship that would influence future usage. This is consistent with other research findings (Chalmers & Luker 1991; De la Cuesta 1994). Health visitors overwhelmed the mothers with so much information because policy dictated that they could only do one home visit,

> On a new birth visit it's not very easy really. I mean it sounds a bit mundane but it's just to be sure she is making a good postnatal recovery, really truly. I mean I ask if they are taking iron tablets and you know and they have made their postnatal appointment and bring the baby to the clinic that means you know you are going to watch the baby. (HV2)

The primary visit did not appear to be a partnership as there was little negotiation, collaboration or parent involvement. Yet the primary visit is similar to what Gallant *et al.* (2002) describe as the initiation of the partnership.

Bidmead and Cowley (2005) say this early stage of the partnership should involve the removal of any discomfort that might be felt when two strangers come together for the first time. Examples of this were seen in the Health Visiting in Partnership Project (Cowley & Almond 2001), where clients offered personal information and the health visitor offered relevant personal disclosure at an appropriate time too. For example, a mother described how overwhelmed she was with her feelings for her baby. The health visitor remarked that when she had hers it was like falling in love with her own baby.

The study found that some health visitors substituted the term relationship for partnership, whilst others said that a relationship was a necessary constituent of a partnership between a health visitor and a client. The key elements of partnership found in Cowley and Almond's (2001) study were:

- trust;
- caring;
- openness;
- disclosure.

These elements seem largely about the interpersonal skills of the health visitor and his or her ability to communicate in a way that enables the mother to be an active participant in the process of receiving care, advice or treatment.

6.3   Pre-requisites for Partnership Working

Even before a partnership can be initiated, health professionals have to have the willingness to work in a partnership manner. Certain beliefs, values and attitudes are needed. Such beliefs or dispositions may be democracy, advocacy and the equality of class, gender, race and age. A pre-requisite for partnership working is having a particular working ethos. An example of such an ethos is *client-centredness* (Little *et al.* 2001; Blank 2004). Whilst some commentators argue the merits of client-centred models these may not automatically be deemed as partnership models. The health professional is required to see themselves not as the sole expert in the partnership but as only one of the experts. The patient or client has their own expertise, for instance how they feel, knowledge of their situation, their past medical history, their past experiences, their needs, and their family or child's needs or behaviours.

Cowley and Almond's (2001) research found that partnership was seen to happen when each party was open to other views,

> You know like some clients will say when they have difficulties with their child sleeping and they just want to tell you all about those difficulties, but are not willing to try and change any pattern of behaviour, and I think she had a willingness that she did want to, she did want to try and change, I think because she was agreed, she said she agreed to come into clinic, and she agreed to do this like sleep diary, and she agreed to try and make these changes. (HV3)

Partnership at times was seen to occur in a relationship of equality – the mother and health visitor were equals. The only unequal element found was the type of knowledge that each party possessed. Health visitors had professional knowledge that gave them the capacity to offer advice and it was this knowledge that the mothers respected and wanted the health visitor to impart. Partnership has connotations of power. It is the recognition of its existence and acceptance that it is held by both parties, that will determine the nature of the partnership,

> Yes because I wouldn't have made any decisions. I would have just carried on as I was, and I wasn't strong enough to say 'well yes you have given me some advice but I don't really want to take it' whereas now you know I have been prescribed tablets but it is my decision not to take them, but she hasn't turned around and said 'well you must take them' she went along with it, you know, at the end of the day, she voiced her views and that, but they weren't views that I felt were like judgmental and 'you know you are doing the wrong thing' you know, 'I am wasting my time coming and speaking to you because you are not basically doing' she's just very, I find her easy to open up to. I think that if you are not one hundred per cent all the time, I do think you need someone like that. (Client 2)

Observations of home visits were illuminating and were vital to understanding the enactment of partnership. Health visitors did not appear powerful and neither did the mothers. In other words neither exerted their power over the other. The common denominators were respect and courtesy. The health visitors were conscious of their status as guests in the clients' homes and acted accordingly. The mothers were welcoming and interested in what the health visitor had to offer.

> The way I would sort of define it would be like a health visitor visiting, say visiting a woman who maybe was having problems, ok they come and give the advice, have a chat about it and then going away, and then following it up as she does, she will phone me, you know, I don't think the partnership is coming in to speak to somebody and discussing it, going away and not following it up, even if you phone them up and the person says well thank you, but I don't want to see you again, I am quite happy as I am. You know, I think you do need to have these follow ups, even if you feel ok, it is nice to know that really there is still somebody there at the end of the phone, down at the clinic that you can trust I suppose. It's just nice to have that, and you know that if things aren't going too well you can just phone them up and she will probably if I didn't go down there, she would probably come round, I know that she would do that. (Client 3)

The partnership literature has at times become sidetracked with the discourse on power in relationships (Gallant *et al.* 2002). There seems to be an assumption that a partnership based on equality is in some ways related to power distributions. Equality in a partnership is about a willingness to share and be open, with mutuality and respect. It is about being non-judgemental and flexible. Knowledge is also not related to power in relation to partnership working. Both partners have power, the professional has been educated and their knowledge is seen as a resource to be given and shared with the partner. The client partner on the other hand has experiential knowledge. Knowledge from the two partners is needed for both parties to understand the situation from multiple perspectives. This acts as a foundation on which agreed decisions can be made, as this extract from an interview with a health visitor client indicates.

> In some ways it has to be not really equal, because I mean, she, you know, she went to college to learn about babies and stuff and I didn't, but I had the baby, and it's my first baby so I don't think I should be equal to her, although I am the mother, and I tend to say I know better, but in some ways you know, I know my baby well, you know, a lot more than she does, because I am the mother, but she knows, she will know so many things that I don't know, and I know things that she doesn't know. So I don't think it should be equal. (Client 2)

Partnership is more than a theoretical model of working – it requires a particular philosophical or moral and ethical attitude. It is, however, more than this, it needs to be practised, otherwise it is mere rhetoric.

6.4   Skills for Working in Partnership

Authors seem to find it easier to wax lyrically about partnership philosophies, beliefs and attitudes than the skills required for partnership working, judging by the paucity of these described in the literature. Nevertheless, public health practitioners, particularly novices, do need to know what skills are needed so they can conduct a self-assessment of their knowledge and skills and then proceed to addressing any deficits. Examples of training to work in partnership with service users have been invisible in the literature. This is surprising given that government policy states the need for public involvement and working in partnership (DH 1997, 1999, 2004b). Given the lack of empirical work on partnership working with service users, the typology of skills offered in Table 6.1 needs to be regarded as the first tentative steps to address this deficit and as the beginnings of a partnership skills model. This typology will need to be amended and updated as knowledge about partnership increases.

Egan (1998) and Heron (2001) provide details about enhancing helping skills. What is evident from Table 6.1 is that many of the skills require the practitioner to engage in a process of reflection to gain awareness of his or her value base and personal philosophy. This process may raise conflicts that come with increasing self-knowledge.

Table 6.1 Skills typology for a partnership working with service users.

Values philosophy attitudes	Skills
Democracy	Gaining information and actively listening to the partner's viewpoint Honesty and trust building Encouraging active participation Enabling partner involvement Allowing partner to have their say
Advocacy	Putting aside one's own views and being prepared to present the partner's views unreservedly Feeling and showing empathy Supporting
Partner centredness	Focusing on the partner's needs rather than professional agenda Flexibility Positive regard for partner's needs Warmth and building partner's self-esteem
Non-prejudicial and non-judgemental	Politeness and acceptance of differences Showing respect for cultural, age, gender or class differences Genuineness and cultural competence Willingness to work together Creating a relaxed atmosphere
Lay expertise	Listening and acknowledging partner's contributions. Sensitive questioning to uncover partner's expertise Genuine regard for partner Being prepared to review own beliefs, values and views Humility
Cooperation	Giving partner time Patience Facilitating contribution, e.g. turn taking in conversation, creating rapport Appropriate self-disclosure and reciprocity
Equality	Showing understanding by gestures and paraphrasing Commitment to sharing responsibility, power, benefits and risks Willingness to relinquish any sense or feelings of power and dominance Willingly sharing information
Joint decision making	Offering own ideas and information Accepting there may be more than one solution Humility Patience Planning together in a relaxed and non-combative way
Negotiation	Facilitating partner to present their ideas before presenting own Repeating this process until an acceptable agreement is reached

Public health practitioners are engaged in promoting the health and wellbeing of the whole population. The skills typology reflects the multicultural composition of the UK and indeed most countries. The partnership working literature has neglected to consider the nature of partnership working in different population contexts. The case study presented below attempts to address this omission and shows how it is possible to work in a three-way partnership; that is the health visitor, a non-English speaking client and a bilingual interpreter.

Case Study Example

Partnership working to improve health and wellbeing: detecting and managing postnatal depression in non-English speaking women

A health visitor receives notification that a family have moved into the area of the city that she covers. The client is married with an 8-week baby. The health visitor determines that the mother may not be English given her name is Surjit Kaur and may well be a Sikh Punjabi. It is a policy expectation that health visitors meet families with children less than 5 years of age on at least on one occasion and to assess all women for postnatal depression within the first 3 months of delivery. A validated tool for screening women who speak Punjabi (Edinburgh Postnatal Depression Scale, EPDS) is available for health visitors (Werrett & Clifford 2006). Little empirical knowledge on how health visitors assess women who have a different ethnic and cultural background to their own is available.

Figure 6.1 shows a flow chart outlining two ways the health visitor could respond. It describes some of the attitudes, skills and cultural knowledge that are required to successfully engage with women who do not have English as their primary language. This is a typical situation that health visitors are confronted with and although it is a hypothetical case it is drawn from research observations and interviews with health visitors assessing minority ethnic women for postnatal depression. However, it has been idealised to demonstrate a partnership approach to this aspect of health visiting. These idealizations are drawn from recommendations provided by participants in the equity project which is in progress. It is a fabricated description because a three-way partnership was not seen during either of the research projects. Due to limitations of space the case study is necessarily brief.

6.5 Constraints and Barriers to Working in Partnership

Table 6.1 outlines the values and philosophies underpinning partnership working with service users. Clearly the absence of these and the related skills would act as barriers to working in partnership. Charles *et al.* (1999) felt that the key barrier to working in partnership is the lack of time and resources that doctors need. A busy waiting room or a clinic may act as a disincentive to working in partnership because, as Table 6.1 indicates, for the two parties to make a contribution, more time is needed than is necessary if the interaction is one-sided. The time taken in a three-way interaction (see case study) requires even more time. The possibility, therefore, is that unless resources are available to allow practitioners to work in this way, practitioners will not be compelled to work in partnership with their clients. Slowie (1999) and Mariotto (1999), however, put forward a persuasive argument, stating that whilst the initial investment is high in terms of time and effort, the long-term benefits of fewer referrals, less morbidity and increased patient empowerment, justify partnership working. Mariotto (1999) cautions, however, that as the public become aware of the limits of medicine and health care practices there may be an exodus to alternative and complimentary treatments. The popularity of complimentary services has increased but it is not known whether this is due to partnership working or an increase in knowledge about the limits of medicine and the crudeness of pharmacological treatments.

As suggested earlier, training in partnership working is needed but this will not be sufficient until local policies also promote this way of working. Managers need to invest in this way of working. The next section examines what health gains are possible from this way of working in the hope that these will influence policy and investment to promote the health and wellbeing of populations.

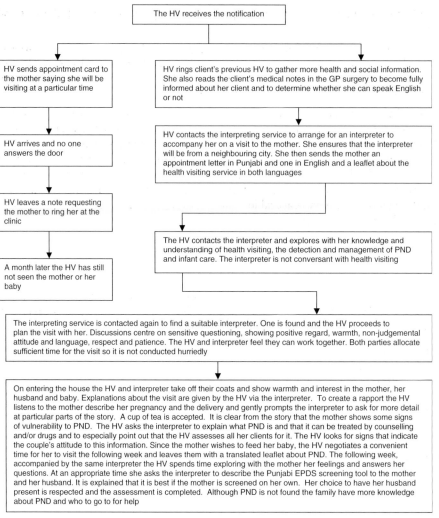

Figure 6.1 Flow chart outlining two ways the health visitor (HV) could respond in the case study. EPDS, Edinburgh Postnatal Depression Scale; PND, postnatal depression.

6.6   Partnership Working to Improve Health and Wellbeing

There are several methodological challenges in finding links between partnership working and health gain, since the concept is poorly understood and has many interpretations. At an intuitive level most public health practitioners would believe that this way of working can only be good for service users. But in today's evidence-based world, funding will not be available until some concrete health gains from partnership working are demonstrable.

The most common claim to health gain arising from working in partnership is empowerment. McIntosh and McCormack (2001) say that if nurses facilitate the development of self-reliance and self-determination, service users will be able to make choices and health-related decisions. In this situation non-compliance is not seen as deviant behaviour but as an act of assertiveness and self-determination. Non-compliance therefore becomes an obsolete term in the realms of partnership (McIntosh & McCormack 2001). Butterworth and Rushforth (1995, p. 378), following a major review of mental health nurses, suggested that working in partnership can be beneficial for nurses as well as for patients:

> The richness and satisfaction that such a partnership can bring, and the potential improvements in the quality of life for people, are profound and exciting: they illustrate and vindicate the role of nursing as a major force in the promotion of good mental health. This partnership can encompass both the nurse's duty of care and an honesty about the powers they hold.

Whilst there is clearly a lack of hard data, it is clear from Table 6.1 that if service users are given the opportunity to make a contribution to their health care, or perceive that their perspective is important, then they are clearly going to feel valued. This can only be good for health.

Returning to Cowley and Almond's (2001) partnership study, some health outcomes were claimed to arise from health visiting in partnership (Almond 2001d). Health visitors' beliefs in the health outcomes of this way of working were largely constrained to medicalised interpretations. They felt that as health outcomes were unmeasurable then they would not count. Nevertheless they felt that partnership working could improve:

- recovery from postnatal depression;
- help in the continuation of breast feeding;
- uptake of preventative services.

Their clients on the other hand were not constrained in how they felt the partnership with the health visitor had helped them (Almond 2001d). The following is a list of the health benefits that were discovered from interviewing 26 health visitors' clients:

- affirmation;
- assertiveness;
- empowerment;
- hope;
- improved relationships;
- increased knowledge;
- increased motivation;
- peace of mind;
- positivity;
- reassurance;
- relief;
- self-confidence;
- successful parenting.

Whilst these might be considered as soft health outcomes since some of them are difficult to measure, they are nevertheless empirically generated insights into the health benefits that can be achieved from partnership working.

Conclusion

The partnership literature is largely theoretically derived and sparse on research. The concept of partnership is diffuse and multidimensional, incorporating the concepts of collaboration, negotiation, involvement and participation. There is no doubt that it is informed by moral and ethical principles and it has a political dimension too. There are examples of political advocacy. Inherent in the varied discourses is the belief that partnership is a good thing. The boundaries between service provider and service user are shifting and stand to shift further if partnership methods are adopted. What is required is less political rhetoric and more investment in partnership working.

The Health Visiting Partnership Project (Cowley & Almond 2001) has sought to address the deficit of research in this field. Whilst it has gone some way to critically analyse and elicit the nature of partnership working and the health gains that can be achieved from this, it is still not clear whether the

Section 2

health visitors were actually working in a way that was markedly different from their 'normal' practice. Two conclusions can be drawn from this. One is that most health visiting practice is in itself partnership working or has most of the attributes of partnership. The health visitors did not undergo any specific partnership training either because it was not deemed necessary or it was not available.

The other conclusion is that since partnership is a multidimensional concept further research is necessary to attempt to differentiate it from practice that is not deemed to be partnership, to determine the outcomes from the two modes of practice. A randomised control trial would lend itself to such an experiment. No dissenting voices about partnership working were found, however cautions about the time this way of working would take did seem to be the concern of a few. Until further empirical studies are done much of the discourses on partnership are at best mere rhetoric. Furthermore, research is required to explore the realities of the service users' experience. Their views are largely missing from the literature.

The literature provokes many questions and leaves most unanswered. It has largely focused on the professional perspective. The service users' role has largely been overlooked. Additionally it has not as yet dealt with whether and how partnership working can have an impact on reducing health inequalities. The partnership research undertaken by Cowley and Almond (2001) was undertaken in a social and economically impoverished area of London, but exploring the links between partnership working and health inequality were beyond the remit of the project. Since the reduction of health inequalities is a major public health activity it seems necessary to explore the contribution partnership working may have with populations whose health is unjustly less good than others. The literature is also devoid of examples of working in partnership with minority ethnic populations.

The concept has been systematically analysed in various contexts but these analyses do not add a great deal to an understanding of the realities of working in partnership. The literature assisted in the development of a skills typology but it could be argued that these are largely hypothetical until they have been tested empirically. Empowerment was a key health gain of partnership working, but whether empowerment is an actual outcome or an aspect of partnership working is open to debate. Or it can be viewed as a philosophical position that drives partnership working.

More research is needed to provide substantive evidence that health care practitioners are willing to adopt the more time consuming and challenging partnership approach to working with service users. The skills typology sets a challenge for debate and further discourses about partnership practice. It will most certainly need further amendment and is provided as a starting point to aid the planning of training in partnership working and as a self-assessment for public health practitioners.

Acknowledgements

Professor Sarah Cowley supervised the Health Visiting in Partnership Project. Thanks go to the Community Health South London NHS Trust who collaborated with the project, team leaders, health visitors and their clients. The project was supported by the Funding Committee of Guy's and St Thomas' Charitable Foundation.

References

Almond P. (2001a) An analysis of the concept of equity and its application to health visiting. *Journal of Advanced Nursing* 37 (6), 598–606.

Almond P. (2001b) What is consumerism and has it had an impact on health visiting provision? A literature review. *Journal of Advanced Nursing* 35 (6), 893–901.

Almond P. (2001c) Approaches to decision-making and child protection issues. *Community Practitioner* 74 (3), 97–100.

Almond P. (2001d) *The search for health outcomes: a qualitative study exploring clients' and health visitors' conceptualisations of health outcomes.* Unpublished MSc community health dissertation, Kings College, University of London.

Almond P. (2007) *A case study of equity in health visiting postnatal depression policy, services and practice.* PhD in progress, University of Southampton.

Arnstein S.R. (1969) A ladder of participation. *Journal of the American Institute of Planners* 35 (4), 216–24.

Bidmead C., Cowley S. (2005) A concept analysis of partnership with clients. *Community Practitioner* 78 (6), 203–8.

Bidmead C., Davies H., Day C. (2002) Partnership working: what does it really mean? *Community Practitioner* 75 (7), 256–9.

Blank A. (2004) Clients' experiences of partnership with occupational therapists in community mental health. *British Journal of Occupational Therapy* 67 (3), 118–24.

Bleker O.P. (2000) Treat patients as you would like to be treated yourself. *British Medical Journal* 320, 117.

Butterworth T., Rushforth D. (1995) Working in partnership with people who use services; reaffirming the foundations of practice for mental health nursing. *International Journal of Nursing Studies* 32 (4), 373–85.

Casey A. (1995) A partnership with child and family. *Senior Nurse* 8 (4), 8–9.

Chalmers K., Luker K. (1991) The development of the health visitor–client relationship. *Scandinavian Journal of Caring Sciences* 5 (33), 33–41.

Charles C., Whelan T., Gafni A. (1999) What do we mean by partnership in making decisions about treatments? *British Medical Journal* 319, 780–2.

Coulter A. (1999) Paternalism or partnership? *British Medical Journal* 319, 719–20.

Cowley S., Almond P. (2001) *Health Visiting in Partnership Project: an investigation of partnership working and decision making in relation to 'extra health visiting' and outcomes of care in Community Health South London NHS Trust*. Project Number R991111. London: Kings College London.

De la Cuesta C. (1994) Relationships in health visiting: enabling and mediating. *International Journal of Nursing Studies* 31, 451–9.

DH (Department of Health) (1997) *The New NHS: modern, dependable*. London: HM Stationery Office.

DH (Department of Health) (1999) *Patient and Public Involvement in the New NHS*. London: HM Stationery Office.

DH (Department of Health) (2004a) *Chronic Disease Management: a compendium of information*. London: HM Stationery Office.

DH (Department of Health) (2004b) *Making Partnerships Work for Patients, Carers, and Service Users*. London: HM Stationery Office.

Egan G. (1998) *The Skilled Helper: a problem-management approach to helping*. London: Brooks Cole Publishing Company.

Fleming V.E.M. (1998) Women and midwives in partnership: a problematic relationship? *Journal of Advanced Nursing* 27, 8–14.

Gallant M.H., Beaulieu M.C., Carnevale F.A. (2002) Partnership: an analysis of the concept within the nurse–client relationship. *Journal of Advanced Nursing* 40 (2), 149–57.

Heron J. (2001) *Helping the Client: a creative practical guide*, 5th edn. London: Sage Publications.

Holman H., Lorig K. (2000) Patients as partners in managing chronic disease. *British Medical Journal* 320, 526–7.

Kawik L. (1996) Nurses' and parents' perceptions of participation and partnership caring for a hospitalised child. *British Journal of Nursing* 5 (7), 430–4.

Kirkham J.S. (2000) Patient partnership is just one aspect of treating patients. *British Medical Journal* 320, 252.

Lalonde M. (1974) *A New Perspective on the Health of Canadians*. Ottawa: Health and Welfare Canada.

Little P., Everitt H., Williamson I. *et al.* (2001) Preferences of patients for patient centred approach to consultation in primary care: observational study. *British Medical Journal* 322, 1–7.

Mariotto A. (1999) Patient partnership is not a magic wand. *British Medical Journal* 319, 783.

McIntosh J., McCormack D. (2001) Partnerships identified within primary health care literature. *International Journal of Nursing Studies* 38, 547–55.

Morse J.M., Mitcham C., Hupcey J.E., Tason M.C. (1996) Criteria for concept evaluation. *Journal of Advanced Nursing* 24, 385–90.

Slowie D.F. (1999) Doctors should help patients to communicate better with them. *British Medical Journal* 319, 784.

Waterworth S., Luker K.A. (1990) Reluctant collaborators: do patients want to be involved in decisions concerning care? *Journal of Advanced Nursing* 15, 971–6.

Watson A.R. (1999) Teamwork is necessary. *British Medical Journal* 319, 719.

Werrett J., Clifford C. (2006) Validation of the Punjabi version of the Edinburgh Postnatal Depression Scale (EPDS). *International Journal of Nursing Studies* 43, 227–36.

WHO (World Health Organization) (1978) *Primary Health Care. Report of the International Conference on Primary Health Care, Alma Ata USSR, 6-12th September*. Geneva: World Health Organization.

CHAPTER 7

Communication and You

Jackie Yardley

Public Health Skills: Communication

- Effective communication: perspective, beliefs and values, environment, rapport, pacing, listening and hearing, language and goal setting
- Communication feedback: conflict, emotion, trance and endings

---

Introduction

> The outcome of any communication is the response you get. (Shapiro 2002, p. 9)

In today's litigious society, complaints to the NHS have increased and most of these complaints hinge around misunderstandings and poor communication (Pincock 2004). The following recommendations (University of Southampton 2002) advocate the need for, and implementation of, communication training. Schools of nursing and midwifery highlight the need for improved communication skills, and approved competency skills are essential for the health professional within their assessment period (NMC 2004). However, communication is a topic that most consider as an easy option, that they are already skilled and knowledgeable and that it is only the more complicated aspects of communication that need addressing – such as anger, the dying patient, aggressive relatives for example. This chapter challenges you to think again. As soon as the communication process is viewed as a series of neat phrases, structures and processes to be adhered to, the complexities and subtleties of the communication process are lost. The challenge will be for you to examine yourself, your presuppositions, prejudices, perspective, beliefs and responses to the communication process. Once you understand your part in the communication process the outcome of any communication will still be the response you receive, however you will have a greater understanding of the meaning of that communication.

Through the use of reflective practice using your own experiences and the checklist provided you will begin to appreciate how, in understanding your contribution to any given interaction, you can affect and influence the response you receive.

- The *aim* of this chapter is to understand how you can influence effective communication and appreciate how your perspective, reactions and responses can affect the desired communication outcome.
- The *purpose* of this chapter is that it focuses on you and asks you to concentrate on your communication experiences.

There are a number of underpinning theories and disciplines influencing this chapter – an eclectic mix of neurolinguistic programming (Young 2001) transactional analysis (Stewart 1999), counselling (Nelson-Jones 2006), psychology (Rungapadiachy 2001) and hypnosis (Yapko 1990). The focus is deliberately related to the practical application of communication skills and not an academic debate.

7.1   Effective Communication

There are certain principles of effective communication that you need to consider: perspective, rapport, pacing and language. However, the basic elements of communication are your baseline skills, be it for a social chat or a professional engagement. These baseline skills are needed to be sure that you can maintain communication rapport – by sitting/standing in the right place, using body language including non-verbal, using open questions and, most importantly, listening and hearing what is being said. It is worth unpacking some of these principles and basic skills, if only to act as a reminder that you already interact in this way or for you to reflect on your present mode of communication.

7.2   Perspective

Your map of the world is not the blueprint for others. What you observe and record will be filtered depending on your interests, observations and need to engage. It is rather like buying a new car and suddenly noticing how many other people drive that car, a fact you never noticed before.

> **Reflective exercise**
>
> If you raise both hands and cover your face, blocking out your vision, there may be chinks of light and images of your surroundings. However, spread your fingers and more of your surroundings come into view but it remains only part of the picture. Often our perspective of a situation mirrors this process, and based on this held view we communicate our message and understanding of the situation.

7.3   Beliefs and Values

Your beliefs and values will also influence your response and reactions to certain situations and in the context of a professional engagement your responses may not be appropriate. If you hold strong views about the legalization of drugs and you are interacting with someone with opposing views, although you may not identify those beliefs your tone of voice, body language and/or facial expression may give a different message. Similarly, if honesty is a high value for you and someone is telling you about a situation where they have lied, and even if the context suggest a valid reason for the lie, you may find any rapport evident at the beginning of the conversation has gone. Being congruent is essential for effective communication and if you are aware of conflicting beliefs and values owning this fact from your perspective may be the best solution; you may need to recognise you will not be the right individual for certain people. This is better than pretending everything is fine because this will break down the communication further; equally, making the other person responsible for the 'problem' exacts a judgemental framework.

7.4   Environment

If you are in a country where you are unable to speak the language you are consciously aware of your communication limitations and you will employ a range of tactics from sign language through to what amounts to a game of charades in order to make yourself understood. Talking more slowly and louder only creates more frustration as there is a total mismatch in rapport and understanding. However, there can be a conviction that there is mutual understanding only to find out later this has not been so. This scenario illustrates awareness at a conscious level of failed communication. In a different environment at work, home and/or social setting where we communicate at a more unconscious level, we make assumptions, stop listening, trance, make judgements and discount on the basis 'they' do not know what they are talking about. Often these communications are not even registered as failed communications as there is a lack of awareness by both parties.

7.5   Rapport

Rapport is the essence of communication and establishing rapport at the outset makes the desired outcome more likely to be achieved.

Reflective exercise

Think of a time when you know there has been a total mismatch in the communication between you and a client or family member. Using Table 7.1 do you understand what happened in that interaction now?

Establishing rapport is more than body language, although clearly it matters if someone is sitting/standing/leaning against a wall that you initially mirror their posture. The tone of your voice also needs to match, however this will be at an energy level. This means if someone is angry you respond with the same urgency; just remember a time when you have felt upset and someone has attempted to calm you down with the soft voice and a 'there, there' – for most people this type of response will leave them feeling even more wound up! Non-verbal messages are important and can include facial expressions, shrugging of the shoulders, tapping the feet, etc.; if we can observe these messages in others they can receive the same signals from us.

7.6   Pacing

Pacing is also an important aspect of effective communication. It can be easy to be ahead of the needs of an individual, and if the scenario is familiar and the possible outcome almost predictable, you may find yourself asking questions that leave the person/s feeling threatened and backed up against a wall, and giving advice that at that stage is inappropriate. Pacing requires sensitivity, observation of cues (body and facial) and awareness of the changes in physiology; for example if someone is feeling angry their breathing may become shallow and fast, their muscles will tense, their body may become rigid

Table 7.1   Reflective exercise checklist: imagine you are watching a video of your interaction. (It may help to close your eyes.)

Checklist	Your responses
What do you see?	
What do you hear?	
What tones of voice are being used?	
What feelings are generated as you watch the video?	
How have you contributed to the situation?	

and there may be signs of perspiration; someone feeling shocked may become facially pale; and someone feeling flustered and/or embarrassed may facially flush. When people are agitated they may pace, and someone who is in shock may be still, rooted to the spot. All these changes are a message to you, remembering that these signs are not the total but are just examples.

Rapport and pacing are interchangeable. For example, someone who is agitated, pacing about and talking loudly requires you at that stage to pace with them and use a more urgent voice; by slowly reducing the pacing about and lowering the tone of your voice, all of the time observing the breathing patterns and any facial cues of the other person, you are able to move to a place where you can sit and listen, keeping your contribution at that point to a minimum. This type of management is known as *matching and mismatching* (Young 2001). Mismatching can be useful when you want to disengage in a conversation. Often people find it difficult to end a conversation; standing up, moving towards a door and reaching for your bag can all give a message that your conversation has ended. Endings will be discussed later in the chapter.

7.7 Listening and Hearing

If you are gathering information from someone in order to make an assessment or to make decisions about a family, you will have used questions to elicit the information you want and your focus will be on the responses. However, in doing that you may miss other vital information. As you hear the response your thoughts will go automatically to the information received and you may process that knowledge, creating an informed decision, according to your understanding, on the next action. This process may be rapid but if the person has continued the conversation you will have missed an aspect of that interaction.

Some useful points to remember are:

- pacing the conversation can help by letting the person know you need to gather some information first and that you will then talk about other issues they may need to raise;
- recording bullet points as an *aide mémoire* may allow you to stay focused;
- let the person know that you need to clarify some points and this will give you an opportunity to check the story.

Some basic principles of listening require you to be attentive (Bayne *et al.* 1998) non-judgemental, empathetic and, if possible, create an environment that is conducive to being focused and you being able to listen to the conversation. The use of paraphrasing and summarizing a conversation can give feedback to the person that you have heard what has been said; it will also give the person/s a chance to reflect and correct. You could say:

- Let me just check I have understood ...
- So, X, Y and Z happened; it seems *to me* that that made you angry? (By using this approach where you own what you are saying, it is less threatening for the person to say, 'No, that is not how it made me feel'.)

If someone repeats the same story over and over to you, you may need to ask yourself why. Does the person feel you have never heard, understood and/or responded in a way acceptable to them? You may need, however, to ask yourself why you have not moved this story to another place – do you need to listen again and encourage a movement forward or a letting go in order to release the pause button?

7.8 Language

By entering into someone else's world you need to check that you are not only listening and hearing but that you respect their map of the world, which will differ from your map of the world. Using and understanding the language used by the individual/s also requires you to explore their meaning of the words used. You will also need to understand the level or intensity of the words used.

Activity

Try this activity to understand this better. Using the example of *sad*, think of your immediate response to the meaning of the word and the level of intensity/impact of that word:

- immediate response: *unhappy*; intensity/impact: *low*;
- immediate response: *dejected*; intensity/impact: *middle*;
- immediate response: *inconsolable*; intensity/impact: *high*.

There is no right or wrong answer but can you see, depending on the meaning and impact of the word from your perception, how it will influence your response and reactions. I have known people hear the word sad and their response has been suicidal.

The only person who knows and understands the meaning of the word is the person who has used it. Ask them: 'You said you feel sad, can you tell me what that means for you?'

Try the following words using the same format as in the example above:

- angry;
- pain;
- lonely.

In conversations we often use surface language simply because it takes too long to go into full detail with all the nuances required for a more in-depth knowledge of the topic in discussion. However, if you add to this *generalizations*, *deletions* and *distortions* (Bandler & Grinder 1975; Hall 2006), the whole significance of the conversation begins to lose its meaning, except possibly to the person imparting the information and even then they may not be aware of how they have changed the message.

There are aspects of generalizations, deletions and distortions that are important; for example when coping with an unpleasant experience you may selectively decide to delete aspects of that incidence from your memory. Equally, you may choose to delete an aspect of your 'health' and if the deletion is maintained it may result in ill health. Deletions can lead to misunderstanding and in some cases cause chaos, damage and/or hurt because a vital aspect of the story is missing. With distortions you may take an aspect of an experience and distort the meaning because it fits with the generalizations you have made or complement the deletions you have used, consciously or unconsciously, in order that you can distort your reality. Films, fiction and theatre are good examples of reality being distorted for entertainment. With generalizations, it will be based on a past experience – there will have been an incident which now means that all people, animals or objects linked to your experience are categorised; so if, for example, you were scratched by a cat it now stands that all cats are dangerous.

Certain questions enable you to reconnect with the deeper structure of the conversation. This requires a more challenging approach and you may find this difficult. However, you would not be alone in your reluctance to engage in the following questions. Understanding your reluctance is important and will be addressed later in the chapter. With generalizations you can ask (using the example of the cat):

- Are all cats dangerous?
- Does every cat behave that way?
- Are there any exceptions?
- Do you know of any cat that has never hurt anyone?

This can be a very useful strategy, especially when working with someone who has low self-esteem and/or has longstanding relationship issues and is convinced another person/s hates him or her.

With distortions and deletions the following questions can elicit another aspect of the story. A disjointed story full of deletions and distortions may be clarified by the following:

- (It's hard) ... Compared to what?
- (Fed up) ... With what?

- I would like to understand more about this situation …
- (He did it) … Did what?
- What evidence do you have …?

Often when people are distressed, confused and stressed their story is a jumble and the story may be told, not as it happened, but like a kaleidoscope with the pattern changing and with certain aspects more important than others. The story is disjointed and with parts of the story missing the above questions may illuminate and bring understanding. In this type of scenario, however, you must remember the principles of pacing.

It is thought that we think in pictures, sounds and feelings (Bradbury 2000) and although we may access all of these, we often display a preference for one. When accessing a thought we will use the language associated with that mode of thinking. There are also eye accessing cues (Bradbury 2000) that will indicate the person's preference; if their eyes are looking up left and right they will be *visual*; eyes level, left and right, often with the head tipped to one side, and they will be *auditory* (often auditory people will be looking down to the left if they are holding an internal dialogue with themselves and to the right if they are checking out their feelings); the feelings (*kinaesthetic*) person looks down right (feelings) and left (to check thoughts about a situation), and there will be the same kinaesthetic response with the person thinking about smells (olfactory) or taste (gustatory). The posture of the predominantly visual person will be upright and their breathing will be quite shallow and they talk quickly with a clear and often loud voice. The auditory posture will be more as if they are on the telephone, with the head tipped to one side; their breathing tends to encompass the full range and their voice is melodic and variable in speed. The kinaesthetic person will have a more rounded appearance and will speak with a much lower voice that will be slower and softer in tone. The language or predicates (Lewis & Pucelik 1992) of the different modes are highlighted. However, remember the only person who knows what is happening, is the person engaged in the experience, so remember to check. Understanding a person's preferred mode by listening to the predicates used can increase rapport when you respond using their preferred system.

Activity

Now try the activity in Table 7.2. When you are looking for other examples you may find one section easier than the others and you may have identified your own preferred mode.

The predominately visual person will often disassociate from a situation, which means they will look on at the scene and describe the incident without engaging in feelings. The kinaesthetic person, on the other hand, will be associated with the situation and will talk about the effects of the situation and their feelings. Can you imagine what happens if these two people discuss the same situation? For one there is a clear picture and little emotion and for the other person the focus is the emotion and little clarity. Neither understands the other because for one there is frustration at the constant questions linked to 'how do you feel' and for the other there is hurt at not being asked 'how do you feel?'

Reflective exercise

Which of the following are you more interested in?

- How someone feels – kinaesthetic.
- Putting together the picture – visual.
- Listening – auditory.

Table 7.2   Predicates: language indicating the preferred system.

	Language example	What others can you think of?
Visual Looking up and left indicates a remembered event. Looking up and right indicates constructing an image and/or reconstructing an experience that happened a long time ago	I see what you mean … I have a vision … In view of their reaction … It looks as if … It's plain to see … My image of what took place is hazy … If you want my perspective … That's a bird's eye view …	
Auditory Looking left (at eye level) indicates a remembered sound and to the right a constructed and/or reconstructed sound If the eyes look down to the left the person is having an internal dialogue with themselves	My engine purrs like a cat … I hear what you are saying … What you have said rings a bell … Tell me your story … You need to listen more … I think this strikes a chord … There she goes again, shouting the odds …	
Kinaesthetic Looking down and to the right indicates a kinaesthetic preference and often the person will access their internal dialogue	Please get in touch with me … I wish I could get a handle on this … I can feel it in my bones … My manager gets me all hot and bothered … For goodness sake get a grip… I feel light headed … I am floating …	

There is no right or wrong and you may use all three approaches, however it does help to explain why sometimes your interaction fails and there is a total mismatch. By listening to the predicates used and the eye accessing cues you can learn to match the person you are communicating with.

7.9   Goal Setting

When working with goal setting there is a need to focus on the desired outcome as people often become focused on what they do not want. You can ask the person to describe the present scenario and their preferred scenario (Egan 1986). You need to encourage the move towards the preferred scenario by asking questions that will encourage the move forward:

- What will you need to do to obtain your goal?
- When would you like to achieve your goal?
- What will that be like when you have reached your preferred scenario?

You should *avoid* the following:

- going back into the present scenario (only do so for clarification);
- using negative language.

It is important to keep the goal in the positive. For example, if someone wants to lose weight by stating it as, 'I want to stop eating so much' the goal is focused on what they do not want and not on what

Table 7.3 Changing language patterns.

Negative	Positive (saying what you want)
You never come to the clinic	We would like to see you at the clinic
Don't forget to take your tablets	Take your tablets twice a day, once in the morning and once in the evening
You must stop eating so much sugar	You will need to eat less sugar

they do want – for example, 'I want to eat more healthily'. Negative messages only encourage us to do the exact opposite; if asked to not think of the colour blue you will find yourself doing just that, thinking of the colour blue! Interestingly we will tell people 'don't worry' when in fact we want to communicate a message of hope. It takes practise to change language patterns and phrases that so easily trip off the tongue; generally we find it easier to construct in the negative than the positive (Table 7.3).

This shift in focus will elicit a much more positive outcome. Another useful question when goal setting can be 'What stops you from achieving your goal?'

Reflective exercise

Think of a goal that you have set for yourself and so far have not achieved and ask yourself, 'What stops me?' Now ask yourself, 'What is the payoff (benefits) for never achieving the goal?' Most people will say at this point that there is no payoff; however, read the following example and ask yourself the question again.

Case Study Example

Rita is constantly stressed at work and frequently burst into tears, her colleagues will take work from her and make a fuss of her, making her a cup of tea and giving her a hug. At home Rita also feels stressed, however no one helps her out and certainly no one gives her a hug or makes a cup of tea. Rita has decided she wants to be more organised at work and that this will cause her to feel less stressed. She has set targets, made lists and planned to create a more effective filing system, however something always manages to stop her from achieving her goal.

What do you think are the positive benefits of her staying as she is?

7.10 Communication Feedback

Instead of viewing a breakdown in communication as failure, think of it as providing you with feedback (Bradbury 2000). This feedback enables you to make changes and enhance your communication skills.

One of the main reasons for a breakdown in the communication process is our need to mind-read and make assumptions. We make tenuous links between one event and its impact on another aspect of life, in other words, cause and effect. Judgements made add to the communication breakdown.

> **Reflective exercise**
>
> Has there been a time when you have made a judgement about a family? You were sure you knew the reasons as to why they were experiencing problems and based on the assumptions made, you created a plan of action? Now use Table 7.4 as you reflect on that time.

Table 7.4　Reflective exercise checklist.

Checklist	Your responses
What evidence did you have to make the decisions you did?	
Did this situation remind you of another individual/family you have had contact with?	
What are the other possible reasons as to why things were the way they were?	
Did you ask the right questions to elicit possible reasons from those involved in the scenario?	

The more experience you have, the easier it is to make judgements about a situation and in many cases your instincts will be correct; however, the only person/s who know/s are those involved. By asking questions you may build a different picture and understanding of the situation. Some of the following questions may be useful:

- What do you think is happening?
- How can you make things different?
- What will you need to change the situation?

By asking these questions you are increasing your understanding of the situation and this will reflect in the way the conversation continues. At the same time you are giving a message to the other person; you are saying to them, 'You have the resources to identify what is happening in this situation and I trust your judgement'. Rapport is increased when the person feels heard and respected for their opinions.

The concept of *transference* and *counter-transference* (Nelson-Jones 2006) can bring understanding to a communication breakdown. Transference of thoughts, feelings and actions come from the individuals you are communicating with. They may have been in the situation they find themselves in before, and the whole scenario generates a negative reaction and they respond to you as if you were part of the problem. Equally, counter-tranceference can come from you, and again the individuals can trigger a response from you to them that is not appropriate. The person may remind you of your mother, someone you never 'got on' with, and your reactions towards that person can create a barrier in the communication because at some level your anger, hostility and/or sadness linked with your mother will be registered by the receiver of your communication. Even if they do not understand what has taken place, people register changes in tone of voice, body language and non-verbal cues. It is possible that the transference/counter-transference might produce a response of attraction or over-caring for the same reasons as above, only this time the recognition is at a positive level. However, this response can also create difficulties in that you become overinvolved and/or your motives are driven by a desire to engage in an inappropriate relationship with the person.

When you are puzzled by a communication breakdown, ask yourself the following questions:

- Does this person remind me of someone I dislike or has caused me distress?
- Does this person remind me of someone I care about or find attractive?
- Have I been in this situation before and was the outcome negative?

Once this understanding is in place, disassociating yourself from the counter-transference enables you to engage in a more productive way.

7.11   Conflict

Case Study Example

Ever since John has worked with the team there has been constant conflict. His dislike of confrontation has caused him stress and anxiety, especially as his manager is on annual leave and he has been asked to chair the next team meeting. The situation is compounded for John by a strong belief that he is unable to handle conflict and conflict is best avoided.

Does this sound familiar?

If you have a dislike of confrontation and you find yourself in a situation that requires you to engage in the dispute, your response may be to sidetrack the conversation and suggest everyone takes time out. Of course this may be appropriate; however, if it acts as an avoidance strategy you may, for example, find you feel frustrated, afraid and agitated. It may help to consider one of the strategies given in Table 7.5. It also helps in a confrontational situation to ask yourself what happens to you and the response/s elicited by that process.

Table 7.5   Conflict.

Question	Strategies
Am I responsible for the situation?	Answer no – depersonalise. The person's anger has to be directed at someone and you are in the firing line, however you are not responsible. You will feel less threatened once you don't own their anger
Can I view this situation in a different way?	Reframe: being non-confrontational means you are more likely to stay calm. This is an asset when communicating in difficult situations

Your thoughts will impact on your feelings and consequently on your behaviour (McDermott & Jago 2001) by challenging your thinking; for example: Why am I afraid? What is the worse case scenario? Is this old behaviour that is not suitable now? By challenging your thinking, you will identify self-limiting

Activity

Try the activity in Table 7.6 to understand this better.

Table 7.6   Activity checklist.

Checklist	Your responses
What thoughts go through your head? *Example:* You start telling yourself you can't handle conflict	
How does that affect you physically? *Example:* Your breathing changes, it becomes shallower	
How does that affect your behaviour? *Example:* You divert the conversation	

beliefs (Dilts *et al.* 1990) and begin to understand that you can allow yourself to engage in a more meaningful way. When there is a conflict between a belief you hold and your behaviour you will usually find the belief will win. Think of a time when you have completed some task and you believe you have made a complete mess of it although someone tells you what a great job you have done. You may even thank them, but your internal dialogue will engage with the belief of self-doubt. If you then think of an old established belief, 'I am useless at dealing with conflict', all the strategies for maintaining that belief will 'kick' in.

Reflective exercise

Think of someone you know who handles conflict well and ask them how they manage to stay calm, in control and objective. Do they stand in a different way or use a different tone of voice? What are their facial expressions like? Now imagine what it would be like if you used some of those strategies.

Sports people use video clips so that they can observe excellence and behaviour that would benefit from change. Sometimes only a minor adjustment is needed, but it favours a positive outcome.

Some conversations lead us to behave as if the other person is a child and we adopt the role of mother (Stewart 1999); this mother role can be critical and/or nurturing. These types of interactions or ego states are often at an unconscious level and, depending on who we are interacting with, we can easily shift from being mother/father, child and/or adult.

The child in us can be spontaneous (natural) or adaptive (Stewart 1999) and it makes it easy for us to behave in a childish way, to rebel and assume the role of not taking responsibility for our actions. Equally, the spontaneous child allows us to be creative and indulgent and this part can motivate the adult part of us to consult the parent about the suitability of the desire and/or action. Rather like transference and counter-transference (Nelson-Jones 2006), you may find yourself in situations whereby you automatically adopt the adaptive child ego state simply because the other person always adopts the critical parent. These types of interactions can be hard to break and in some cases interfere with long-term relationships.

Activity

Now think of some work relationships and complete the activity in Table 7.7.

Table 7.7   Activity checklist.

Checklist	Your responses
Which ego state/s do you adopt?	
Does it matter? If so how does it matter?	
Does it help you to understand why some relationships leave you feeling uncomfortable?	
How can you change your approach?	

The last question in Table 7.7, 'How can you change your approach', is important because so often when we are communicating with someone – especially if we consider ourselves more knowledgeable and/or skilled – we expect the other person to make changes based on our knowledge, beliefs and perception of what is best for them. Tension occurs when there is an undesirable outcome based on our beliefs. The only person who can make a change is the person him/herself; some will agree to change and may even engage in the approved behaviour, but this will be short-lived if that change has not been part of their own pattern of change. This is where goal setting (see Section 7.9) can be useful. It also means there is a need for behavioural flexibility on your part. What happens when change is essential for survival, be that social, physical or emotional? You may still have to accept that the other person/s have the right to make decisions you do not agree with. If someone has decided to withdraw from their treatment, you can only put forward your point of view. Accepting their decision can be hard but you can maintain your integrity and point of view and still engage in professional dialogue with the other person/s. This requires you to disengage from the emotion of the situation.

7.12   Emotion

Some people, especially those who are more kinaesthetic, heavily invest in a one to one or even family interaction and become hurt, upset, angry or frustrated when the family either refuses the suggestions made or, worse still, they are rejected by the individual or family. The focus again has to be on self and, not with the voice of the critical parent but through reflection, understanding as to why there has been a breakdown in the relationship.

Reflective exercise

Think of a time when you have invested a lot of energy, time and emotion and ask yourself these very difficult questions:

- Who was it for, you or the other person?
- Does it matter to you that you are liked?
- Do you criticise yourself?
- Do you feel a 'failure' in some way?

The questions in the reflective exercise box are important in helping you understand why it can be very painful if there is a sense of rejection in a professional relationship. You may want something from that person that they can not give. When an interaction runs smoothly it can make you feel 'good' or 'valued'; however as soon as the reverse happens feelings of 'failure' can creep in. Only you can make you feel 'good', the rejecting family are all in their own world and absorbed by their present and future. Sometimes you are the safest person for them to 'kick' as they also feel anger, fear and frustration and their sense of helplessness may cause the friction. It can be difficult to stay engaged when this happens, however a quick mental check can enable you to remain single-minded:

- Are you responsible for the outburst and/or complaint?
- If you are responsible, talk about it; if not, disassociate yourself from the incidence – that is, depersonalise.
- Tell yourself you just happened to be available as a metaphorical kicking bucket.

Above all ask yourself if you are safe in the situation and, if not, *leave*!

7.13   Trance

Everyone trances (Yapko 1990), it is one way of managing daily living. The problem with going into a trance is that you are unaware of what else is happening, conversation details are missed, body language is lost in the moment you allowed your mind to travel somewhere else. Misunderstandings take place, information given is not registered. Just as you can trance out, so can the receiver of the information. If you are giving information that has an impact on that person's life or family, they too may be lost in their own thoughts. Given the right trigger, you can find yourself focusing on your issues and not those of the person/s you are interacting with.

Reflective exercise

Think of the last time you were on an enjoyable holiday, see what you see, hear what you hear and feel what you feel. Spend time remembering that experience, maybe you can see the clear blue sky, hear the waves lapping in and out and you can feel the heat of the sun. In that space of time you have been day dreaming, entering into a trance.

Activity

The activity in Table 7.8 asks you to consider certain situations you may have found yourself in, highlighting how easy it is to trance!

Table 7.8 Activity checklist.

Checklist	Your responses
Have you ever been reading a book and read the same page over and over and let your mind wander?	
Have you had a conversation with someone knowing how they will respond and stopped listening to them?	
Have you ever been in a lecturer and remembered you forgot to post a letter, or forgot to take the meat out of the freezer and started planning your alternative meal?	

The list of potential trance situations is endless and we have all done it. However, staying focused is essential especially if the other person is already preoccupied – the pace will need to be slower, the questions asked should explore the understanding held by the individual/s, so that any gaps in knowledge and understanding due the lapses on their part can be identified.

7.14 Endings

Case Study

Ellie dreaded going in to see Mrs Smith as this was going to be her last visit and she found endings very difficult. Mrs Smith reminded Ellie of her mother and she enjoyed their conversations; however she knew that their professional relationship was completed. Mrs Smith had implied that she could always pop in for a cup of tea anytime she liked and would really miss her and Ellie found this even more difficult. She was concerned Mrs Smith would dislike her if she did not visit for a chat.

Have you ever been in this situation?

A lot of people find ending a conversation difficult and there can be a number of reasons as to why it can be hard. Remembering this chapter has been about you, you will know that once again you are being asked to examine yourself. Think of the last conversation you had where you found it difficult to end the interaction.

Activity

The activity in Table 7.9 may help you end difficult conversations.

Table 7.9 Activity checklist.

Checklist	Your responses
Was it a difficult conversation where from your perspective you had not achieved your desired outcome? *Record your thoughts and feelings on why it was difficult*	
Was it an easy conversation where you wished you could spend even more time with the person/s? *Record your thoughts and feelings on why it was difficult*	
What do you think people will think of you if you end a conversation that still has many lose ends and no answers? *Record your thoughts and feelings on why it was difficult*	
Do you trust your own professional decision to end a conversation – if not why not? *Record your thoughts and feelings on why it was difficult*	
Does it matter if people like you? *Record your thoughts and feelings*	

Your answers in Table 7.9 will provide insight as to why you may or may not find it difficult to end a conversation and your solution to the answer will be the best.

The one rule that is worth considering when dealing with endings is to not ask if there are any other issues that the person needs to discuss because this will only open up the conversation again. These are other useful considerations:

1. Making some ground rules at the beginning can be one useful way of managing the time and endings. If you have only 10 minutes state this at the beginning.
2. You can say 'I only have another 5 minutes, are there any questions about our conversation you would like to ask?'
3. Acknowledge there has not been enough time and set up another date and time when you can talk.
4. If you are sitting, stand up, and if standing move to the door. Make some movement.

Conclusion

There are many areas of communication, with technology, media, theatre and narrative being just a few. However, this chapter has focused on you and how, by understanding yourself, you can begin to appreciate the role you play in the communication process. There has been a deliberate absence of issues related to race, gender, age and culture because tokenistic mention (in my opinion) is of low value. The same can be said of mental health issues and learning disabilities as they are not ignored but respected by knowing you are able to explore these issues in the depth required for your needs. It is important to recognise and value your contribution to the communication process and to recognise your skills and knowledge and the role it plays in your daily interactions.

> If you always do what you have always done you will always get what you have always got. (O'Connor & Seymour 1993, p. 9)

References

Bandler R., Grinder J. (1975) *The Structure of Magic. A book about language and Therapy.* California: Science and Behavior Books.

Bayne R., Nicolson P., Horton I. (eds) (1998) *Counselling and Communication Skills for Medical and Health Practitioners.* Leicester: BPS Books, the British Psychological Society.

Bradbury A. (2000) *Develop Your NLP Skills*, 2nd edn. St Ives: Kogan Page.

Dilts R., Hallbom T., Smith S. (1990) *Beliefs. Pathways to health and well-being.* Portland, OR: Metamorphous Press.

Egan G. (1986) *The Skilled Helper. A systematic approach to effective helping.* Pacfic Grove, CA: Brooks/Cole Publishing Company.

Hall L.M. (2006) *Communication Magic. Exploring the structure and meaning of language.* Barking, Essex: Crown House Publications.

Lewis B., Pucelik F. (1992) *Magic of NLP Demystified. A pragmatic guide to communication and change.* Portland, OR: Metamorphous Press.

McDermott I., Jago W. (2001) *Brief NLP Therapy.* London: Sage Publications.

Nelson-Jones R.C. (2006) *Theory and Practice of Counselling and Therapy*, 4th edn. London: Sage Publications.

NMC (Nursing and Midwifery Council) (2004) *The NMC Code of Professional Conduct: standards for conduct, performance and ethics.* London: Nursing and Midwifery Council.

O'Connor J., Seymour J. (1993) *Introducing NLP Neuro-Linguistic Programming. Psychological skills for understanding and influencing people.* London: Aquarian/Thorsons.

Pincock S. (2004) Poor communication lies at the heart of NHS complaints, says ombudsman. *British Medical Journal* 328, 10.

Rungapadiachy D.M. (2001) *Interprofessional Communication and Psychology for Health Care Professionals. Theory and practice.* Oxford: Butterworth Heinemann.

Shapiro M. (2002) *Understanding Neuro-Linguistic Programming in a Week.* Impression No. 10. London: Hodder & Stoughton.

Stewart I. (1999) *Eric Bern.* London: Sage Publications.

University of Southampton (2002) *Programme Specification for the MSc/BSc in Public Health.* Southampton: School of Nursing and Midwifery, University of Southampton.

Yapko M.D. (1990) *Trancework. An introduction to the practice of clinical hypnosis*, 2nd edn. New York: Brunner/Mazel Publishers.

Young P. (2001) *Understanding NLP. Metaphors and patterns of change.* Barking, Essex: Crown House Publishing.

Section 3

Public Health Policies and their Impact on Practice

Section 3 Introduction: Public Health Policies and their Impact on Practice

Key Public Health Skills

- Policy and strategy development and implementation to improve health and wellbeing
- Strategic leadership for health and wellbeing
- Promoting and protecting the population's health and wellbeing
- Research and development to improve health and wellbeing

This section identifies the skills that practitioners need to understand, interpret, analyse and implement policy in order to influence those policies affecting health. Acting both collaboratively and independently within a multiagency, interprofessional team, practitioners can provide leadership on public health issues. Part of this role relies on their ability to self-assess as a way of ensuring a focus is kept on performance and continuous improvement in the delivery of public health activity. Practitioners must understand the skills required for strategic leadership and should be involved in strategic planning, providing and evaluating practice and multiagency, interprofessional interventions to meet the health and health-related needs of communities, groups, families and individuals.

By developing these skills, practitioners are well placed to participate in developing initiatives to protect and promote health and to prevent ill health in the general public. In applying professional judgements to decision making within public health activity, such initiatives must address the differing needs of the public as well as aiding continuing community, group, family and individual functioning. The ability to understand, interpret and analyse complex situations and determine the most appropriate way to respond to identified health needs is a crucial part of this process.

Introduction to Chapter 8

Public Health Skills: appraisal

- Policy: the range of meanings
- Public health policy frameworks: health improvement, tackling health inequalities and management of long-term/chronic conditions

- Analysing policy: key models and approaches
- Influencing policy: implications for practitioners

At the heart of Chapter 8 is the assumption that public health practitioners who are confident in their knowledge and understanding of policy are better able to influence policy. The chapter therefore aims to develop readers' awareness of policy and public health policy and to introduce them to some key concepts and skills for policy analysis. Overall, the focus is on policy and strategy development and implementation to improve health and wellbeing. The main focus of this chapter is therefore on the appraisal and influence of policies.

Introduction to Chapter 9

Public Health Skills: strategic leadership

- Strategic analysis: SWOT analysis, PESTEL analysis, needs assessment and stakeholder analysis
- Strategic choice: revising the mission statement, identifying strategic options, and evaluating and selecting strategic options
- Strategic implementation: communicating the strategy, organizational structures in place, aligning culture and strategy, reviewing progress and amending the strategy

Chapter 9 is designed to help the reader develop a public health strategy. The chapter explores the three main elements to strategic management and offers a review of current public health services using strategic analysis tools. The authors make reference to earlier chapters on needs assessment and provide a critique of stakeholder analysis in this context. Strategic choice is discussed in relation to the options for developing a public health strategy and processes for implementing the strategy outlined. The main focus of this chapter is strategic leadership and the application of leadership skills.

Introduction to Chapter 10

Public Health Skills: interpretation and application of policy legislation into practice

- Environmental health protection: health and safety in the wider community (occupational and private life)
- Infection control
- Interpreting codes of practice with regard to the environment and wider community

Chapter 10 is about health protection. The chapter views health protection as a branch of public health which seeks to protect the public from, or limit exposure to, hazards that may be harmful to health. In discussing the various aspects of health protection the authors are concerned with the prevention, investigation and control of infectious diseases as well as environmental hazards. The hazards relate specifically to:

- food, water, air and environmental quality and safety;
- the transmission of communicable diseases;
- outbreaks and other incidents that threaten public health.

Environmental hazards can be chemical (including poisons and pharmaceuticals) or radiological (including ionizing and non-ionizing radiation). Communicable hazards are infectious agents capable of causing disease in humans that are transmitted from one person to another. The chapter concludes with the role of the public health nurse in dealing with an outbreak/incident management, thus highlighting the importance of readiness for emergency situations that may impact on human health including acts of terrorism and the deliberate release of hazardous agents.

Introduction to Chapter 11

Public Health Skills: analysis and interpretation

- Evidence-based practice: critiquing evidence, implementing and evaluating practice
- Processes for evidence-based public health: recognizing an information need and asking questions
- Searching for evidence: critically appraising selective evidence and synthesizing the evidence
- Using evidence to inform public health practice: approaches to implementing evidence in public health practice and evaluating the impact of evidence on public health practice

Chapter 11 explores how evidence is used as part of research and development for nurses working in the field of public health. The chapter is based on the premise that evidence is important for public health practice where the purpose is to ensure that preventing ill health, promoting health and managing treatment and services are of high priority and improve health outcomes for client groups. The reader is taken through the process required to undertake evidence-based public health and is able to evaluate these in the context of their own field of public health practice.

CHAPTER 8

Appraising and Influencing Health Policy and Strategy

Sue Toward

Public Health Skills: Appraisal

- Policy: the range of meanings
- Public health policy frameworks: health improvement, tackling health inequalities and management of long-term/chronic conditions
- Analysing policy: key models and approaches
- Influencing policy: implications for practitioners

Introduction

At the heart of this chapter is the assumption that public health practitioners who are confident in their knowledge and understanding of policy are 'better equipped to influence it in their working lives' (Buse *et al.* 2005, p. 2). The chapter therefore aims to develop readers' awareness of policy and public health policy and to introduce them to some key concepts and skills for policy analysis. Overall the focus is on the occupational standards principle of public health practice: 'policy and strategy development and implementation to improve health and well being' (NMC 2004, Skills for Health 2004).

The chapter begins with a discussion of the widely used terms 'policy' and 'health policy'. The public health policy framework since 1997 is then summarised. There follows an exploration of some models for analysing policy which are applied to the November 2004 White Paper *Choosing Health* (DH 2004a). The chapter concludes with some reflections on the implications for practitioners seeking to contribute to policy development.

8.1 Policy: The Range of Meanings

As Colebatch has contended, the meaning of the concept of policy tends to be 'assumed rather than explored' (Colebatch 2002, p. 5). If we suspend a tendency to assume in favour of exploring, we discover a range of possible definitions of policy. While Hogwood and Gunn (1984) identified 10 meanings of the term, Colebatch (2002) postulates five. These can be summarised as follows:

1. Government decisions, actions and activities.
2. Specific commitment.
3. Routine practice and procedure.

4. Broad orientation.

5. Statement of values.

The first definition – policy as government decisions, actions and activities – is arguably the most familiar one. In our system of representative government it reflects an expectation on the part of the electorate that governments should take decisions and engage in fields of activity shaping national life, for example by addressing a range of social, economic and environmental problems. Governments are given authority – the right to influence others (Buse *et al.* 2005) – and this is argued to legitimate policy.

The idea of policy as a specific commitment flows from Colebatch's first definition (Colebatch 2002). In the run up to a general election, political parties set out in a manifesto their priorities for government. These priorities are translated into programmes and goals, often expressed as targets, in subsequent policy statements. For example, a raft of targets or specific commitments accompany the two public health priority areas – population health improvement and supporting people with long-term conditions – identified by the Labour government re-elected in 2005 (DH 2006a). The extent to which a government delivers on commitments or achieves the targets it sets is a key way of judging a government's performance or of holding it to account.

Policy commitments made by government are highly likely to impact on the routine practice of, and procedures followed by, public servants. These can be seen as local policies set within the overall framework provided by government. The targets and measures associated with the government's two other health policy priority areas – access to services and patient/user experience (DH 2004b, 2006a) – exert a profound influence on the day to day work of health professionals. Their routine practice and the procedures they follow have to align with these priorities. In an organizational context, boundaries are set for decisions and actions, implying order, system and consistency (Colebatch 2002).

The last two definitions of policy in the Colebatch framework – broad orientation and statement of values – can be considered together. Overall they suggest the idea of policy as setting overall direction within an ideological framework. Traditional left and right ideological differences in health policy tend to become apparent when we locate policy makers' position on the 'state versus market' continuum. According to Lewis and Dixon (2005), at one end of this spectrum we find the traditional left's model of a 'nationally planned, owned and provided service, governed from the centre'. At the other extreme lies the right wing blueprint of a wholly market-based health system.

What is striking about the health policy of new Labour – that is, of the government which came to power in 1997 – is that it tends to reject the traditional left ideological position in favour of the values associated with the right. As Lewis and Dixon (2005) also argue, new Labour has gone further than previous Conservative governments in embracing market-style incentives and mechanisms for health care. This may seem paradoxical given new Labour's explicit rejection in the 1990s of traditional left and right positions, embodied, respectively, in 'old' socialism and the 'new right' ideology pursued by Margaret Thatcher's three administrations. The idea at the heart of the new Labour 'project' was that of the so-called 'Third way', neither left nor right but a kind of synthesis of the two with an emphasis on 'what matters is what works'. Grayson and Gomershall (2003) suggest that evidence-based policy, which is discussed in more detail in Section 8.4.6 has helped to fill the gap: 'a kind of non-ideological ideology of pragmatism with which nobody can reasonably disagree'.

Notwithstanding the emergence in the 1990s of 'Third way' thinking in policy making, it is important to look for the broad orientation or value base of government decisions, actions and specific commitments. In analysing a major policy statement such as *Choosing Health* (DH 2004a) we need to acknowledge that the various meanings of policy identified by Colebatch (2002) coexist or overlap. This is also apparent in Easton's definition of policy as a 'web of decisions and actions that allocate ... values' (Easton, cited in Ham 2004, p. 113). This straddles at least two of Colebatch's definitions of policy and also conveys the important idea that policy rests on authority.

Colebatch's point which provided the starting point for our discussion of the concept of policy – that the meaning tends to be assumed rather than explored – is relevant also when we come to consider the term 'health policy', already used several times in this chapter. It is to this specific area of policy that we now turn.

8.2   Health Policy: Two Distinct Meanings

Health policy is an area of *social policy*, a term that encompasses policy decisions and actions influencing welfare or intended to combat social problems in society. The policy areas traditionally included within this definition of social policy are health, social security, personal social services, education and housing. As far as health policy is concerned, Hunter (2003) has convincingly argued that the term has two distinct meanings. These are, first, health care policy and, second, policy for health or public health policy.

The central preoccupation of *health care policy* is with the delivery and resourcing of health care services. It is concerned with how a range of resources – human, organizational and financial – are used to 'rescue' people who are ill, regardless of the cause(s) of their illness (Hunter 2003, p. 5). In practice, health care policy tends to be dominated by issues arising from the treatment and care of patients in acute hospital settings. These types of health care facilities or resources lie 'downstream' to the causes of illness, for example those arising from the conditions that shape individual and population health (Hunter 2003).

Nine key themes which have shaped health care policy in recent years are discussed elsewhere (Toward & Maslin-Prothero 2007). The themes contrast markedly with the central concerns of *policy for health*, which is focused on improving the health of a whole population and tackling various types of health inequality. Population health and health inequalities are seen in the context of a range of social, environmental and economic factors that affect health and lie 'upstream' to health services. Policy for health is thus concerned with wider notions of health and its determinants and potentially cross-cuts many policy areas. This implies that in order to understand the policy for health/public health policy framework we have to survey a broad sweep of policies. The starting point for our overview is 1997, when the first new Labour government was elected.

To make this task manageable, we will concentrate on three key themes or priorities shaping policy for health. Two of these have already been highlighted as health improvement and tackling health inequalities. A third theme – the better management of long-term or chronic conditions – will also be considered. These three themes, and some of the policies they have given rise to, are explored in more detail below.

8.3   The Public Health Policy Framework Since 1997

8.3.1   Health improvement

The new government's first health White Paper *The New NHS: modern, dependable* (DH 1997) was published within months of its landmark election victory in May 1997. From a public health perspective, the legislation which followed – the 1999 Health Act – is notable because of the emphasis it places on health improvement. Health authorities were given a public health leadership role that included responsibility for developing health improvement programmes. These are plans to improve the health of the whole population but also for targeting specific sections of the community with the most challenging health needs (Baggott 2000). Local authorities also acquired new statutory responsibilities, for example to contribute to plans for improving health and health care, to cooperate with local NHS bodies in health improvement activities and to promote the 'economic, social and environmental well being of their areas' (Baggott 2000, p. 107).

The 1999 Health Act also led to the replacement of GP fund holding, a Conservative reform and an aspect of the controversial purchaser–provider split (Secretary of State for Health 1989), by a system focused more explicitly on health improvement. All primary care services were reorganised into Primary Care Groups (PCGs) which later evolved into Primary Care Trusts (PCTs). The main functions of PCGs were to improve the health of their community, to develop and integrate primary and community care services in their area, and to take on a role in the commissioning of hospital services. The principle of primary care-led commissioning was thus retained, despite the abolition of GP fund holding.

Section 3

For all the controversy generated by Margaret Thatcher's market-style reforms of health care such as GP fund holding, it is important to acknowledge policy developments under the Conservatives that were concerned with health improvement. Two examples suggest some degree of policy continuity between the Conservatives and Labour and serve to underline that policy makers – in this case the Labour government elected in 1997 – rarely, if ever, start with a blank canvas in policy terms.

The first example is provided by the way in which, under the Conservatives, population health improvement and health gain emerged over time as key principles to guide GP fund holder and District Health Authority purchasers in their priority setting and decision making. Second, it was a Conservative government that published, in 1992, the White Paper *The Health of the Nation*, the first ever health strategy in England (Secretary of State for Health 1992). The emphasis of the strategy was on improving and maintaining health, not simply health care. Five priority areas – coronary heart disease and stroke, cancer, mental illness, HIV/AIDs and sexual health and accidents – and associated objectives and national targets were identified.

This target setting approach was continued under Labour and is evident in the health strategy that succeeded *The Health of the Nation* (Secretary of State for Health 1992). This is somewhat confusingly entitled *Saving Lives: our healthier nation* (Secretary of State for Health 1999). Labour's strategy concentrated on four (not five) key areas – coronary heart disease and stroke, cancer, mental illness and accidents – and set just four targets instead of 27. The new strategy was criticised for a number of reasons: first, because sexual health had been dropped as a key area; second, because of the predominantly disease-based approach of the strategy; and third, because of the phrase 'saving lives', which tended to bring the strategy within the health care model (arguably a weakness also of the 1992 *The Health of the Nation* policy statement; see Hunter 2003).

Notwithstanding these criticisms, after a decade of Labour government, health improvement has persisted as a major theme in health policy and, indeed, across other policy areas. As we have already seen, it has been identified as one of four national priority areas (DH 2004b, 2006b). It also runs through the reports produced by the Wanless review team (Wanless 2002, 2004). These provide the background to or context for the government's public health White Paper *Choosing Health* published in November 2004 (DH 2004a). This is analysed in more detail below.

In summary, then, it is helpful to think of health improvement as a key theme cross-cutting a wide range of policy areas, evident in such initiatives as health impact assessment and local area agreements based on partnership working. The multisectoral dimensions of policy are also underlined by the second policy for health, tackling health inequalities. It is to this theme that we now turn in more detail.

8.3.2   Tackling health inequalities

The emphasis since 1997 on reducing health inequalities is best seen in the context of a concerted push to tackle wider socioeconomic inequalities, amounting to a constellation of disadvantage and underpinning what is arguably the most powerful explanation of health inequalities. The push to tackle socioeconomic deprivation has involved a multiple and complex policy response in and across virtually all government departments. Hunter (2003) notes that the Treasury, under the Chancellor of the Exchequer, has assumed a key role in developing measures, for example the tax credit system, to tackle poverty, particularly as it affects children. Other initiatives to reduce socioeconomic inequalities have been usefully classified by Hunter under three headings: employment-related, area-focused and initiatives to tackle social exclusion. Employment-related developments include the 'Welfare to work' programmes and the national minimum wage. Health Action Zones and Sure Start are examples of area-focused initiatives, while the National Strategy for Neighbourhood Renewal, the 'New deal for communities', is a strategy for tackling social exclusion. A key recommendation of the 1998 Independent Inquiry into Inequalities in Health led by the former Chief Medical Officer Sir Donald Acheson (Independent Inquiry into Inequalities in Health 1998) was that all policies likely to have an impact on health should be assessed in terms of their impact on health inequalities. This suggests something of a 'litmus test' for the initiatives for tackling socioeconomic inequalities briefly reviewed above.

Revealingly, of the Acheson Inquiry's 39 recommendations on tackling health inequalities, only three directly concerned the NHS or came within the sphere of what has been termed health care policy. None the less, politicians have continued to exhort the NHS to play its part in reducing health inequalities. Hunter (2003, p. 59) has detected the 'language of health inequalities and social equity' in the strategy in *Saving Lives: our healthier nation* (Secretary of State for Health 1999). While the 10-year strategy set out in *The NHS Plan* (DH 2000) is focused on health care policy, it does contain a short chapter on public health (chapter 13: 'Improving health and reducing inequality'). However, the chapter acknowledges that because of the wider determinants of ill health and inequality, 'the NHS cannot tackle health inequalities alone' (DH 2000, p. 111). It calls for new partnerships at local level – which eventually emerged as Local Strategic Partnerships – to tackle inequality.

Arguably of greater significance in *The NHS Plan* chapter on public health is the announcement of the government's commitment to developing national targets for health inequalities. These were subsequently announced in March 2001 and are set out under priority 1 ('Improve the health of the population') in the 2004 *National Standards, Local Action* document (DH 2004b) and reiterated in the 2007/8 NHS operating framework (DH 2006a). Progress towards achieving the targets was reported on in the 2006 *Department of Health: Departmental Report* (DH 2006b). It should be noted, however, that other health improvement targets, for example those for reducing mortality from cardiovascular disease and cancer, are also formulated in terms of tackling health inequalities (Table 8.1).

Hard on the heels of *The NHS Plan*, two further policy statements on public health appeared in the summer of 2001. These were *Tackling Health Inequalities* (DH 2001a) and *Vision to Reality* (DH 2001b). The first document was a consultation on the action needed, focusing on six priority themes, to achieve the two national health inequalities targets announced in March 2001. *Vision to Reality* was a review of progress on public health policy implementation since the 1998 Acheson Inquiry. Hunter (2003) offers a lively critique of both documents.

Table 8.1 Public service agreement (PSA) targets and measures for health inequalities. *Source*: DH (2006b).

PSA Target	Measure
Target 2 Reduce health inequalities by 10% by 2010 as measured by infant mortality and life expectancy at birth	Mortality in infancy by social class: the gap in infant mortality between 'routine and manual' groups and the population as a whole Baseline is average of 1997, 1998 and 1999
	Life expectancy by local authority: the gap between the fifth of areas with the 'worst health and deprivation indicators' (the spearhead group) and the population as a whole Baseline year is average of 1995, 1996 and 1997
Target 3 Tackle the underlying determinants of health and health inequalities by:	
• Reducing adult smoking rates to 21% or less by 2010, with a reduction in prevalence among routine and manual groups to 26% or less	Smoking: reduction in numbers of adult (26 %) and routine/manual (31%) groups of smokers (2002–03 baselines). Prevalence from General Household Survey
• Halting the year on year rise in obesity among children under 11 by 2010, in the context of a broader strategy to tackle obesity in the population as a whole (joint target with the Department for Education and Skills and the Department for Culture, Media and Sport)	Obesity: Prevalence of obesity as defined by national BMI percentile classification for children aged between 2 and 10 years (inclusive) measured through the Health Survey for England Baseline year is weighted average for 3-year period 2002–2004
• Reducing the under-18 conception rate by 50% by 2010, as part of a broader strategy to improve sexual health (joint target with the Department for Education and Skills)	Teenage conceptions: the under-18 conception rate is the number of conceptions to under 18-year-olds per 1000 females aged 15–17 Baseline year is 1998 (ONS conception statistics).
BMI, body mass index; ONS, Office for National Statistics.	

Section 3

The second public health priority area in the *National Standards, Local Action* document (DH 2004b) and set out also in the 2007/8 operating framework (DH 2006a) is identified as 'Supporting people with long term conditions'. It is to this, our third theme shaping policy for health, that we now turn.

8.3.3 Better management of long-term and chronic conditions

Chronic conditions have been defined as 'disease which current medical interventions can only control, not cure. The life of a person with chronic disease is forever altered – there is no return to normal' (DH 2004c, p. 3). In the UK an estimated 17.5 million people suffer from chronic conditions which require long-term care and advice. The most common such conditions are asthma, dementia, diabetes, hyperlipidaemia and hypertension (Pereira Gray, 2003).

Given the enormous challenge posed by chronic disease in the UK, it is perhaps surprising that it is only relatively recently that long-term or chronic conditions have started to move up the health policy agenda. There are now definite signs of a changing climate bringing this, our third policy for health theme, to the fore. Four developments, all of which have major implications for health professionals, underline this.

The first of these is government's investment in and roll out of the Expert Patient Programme (EPP) (DH 2001c). According to *The NHS Improvement Plan*, full roll out of the EPP by 2008 will enable 'thousands more people with long term conditions to take more control of their health' (DH 2004d, p. 34).

Second, there has been investment in the development of chronic disease management (CDM) models in primary care settings. Some of this work has been led by American companies, for example Evercare and Kaiser Permanente. An example of a CDM model is reproduced in Figure 8.1.

It is envisaged that the community matron role will be focused on the case management of patients with highly complex conditions; that is, those assessed to be occupying the apex of the triangle in Figure 8.1. Community matrons will identify people at greatest risk and work in partnership with them to secure the better management of their long-term condition(s) as well as to prevent hospital admission. Overall, the community matron role will be key in delivering the first part of the national target for supporting people with long-term conditions : 'to improve health outcomes for people with long term conditions by offering a personalised care plan for the most at risk vulnerable people' (DH 2004b, 2006c). Also of significance is the second part of this target: 'to reduce overall emergency bed days by 5% by 2008 through improved care in primary care and community settings for people with long-term conditions' (DH 2006c, p. 26). It is worth noting that this part of the target is expressed

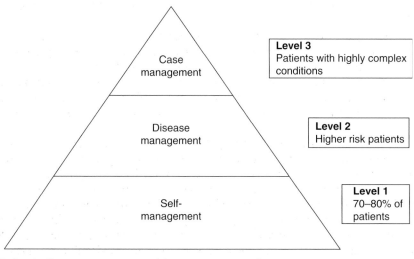

Figure 8.1 A chronic disease management model. *Source:* DH (2004d).

in terms of the acute hospital sector, illustrating the knock-on effect of policy for health on health care policy.

The fourth development which supports the idea that the 'policy spotlight' is increasingly focused on the better management of long-term/chronic conditions was the publication, in 2005, of the *National Service Framework for Long-Term Conditions* (DH 2005a). National Service Frameworks (NSFs) set out national standards along with key interventions, targets and plans for implementation. Primary care and other trusts are expected to implement NSFs, and their progress in doing so is monitored by the Healthcare Commission (www.healthcarecommission.org.uk). In overall terms, NSFs are used as benchmarks for the quality of care provided. If a disease area, condition or client group becomes the subject of an NSF, this tends to result in it receiving a much greater level of managerial attention.

The above review of key themes shaping policy for health has not assessed the significance of the 2004 White Paper *Choosing Health* (DH 2004a). The next section of this chapter sets out a summary of the White Paper. This is followed by an overview of some key models for policy analysis, which are explored in relation to *Choosing Health*.

8.3.4 *Choosing Health*: a summary

Summarizing a White Paper as complex and wide ranging as *Choosing Health* (DH 2004a) presents a considerable challenge. In over 200 pages it sets out a raft of measures and initiatives; so many, in fact, that Klein has argued the White Paper 'gives the impression of being a trawl through Whitehall in which departments were asked to put any policies with a possible bearing on health into the pot' (Klein 2005, p. 65). He goes on to point out that the 'catalogue of interventions, actual or planned, spans a whole range of government activities and interests'. Some of these concern the NHS – for example specific health promotion initiatives – but many are associated with other policy areas and will be the responsibility of non-NHS agencies or organizations.

So a key principle running through the White Paper is that the NHS should improve health and prevent disease, not just provide treatment for those who are ill. The NHS will increasingly focus on supporting individuals to make and maintain healthy choices. Certain groups of people, who may find it difficult to choose healthy lifestyles, come in for particular attention. These include children and young people, adults with social care needs, people in prison, people with mental health problems, or people who are at risk in some way, for example because of obesity, alcohol abuse or their sexual behaviour. The White Paper stresses that the whole NHS workforce will be involved in health improvement activities, and sets out how the roles of some health professionals (for example health visitors, school nurses and community matrons) will be developed. Community matrons will be able to refer to a new 'breed' of health worker, *health trainers*, whose job will be to provide advice to individuals about how to improve their lifestyles. They will be drawn from the local community and accredited by the NHS.

Other key principles shaping the new approach to public health set out in the *Choosing Health* White Paper are stated as informed choice, personalization and working together. The principle of informed choice recognises that people want to be able to make their own decisions about choices that affect their health and to have good quality information to help them to do so. Personalization implies tailoring support to the realities of individual lives, while the working together principle underlines that progress depends upon effective partnerships across communities and agencies with individual patients or clients.

The principles that underpin *Choosing Health* are expected to shape the role and activities not just of the NHS but also to permeate government decisions and actions, at both national and local level, which have a bearing on health (Klein 2005). The emphasis is on the government, communities and the NHS together supporting people to make 'better' – that is healthier – choices for themselves and their families' health. The government acknowledges that legislation is necessary (as in the case of smoking in public places) to enable it to discharge its duty to protect people's health from the actions of others. It has another key role in improving the quality of information available to people in order to help them in their health choices, for example through mounting a national campaign targeting those at risk of sexually transmitted infections or unplanned pregnancies. Other government interventions include action to safeguard children's health, including curbs on the promotion of unhealthy food to children, and working with the food industry to develop a system for the clear, unambiguous labelling of the nutritional content of food.

Overall, the *Choosing Health* White Paper explicitly acknowledges that the NHS cannot solve all health-related problems on its own. Responsibility for improving population health and tackling health inequalities is widely shared across consumers, national and local government, industry, employers, the NHS and other statutory agencies. It is interesting to consider whether this major policy statement strikes the right balance in terms of what is expected of, and the responsibilities which are given to, the key stakeholders for public health improvement that have been identified. Having posed this question, it is appropriate now to move on to consider some key approaches to analysing policy.

8.4   Analysing Policy: Key Models and Approaches

The key approaches to policy analysis explored in this section are drawn from several texts (Hudson & Lowe 2004; Wait 2004; Buse *et al.* 2005; Spicker 2006). After an introduction to some important concepts in policy analysis, the approaches are summarised and then explored in relation to *Choosing Health* (DH 2004a). The emphasis here is to illustrate and provide examples rather than to be exhaustive in the analysis. Overall, the aim is to develop readers' awareness, skills and confidence to enable them, in time, to influence policy in practice.

The analytical framework for policy developed by Walt and Gilson (1994) and reproduced in Buse *et al.* (2005, p. 8) and in Figure 8.2 is a useful introduction to key concepts in policy analysis. The triangle highlights four 'components' of policy and the interrelationships between them. The components are content, context, the process(es) by which policy is made, and the role of key actors in policy making. *Content* is the substance or the 'what' of policy, while *context* points to the wider environment – political, economic, social, cultural or historical – shaping policy and its implementation. *Process* refers to the way in which policy is initiated, formulated, negotiated, communicated, implemented and evaluated (Buse *et al.* 2005). Finally, *actors* are the individuals, professional groups, lobbyists, agencies and organizations (both state and non-state) involved in shaping policy.

As already indicated, the four components of the Walt and Gilson model interact – an important dynamic to consider. The model can be used either for: (i) retrospective analysis, to help understand past policy in terms of content and through all the stages of the policy process (see above); or (ii) prospectively, that is to look forward and plan for a particular policy or how to change existing policy.

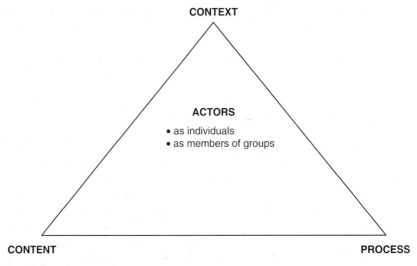

Figure 8.2   The policy analysis triangle.

Retrospective analysis is also referred to as 'analysis *of* policy', while prospective analysis can be described as 'analysis *for* policy' (Buse *et al.* 2005; Spicker 2006).

The policy process is broken down by Buse *et al.* (2005) into four distinct stages which provide a framework for the analysis of *Choosing Health* (DH 2004a). The four stages are:

1. *Problem identification and issue recognition*: examines the wider context and why and how issues come to the attention of policy makers and get onto the agenda.
2. *Policy formulation*: discusses which actors are involved in developing policy, and how policies are drawn up, agreed and communicated.
3. *Policy implementation*: explores whether policies are changed on implementation and, if so, the impact this has on policy outcomes.
4. *Policy evaluation*: monitors whether a policy achieves its objectives and identifies any unintended consequences.

As well as noting the four stages of the policy process, it is helpful to think of it as having three layers. Hudson and Lowe (2004) identify these as macro, meso and micro. These will also be explored in more detail below in relation to the *Choosing Health* White Paper (DH 2004a). Another framework – rational and political models of policy – is useful for analysing decision making throughout the policy process and the policy implementation stage. We will return to this framework as well.

Having introduced some key concepts and general frameworks for policy analysis, we now move on to consider and apply some more specific approaches. These are derived from the four components of the policy analysis triangle. We will start with a content-based analysis of *Choosing Health* (DH 2004a) before progressing to an exploration of context, actors, implementation and evaluation using the policy process model.

8.4.1 Content-based analysis

This approach involves analysing policy in terms of its content or the 'what' of a policy statement or document. One way of doing this is to use a framework that highlights the various meanings of policy. As we have seen, Colebatch identifies five possible definitions (Colebatch 2002). So if we apply the Colebatch framework to *Choosing Health* (DH 2004a), which policy definition(s) are in evidence?

Klein's incisive comment that *Choosing Health* embodies a 'hopeful scattergun approach' (Klein 2004, p. 65), implying policy activism or overload not amounting to a coherent strategy, draws us initially to consider the White Paper in terms of government decisions, actions and activities – the first definition of policy in Colebatch's framework. Even a cursory reading of *Choosing Health* reveals a mass of government decisions, which have implications at both national and local government level, affecting the actions and activities of a wide range of agencies and organizations with a role in implementing the White Paper. Some of the actions and activities that will result have been identified above; others include a new NHS Direct service, children's centres, the extended schools' initiative, and plans to improve nutrition in schools, develop cycle training for children, establish a network of health champions, promote corporate citizenship across the public sector and to develop specialist obesity services in every PCT.

Moving on to Colebatch's second definition of policy as specific commitment, *Choosing Health* provides many examples of commitments made. These tend to be printed in bold type and are therefore easy to find. For example, in Chapter 6 'A health promoting NHS', paragraph 80, we find the statement 'We will accelerate implementation of a national screening programme for chlamydia, to cover the whole of England by March 2007' (DH 2004a, p. 147). Annex B of the White Paper is entitled 'Making it happen' and this sets out the actions that will be taken in three areas – evidence and information, workforce capacity and capability, and systems for local delivery – to put in place a robust framework for delivering on the commitments in the White Paper. A major follow-up document to the White Paper published in March 2005 *Delivering Choosing Health: making healthier choices easier* (DH 2005b) provides more detail on national, local and regional delivery as well as referencing each *Choosing Health* commitment in so-called 'delivery tables'. These allocate responsibility, identify mechanisms for accountability and give dates for delivery. What this illustrates overall is that 'policy' is unlikely to be found in its entirety in a single policy statement; in this case in the White Paper published in November 2004. When we consider the wider context for *Choosing Health* below, we will see the importance of developing an understanding not only of what led up to, but also of what follows, a particular policy statement.

The third definition of policy in the Colebatch framework is policy as routine practice and procedure. There are many ways in which the implementation of *Choosing Health* will impact on, say, the day to day work of health professionals and others. For example, school nurses will have a key role to play in implementing children's health guides as part of the new child health promotion programme. A national health competency framework will give NHS staff the training and support they need to develop their understanding of and skills in promoting health. Health improvement advice will increasingly be linked to routine clinical practice.

Taking the policy definitions of broad orientation and statement of values together, the summary of *Choosing Health* provided above identified several key principles underpinning the White Paper. Without reiterating these here, they do reveal the government's overall direction and value base for its 'new' approach to public health. Klein concedes that there is an overall philosophy shaping *Choosing Health*, which he describes as 'a sophisticated attempt to balance the spheres of state action (the nanny state) and individual responsibility, avoiding both social determinism and atomistic individualism' (Klein 2005, p. 65). It is worth pondering the underpinning principles set out in the White Paper in the light of this statement.

The second component of Walt and Gilson's (1994) policy analysis triangle that we will be considering in relation to *Choosing Health* is context. It is useful at this point to remind ourselves about the key aspects of the policy process model as it is this model that will help structure not only our consideration of the wider context of the White Paper but also the remainder of our analysis.

8.4.2   Context

According to the policy process model, policy is best understood not as a product – for example a package of decisions or specific commitments – but as a process. As highlighted also by the policy analysis triangle, it is important not only to grasp the content of policy but also to analyse other essential components: 'the actors involved, the processes needed to implement change and the context or processes (social, political, cultural, economic, historical) which may explain why policy outcomes were not achieved' (Wait 2004, p. 22). As we have also seen, Hudson and Lowe (2004) identified three layers in the policy process. At a macrolevel, analysis deals with the wider context or environment in which policy is initiated and developed. This reminds us of the first two stages of the policy process identified by Buse *et al.* (2005): problem identification/issue recognition and policy formulation. So we can now turn in more detail to the wider context of *Choosing Health*. Why and how did public health issues get onto the agenda, and how was policy formulated?

Two aspects of the context surrounding the White Paper are worth underlining. The first is provided by the evidence on health – or perhaps more accurately ill health – trends and associated risk factors such as high blood pressure and cholesterol, obesity, physical inactivity and the abuse of alcohol, tobacco and other substances in the UK (see, for example, Wanless 2003; United Kingdom Health Statistics 2006). While the government tends to couch its response in *Choosing Health* to trends in the nation's health in terms of the need to meet 'new challenges' (p. 9), there seems little doubt about the growing concern among politicians and in Whitehall about the nation's health. As Buse *et al.* (2005, p. 72) point out, 'a perceived crisis is one reason why policy windows open'.

Linked to this is the background to *Choosing Health* provided by the Wanless reports (Wanless 2002, 2004). In 2001, the Chancellor of the Exchequer commissioned a major review to examine future health trends and the resources required over the next 20 years to close gaps in performance and deliver the NHS plan (DH 2000). The review team was led by Sir Derek Wanless, former chair of Nat West Bank. The first Wanless report, published in April 2002, *Securing Our Future Health*, sets out an assessment of the resources required to deliver high quality health services in the future. Three scenarios – solid progress, slow uptake and fully engaged – are described, illustrating the considerable difference in how much the NHS is expected to cost in the future depending on how successfully health services become more productive and efficient, and the extent to which people become more fully engaged with their own health. 'Full engagement', the least costly and therefore the most affordable scenario, implies the need to reduce demand by enhancing the promotion of good health and disease prevention.

Following the publication of his first report, Sir Derek was invited, in April 2003, to prepare a further report on the public health aspects of the fully engaged scenario. His 2004 report considers the extent to which current policy is consistent with the public health developments implied by the fully engaged scenario. The focus of the review is on prevention, the wider determinants of health and the cost-effectiveness of action that can be taken to improve the health of the whole population and to reduce health inequalities.

Choosing Health, published in November 2004, is arguably the government's response to the two aspects of context – broadly speaking epidemiological and economic – we have identified. However, as Buse *et al.* (2005, p. 176) suggest, 'epidemiological or economic facts do not simply speak for themselves in setting priorities but will be used or not depending on political processes'. This implies that politics acts upon or interprets aspects of the context. Politics cannot be neutralised when it comes to policy or policy development nor can it be taken out of the response of commentators or of the media. For example, critics of *Choosing Health* argued that the policy failed to reflect the promise of Wanless and downplayed the impact of wider societal inequalities on health status (McDonald 2006). Notwithstanding these criticisms, *Choosing Health* can be seen as the start of a shift along the continuum of health care policy at one end, towards policy for health at the other. If this shift fails to maintain its direction and momentum, the long-term affordability of the NHS is in question. Attention has already been drawn to the fact that Wanless' fully engaged scenario is the least costly of the three he posits.

Having explored aspects of the macrolevel context, we turn now to the opposite extreme: the microlevel of the policy process. This is the level that 'deals with the most basic unit of society: *individual people*' (Hudson & Lowe 2004, p. 8). As we have already noted, the term 'actor' is commonly used to refer not only to individuals but also to professional groups, lobbyists, agencies and organizations (both state and non-state) that influence policy. Actors are a component of the policy analysis triangle and it is important to consider their role at each stage of the policy process.

8.4.3　Actors

Analysing the role of actors at the microlevel entails exploring the impact that particular people (politicians, special advisers, civil servants, health professionals, consumers, representatives of big business, trade unionists and even celebrities) have in formulating policy and/or influencing its final outcome, for example at implementation stage. As far as *Choosing Health* is concerned, several examples serve to underline the influence exercised by actors in the policy process, for example the policy proposals for improving the nutritional content of school food, signposting food on the front of packaging to encourage healthy eating, and on smoking in public places.

For all the measures set out in *Choosing Health* to improve nutrition in school meals, it is arguably the celebrity chef Jamie Oliver – not formally involved initially in designing policy – whose campaigning will have the greatest long-term impact.

On food packaging, the lack of progress made by the government with its aim of introducing a standard system for signposting food, demonstrates the influence of food suppliers and retailers as actors on the policy which finally emerged. As reported in *The Independent* (Akbar 2006), six major food suppliers have rejected the traffic light labelling scheme developed by the Food Standards Agency. Instead they have opted for their own system(s) based on recommended guideline daily allowances of key nutrients. Ultimately the coexistence of different schemes may be confusing for the consumer and undermine the overall objective of encouraging healthier eating through more informative labelling.

The third example to illustrate the role of actors in the policy process is provided by the political wrangle over smoking in public places. According to the political model of policy, policy is a 'bargained outcome', the result of 'an essentially political activity (policy making) in which the values, judgements and preferences of individual actors enter into all stages of play' (Wait 2004, p. 22). *Choosing Health* signalled the government's intention to 'shift the balance significantly in favour of smoke free environments' (DH 2004a, p. 99) and to legislate for a total ban on smoking in all enclosed public places, workplaces, restaurants and pubs and bars serving food. However, according to the original proposal, 'other pubs and bars will be free to choose whether to allow smoking or to be smoke-free' (DH 2004a, p. 99). This 'reprieve' for pubs and bars not serving food was explained at the time in political and personality terms: it reflected the views of the then Secretary of State for Health, Dr John Reid. However, as a result of intense lobbying, for example by the public health community, changing public opinion, and the appointment of a new Secretary of State for Health, Patricia Hewitt, who held less entrenched views on the matter, MPs were given a free vote. A very decisive majority of 200 voted in favour of a total ban on smoking in public places (see http://news.bbc.co.uk/1/hi/uk_politics/4714992.stm).

So the original policy on smoking in public places, as articulated in *Choosing Health* (DH 2004a), is not the policy the government eventually legislated for. The political model of policy offers an explanatory framework for this. It will always be a political decision as to where government policies and actions should lie on the continuum between, on the one hand, 'nanny statism' and, on the other, unfettered 'atomistic individualism' (Klein 2005, p. 65). Notwithstanding this, it is important to acknowledge the role the state has played and can play in bringing about public health improvements (Jochelson 2005). The range of policy instruments or approaches available to states to change the pattern of what people do are usefully identified by Spicker (2006, p. 106).

The political model of policy thus conveys something of the complex interplay or even power struggle between 'policy objectives, goals, players and policy content' (Wait 2004, p. 22). This is in contrast to the rational or rational – comprehensive model of policy making which draws a linear connection between six stages. Spicker (2006, p. 33) identifies these as: assessment of the environment, identification of aims and objectives, consideration of the alternative methods that are available, selection of methods, implementation, and evaluation. The latter two stages, also highlighted by the policy process model, are explored in more detail below. For now, it is worth noting that the rational model, in implying that policy must invariably precede and lead to action, can be viewed as a 'normative' or ideal type of process. For all the oversimplification of policy and policy making it entails (Buse *et al.* 2005; Spicker 2006), the point of such a model, as Hogwood and Gunn (1984) suggest, is to pose the question 'How *would* policies be made if policy-makers pursued and were capable of complete rationality?' However, as has already been suggested in relation to *Choosing Health*, policy makers in the so-called 'real world' rarely, if ever, start with a clean slate (Wait 2004). Instead there is a raft of existing policies from which they can make only incremental changes in the light of political realities. Lindblom (1979) describes this as 'disjointed incrementalism'. In addition, the reality for policy makers is that 'the means and ends of policy making are likely to be derived in parallel, yet unrelated processes', making it very difficult to establish causality between two parts of the policy process (Wait 2004). The best policy makers can be expected to do is to muddle through guided by trial and error (Hudson & Lowe 2004).

To return now to implementation, we have already seen that this is a stage not only of the rational model of policy making but also of the four-stage policy process model (Buse *et al.* 2005). It is explored in more detail below.

8.4.4   Implementation

Analysing the implementation of policy involves looking at the changes following, or the consequences of, policy decisions. Is there a gap between what was planned and what actually occurred as a result of policy? In recent years governments have focused increasingly on delivery, for example devising systems that increase the likelihood that policies will be implemented as intended. Information on the impact of policies must be available to demonstrate that policies are making a difference to people's lives. This has been described as a 'top-down' approach to implementation which connects closely to the rational model of the policy process (Buse *et al.* 2005). The *Choosing Health* delivery plan, consisting of quantitative targets with explicit achievement dates and a clear accountability framework, is arguably an example of a top-down approach to implementation. Policy execution is seen as a predominantly 'technical, administrative or managerial activity' (Buse *et al.* 2005, p. 122).

There are, however, several compelling reasons why implementation cannot be viewed purely as a technocratic exercise. First, the implementation of policy is shaped by changes in the context. In the case of *Choosing Health*, there is growing evidence that implementation is being knocked off course because of the difficult resource climate in the wider NHS (Carlisle 2006). Money earmarked for new public health initiatives is being diverted to tackle organizational deficits, particularly in the acute sector.

The second reason for questioning the top-down view of implementation becomes apparent if we apply microlevel analysis to policy at the sharp end, that is at the point of implementation when it is finally delivered by and through the myriad actions of, say, public servants. As Hudson and Lowe argue, from this perspective of the 'bottom end' of the process, it may be that the policy maker's 'policy' is not being delivered. Instead what emerges is a 'different policy made up by street-level bureaucrats … which becomes de facto the real policy' (Hudson & Lowe 2004, p. 9). Given the myriad actions and actors involved in implementing *Choosing Health*, it is important, albeit very challenging methodologically, to assess whether the raft of policies undergo change on implementation and, if so, the impact this has on policy outcomes. This leads us into a consideration of the evaluation stage of the policy process.

8.4.5 Evaluation

Buse *et al.* (2005) have defined evaluation as 'research designed specifically to assess the operation and/or impact of a programme or policy in order to determine whether it is worth pursuing'. Does the policy achieve its objectives or are there any unintended consequences? What distinguishes summative from formative evaluation is the timing of the research. Summative evaluation, which fits into the classical rational approach, is retrospective. Its aim is to produce an overall verdict on a policy post-implementation, for example in terms of the costs and benefits. The findings of the evaluation are then fed into policy reform in order to improve effectiveness (Hudson & Lowe 2004). In contrast, formative evaluation assesses how a policy is being implemented with a view to changing or adjusting policy to improve its implementation. In other words, the formative approach to evaluation looks to guide policy as it develops.

Researchers tasked with evaluating public health policies face considerable challenges. For example, a key priority in the *Choosing Health* White Paper is to tackle obesity in the population as a whole. A specific target is set for the under 11 age group: 'to halt the year-on-year rise in obesity among children under 11 by 2010' (DH 2004b). It is also implied that responsibility for achieving the target and the underlying objective will be shared jointly by the government departments with responsibility for health, education and sport. An extensive number of programmes or courses of action across different government departments and levels of government for achieving the objective are set out in the White Paper. But how will we assess the effectiveness of this disparate collection of initiatives and mechanisms, or pinpoint the way they may have contributed individually as well as collectively to the achievement of the target? These are important questions relating to the evidence on effectiveness of public health interventions, and we shall return to them when we look at evidence-based policy below.

The sheer difficulty of evaluating public health activities is further underlined when we consider a statement in the Secretary of State's foreword to the White Paper. Here we are told that 'the success of the strategy will be measured first in the increased number of healthy choices that individuals make, and then in the lives saved, lengthened and improved in quality' (DH 2004a, p. 7). Searching questions need to be asked about how these things can be measured and any 'successes' confidently attributed to a particular public health strategy or initiative. As Buse and colleagues argue, a challenge faced by policy makers lies in knowing 'whether the fact that an evaluation fails to show a programme achieving the results intended is due to the intrinsic methodological difficulty of disentangling the specific contribution of the programme from other factors, or whether the programme has genuinely failed to meet its objectives' (Buse *et al.* 2005, p. 166). They go on to suggest that this is particularly likely to be the case with policies designed to address complex and multicausal 'wicked issues' (Hunter 2003), for example inequalities in life expectancy rooted in the constellation of disadvantage generally held to arise from wider social and economic conditions.

Making real progress in population health improvement or tackling health inequalities is almost certain to involve a longer timescale than the one normally available to politicians, who typically operate over a 4–5 year period. If a particular public health policy or a collection of policies do not achieve the expected outcomes over the time period being assessed this does not necessarily mean the policies

Section 3

will be judged ineffective in the longer run. For these reasons, evaluation research to assess the impact of public health policy has many challenges to address.

8.4.6 Evidence-based policy

To conclude this section on evaluation, we now move on to consider evidence-based policy (EBP). This is another formulation of the rational, linear approach to policy development and one that has been gaining ground since the latter part of the 1990s. Key to this approach is the assessment of past policies to inform decision-makers' thinking at the policy-making stage (Hudson & Lowe 2004) and also the appraisal of the quality of policies before implementation.

Policies may be ineffective not only because of problems at the implementation stage, but also because they are poor policies. The EBP model assesses whether the policy is underpinned by systematic, empirical evidence and cogent argument. In the case of public health policy, what is the scale of likely health benefit? Is there any possibility the policy might do harm? What about ease and cost of implementation? (Wait 2004).

Given the sheer number of initiatives and interventions set out in the *Choosing Health* White Paper, it seems legitimate to ask questions about the underpinning evidence base. For example, what evidence is there for the effectiveness of the health trainer approach, being piloted initially in the poorest communities (spearhead PCTs), or for personal health kits for developing personal health plans? Even if public health interventions do have a strong evidence base, Kelly (2004, p. 1) has argued that such evidence of effectiveness 'only in very exceptional circumstances prescribes precisely which policies or practices should be implemented'. This tends to be because interventions assessed by systematic reviews (the piloting of health trainers?) are generally implemented under controlled scientific and well resourced experimental conditions. They may not be as effective under non-experimental, routine service delivery circumstances.

There are, however, some indications in *Choosing Health* and the delivery plan which followed it in 2005, that the government recognises the need to develop a strong evidence base. For example, on p. 141 of *Choosing Health*, we read that the Department of Health has commissioned the National Institute for Health and Clinical Excellence to prepare definitive guidance on prevention, identification, management and treatment of obesity. Furthermore annex B includes a section on evidence and information that suggests a commitment to developing an evidence base for public health interventions and their cost-effectiveness, for example guidelines on children's exercise referral and occupational health. In addition, *Delivering Choosing Health* (DH 2005b) identifies 45 'big wins', key interventions that the evidence and expert advice suggest will make the biggest impact on health in the shortest period of time.

Our exploration so far of approaches to analysing policy has drawn on components of the Walt and Gilson policy analysis triangle, and on concepts derived from the four stages of the policy process model. We have also considered rational and political models of policy and two out of three of Hudson and Lowe's layers of the policy process. It is hoped that this application of the various policy analysis approaches to the *Choosing Health* White Paper has provided some insights into the strengths and shortcomings of the approaches. Much fuller assessments can, however, be found in Hudson and Lowe (2004), Buse *et al.* (2005) and Spicker (2006).

Activity

Drawing on the work of Hudson and Lowe (2004), Buse *et al.* (2005) and Spicker (2006), write your own definitions of the rational and political models of policy. What are the main strengths and shortcomings of the models? Make some notes and start to develop a critique. Is the main approach to policy analysis explored in each of the three texts predominantly a rational or political one?

Additional analytical frameworks, particular to *Choosing Health*, can be drawn from the Wanless reports which were widely praised by commentators. Two frameworks repay further study. The first of these is suggested by the Wanless definition of public health as 'the science and art of preventing disease, prolonging life and promoting health through the organised efforts and informed choices of society, organisations, public and private, communities and individuals' (Wanless 2004, p. 3). This is a more widely drawn definition and one that makes more explicit the range of different stakeholders in public health improvement than the much quoted definition from the Acheson report on public health: 'the science and art of preventing disease, prolonging life and promoting health through the organised efforts of society' (Acheson 1988). The analytical framework which is suggested is one that explores who should be doing what to bring about population health gain. What levers can be used, and who should be holding them? What is the evidence base which should underpin decisions about roles and responsibilities for population health improvement? Wanless, in chapters 7 and 8 of the 2004 report, discusses these questions; it is helpful also to explore *Choosing Health* in terms of stakeholder roles and levers.

The second additional analytical framework, again from Wanless (2004), is based on the four types of 'failure that afflict decisions about preventative health and health care'. These are information failures, incomplete appraisal of costs and benefits, social context failures and health inequalities. These four types of failure prompt important questions in relation to *Choosing Health*. What policy recommendations in *Choosing Health* will address information failures stemming, say, from insufficient information, confusing messages or through misunderstanding of information about health? What measures in the White Paper are concerned with addressing social context failures – unhelpful environments that may make it difficult for individuals to choose healthy options – or with tackling health inequalities? We have already noted the view put forward by some commentators that *Choosing Health* fails adequately to acknowledge or address health inequalities. So as far as this issue is concerned, is *Choosing Health* an example of non policy making or, at best, of symbolic policy making? After all, the most significant thing about a policy can be what it fails to say, or the inadequacy or weakness of its response to a particular issue.

8.5   Influencing Policy: Implications for Practitioners

The foregoing analysis underlines the importance of practitioners developing their knowledge and understanding of policy in order to 'influence it in their working lives' (Buse *et al.* 2005, p. 6). To exert such influence, it seems particularly important for practitioners to develop their confidence and skills in three key areas:

- strategic thinking and political skills;
- communication;
- research (Spicker 2006).

8.5.1   Strategic thinking and political skills

As we have seen, the policy analysis triangle and the policy process model explore policy as interplay between content, context, process(es) and actors. This underlines how important it is for practitioners to be aware not only of the content of policy but also of the macrolevel wider context, and the political and power dimensions of policy. The NHS Leadership Qualities framework (www.nhsleadershipqualities.nhs.uk) identifies the ability to scan and analyse the wider environment as a characteristic of an effective leader. Public health practitioners need to understand the wider context for their practice and to be able to assess the impact of key trends and political developments in the external environment on their practice and procedure in the future. A variety of tools can be used to undertake this sort of strategic analysis, for example PEST (political, economic, sociocultural and technological) analysis and Porter's five forces model (Sutherland & Canwell 2004).

Activity

Identify a locally developed policy or strategy for improving health and wellbeing (e.g. a PCT obesity strategy). Explore the wider context for the local policy you have selected and analyse the policy using some of the concepts and frameworks explored in this chapter. You may also wish to refer to Spicker's checklist for policy analysis (Spicker 2006, pp. 181–3) and Chapter 10 'Doing policy analysis' in Buse *et al.* (2005). What are the implications of the policy you have analysed for your work/practice area and role?

8.5.2   Communication

In addition, at the meso- and micro-levels of the policy process, practitioners need to see themselves as actors able to influence policy as it is formulated and at the sharp end of implementation. The meso-level is the third layer or middle part of the policy process identified by Hudson and Lowe (2004). Meso-level analysis deals with '*how* policies come to be made, *who* puts them on the policy agenda, and the *structure* of the institutional arrangements in which policy is defined and eventually implemented' (Hudson & Lowe 2004, p. 9). At the meso-layer, for example within a PCT or working across boundaries with a local authority or voluntary sector organization, practitioners need to be familiar with and confident in negotiating or navigating what can be described as the 'institutional architecture', different organizational cultures and processes for policy making and implementation. This entails confident communication skills as well as political awareness. Practitioners should also be aware of the scope to influence policy by exercising their professional judgement and expertise at the implementation stage, usually at the micro-level of the policy process. There will always be tensions in a devolved health care system where many policies, targets and objectives are determined centrally yet policy implementation is devolved to the local level, emerging, for example, in routine practice and procedure. However, it could be argued that practitioners need to have more confidence that results and experience on the ground can 'drive policies at all levels as they emerge' (Wait 2004, p. 24). The balance needs to be shifted away from a top-down to more of an assertive bottom-up mindset on policy implementation, which is underpinned by a belief that practitioners can exert influence and effect change.

8.5.3   Research skills

The policy analysis triangle and the policy process model highlight the importance of developing research skills in order to be able to gather, organise and analyse health policy data. For example, assessing the wider environment could involve both quantitative and qualitative techniques (Spicker 2006). The quality of policy analysis at all stages of the policy process model depends on the accuracy, comprehensiveness and relevance of the information collected (Buse *et al.* 2005).

Finally, in terms of EBP, as Chapter 11 reminds us, there is an evergrowing expectation that practice, and indeed policy, should be based on systematic, empirical evidence. Despite the methodological challenges this may pose, it is vital that practitioners should be skilled in handling, assessing and interpreting the evidence base. Confidence in doing so will greatly enhance their ability to contribute to the design, implementation and evaluation of policy.

Conclusion

In the book *Strategy Bites Back*, Mintzberg *et al.* (2005) discuss strategic thinking in terms of seeing, describing strategic thinkers as 'visionaries' with the ability to see in seven different directions. These are: seeing ahead, seeing behind (understanding the past), seeing above (making out the big picture), seeing below (finding the 'gem' of an idea that has the potential to change an organization), seeing beside (thinking laterally and creatively), seeing beyond (putting ideas in context and constructing the future) and, finally, seeing it all through (implementing the strategy). Practitioners who develop this sort of visionary thinking as well as political, communication and research skills, will grow in confidence about their ability to contribute to policy and strategy development and implementation, the fifth principle of public health practice (NMC 2004). It is important not to lose sight of the underlying purpose of doing so: to improve health and wellbeing. This should be the goal of all public health practice and is the compelling reason why practitioners should strive to influence policy throughout their working lives.

References

Acheson D. (1988) *Public Health in England*. London: HM Stationery Office.

Akbar A. (2006) Food giants criticised for rejecting traffic light warnings on nutrition. *The Independent* 8 June, 15.

Baggott R. (2000) *Public Health Policy and Politics*. Basingstoke: Palgrave.

Buse K., Mays N., Walt G. (2005) *Making Health Policy*. Understanding Public Health Series. Maidenhead: Open University Press.

Carlisle D. (2006) Healthier lives but ever-widening inequalities: what price progress? *Health Service Journal* 16 Nov, 14.

Colebatch H.K. (2002) *Policy*. Maidenhead: Open University Press.

DH (Department of Health) (1997) *The New NHS: modern, dependable*. London: HM Stationery Office.

DH (Department of Health) (2000) *The NHS Plan: a plan for investment, a plan for reform*. London: HM Stationery Office.

DH (Department of Health) (2001a) *Tackling Health Inequalities. Consultation on a plan for delivery*. London: Department of Health.

DH (Department of Health) (2001b) *Vision to Reality*. London: Department of Health.

DH (Department of Health) (2001c) *The Expert Patient: a new approach to chronic disease management for the 21st century*. London: Department of Health.

DH (Department of Health) (2004a) *Choosing Health: making healthier choices easier*. London: HM Stationery Office.

DH (Department of Health) (2004b) *National Standards, Local Action. Health and social care standards and planning framework 2005/06 – 2007/08*. London: Department of Health.

DH (Department of Health) (2004c) *Chronic Disease Management. A compendium of information*. London: Department of Health.

DH (Department of Health) (2004d) *The NHS Improvement Plan: putting people at the heart of public services*. London: HM Stationery Office.

DH (Department of Health) (2005a) *National Service Framework for Long-Term Conditions*. London: Department of Health.

DH (Department of Health) (2005b) *Delivering Choosing Health: making healthier choices easier*. London: Department of Health.

DH (Department of Health) (2006a) *The NHS in England: the operating framework for 2007/08*. London: Department of Health.

DH (Department of Health) (2006b) *Department of Health: departmental report 2006*. London: Department of Health.

DH (Department of Health) (2006c) *Supporting People with Long Term Conditions to Self-Care: a guide to developing local strategies and good practice*. London: HM Stationery Office.

Grayson L., Gomershall A. (2003) *A Difficult Business: finding the evidence for social science reviews*. ESRC UK Centre for Evidence Based Policy and Practice Working Paper No. 19. London: Queen Mary, University of London. http://www.evidencenetwork.org.

Ham C. (2004) *Health Policy in Britain*, 5th edn. Basingstoke: Palgrave Macmillan.

Hogwood B., Gunn L. (1984) *Policy Analysis for the Real World*. Oxford: Oxford University Press.

Hudson J., Lowe S. (2004) *Understanding the Policy Process*. Bristol: Policy Press.

Hunter D. (2003) *Public Health Policy*. Cambridge: Polity Press.

Independent Inquiry into Inequalities in Health (1998) *Report of the Committee Chaired by Sir Donald Acheson*. London: HM Stationery Office.

Jochelson K. (2005) *Nanny or Steward? The role of government in public health*. London: Kings Fund.

Kelly M. (2004) *The Evidence of Effectiveness of Public Health Interventions – and the Implications*. Oxford: Health Development Agency Evidence Briefing.

Klein R. (2005) *Transforming the NHS: the story in 2004*. In: *Transforming the NHS: the story in 2004* (eds Powell M., Bauld L., Clarke K.). Social Policy Review No. 17: Analysis and debate in social policy, 2005. Bristol: Policy Press.

Lewis R., Dixon J. (2005) *NHS Market Futures. Exploring the impact of health service market reforms*. London: Kings Fund.

Lindblom C.E. (1979) Still muddling through. *Public Administration Review* 39 (6), 517–25.

McDonald R. (2006) Chapter 2 In: *Creating a Patient-led NHS: empowering 'consumers' or shrinking the state?* (eds Bauld L., Clarke K., Maltby T.). Social Policy Review No. 18: Analysis and debate in social policy, 2006. Bristol: Policy Press.

Mintzberg H., Ahlstrand B., Lampel J. (eds) (2005) *Strategy Bites Back*. Harlow: FT Prentice Hall.

NMC (Nursing and Midwifery Council) (2004) *Standards of Proficiency for Specialist Public Health Nurses*. London: Nursing and Midwifery Council.

Pereira Gray D. (2003) 2020 vision. *Health Service Journal* 2 Oct, 18–19.

Secretary of State for Health (1989) *Working for Patients*. London: HM Stationery Office.

Secretary of State for Health (1992) *The Health of the Nation: a strategy for health in England*. London: HM Stationery Office.

Secretary of State for Health (1999) *Saving Lives: our healthier nation*. London: HM Stationery Office.

Skills for Health (2004) National Occupational Standards for the Practice of Public Health. Bristol: Skills for Health. www. skillsforhealth.org.uk.

Spicker P. (2006) *Policy Analysis for Practice. Applying social policy*. Bristol: Policy Press.

Sutherland J., Canwell D. (2004) *Key Concepts in Management*. Basingstoke: Palgrave Macmillan.

Toward S., Maslin-Prothero S. (2007) The impact of health and social policy on the planning and delivery of nursing care. In: *Principles of Professional Studies in Nursing* (eds Brown J., Libberton P.), pp. 113–34. Basingstoke: Palgrave Macmillan.

United Kingdom Health Statistics (2006) *United Kingdom Health Statistics*. UKHS No. 2 Health and Care Theme. www.statistics.gov.uk/statbase/Product.asp?vlnk=6637 (accessed 21 Feb 2007).

Wait S. (2004) *Benchmarking. A policy analysis*. London: Nuffield Trust.

Walt G., Gilson L. (1994) Reforming the healthcare sector in developing countries: the central role of policy analysis. *Health Policy and Planning* 9, 353–70.

Wanless D. (2002) *Securing Our Future Health: taking a long term view. Final report*. London, HM Treasury.

Wanless D. (2003) *Securing Good Health for the Whole Population. Population health trend*. London: HM Stationery Office.

Wanless D. (2004) *Securing Good Health for the Whole Population. Final report*. London: HM Stationery Office.

CHAPTER 9

Strategic Leadership for Health and Wellbeing

Yvette Cox and Mark Rawlinson

Public Health Skills: Strategic leadership

- Strategic analysis: SWOT analysis, PESTEL analysis, needs assessment and stakeholder analysis
- Strategic choice: revising the mission statement, identifying strategic options, and evaluating and selecting strategic options
- Strategic implementation: communicating the strategy, organizational structures in place, aligning culture and strategy, reviewing progress and amending the strategy

Introduction

This chapter aims to help the reader to develop a public health strategy. The purpose of a strategy is to provide direction for public health and to ensure that available resources are used to best advantage to meet the changing needs of the population. Formulating a strategy also enables a matching of the public health activities to the environment in which it operates, taking into account social indicators of health and the broader strategies set by government (Rowe 2002). Most texts on strategic management are aimed at commercial companies, with the emphasis being on enabling a company to gain a competitive advantage over its rivals. Within the public sector, strategic decisions aim to improve efficiency in order to develop or retain services on a limited budget (Johnson *et al.* 2005). It remains important to ensure that there is a fit between the services provided and the needs of the population. Strategy formulation enables the identification of the different needs of clients, with a view to tailoring the services to meet the needs of each group or to focus its resources on one particular group (Clegg *et al.* 2005).

9.1   Strategic Management

There are three main elements to strategic management (Johnson *et al.* 2005):

1. *Strategic analysis*: review of current public health and identification of changes required.
2. *Strategic choice*: options for delivering public health.
3. *Strategy implementation*: putting the strategy into action (managing the change) (Figure 9.1).

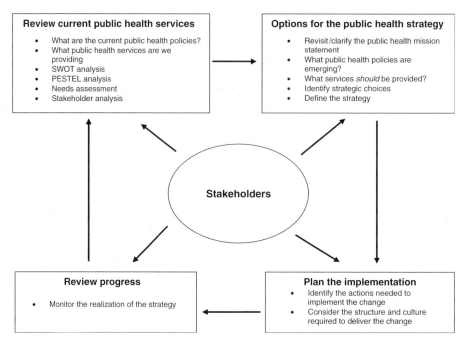

Figure 9.1 Developing a public health strategy.

In order to develop a public health strategy data are needed on such factors as local demography, age and cause of death, incidence and prevalence of disease (Rowe 2002). Data can be collected from a huge variety of places, e.g. the public health common dataset, the Office of National Statistics, local authorities and annual public health reports.

The aim of the public health strategy is to improve wellbeing and quality of life through health programmes that aim to reduce the impact of disease and disability on the local population (Rowe 2002). The strategy should identify gaps in public health services and provide a plan for how services can be developed in order to bridge the gap.

9.2 Strategic Analysis: Review of Current Public Health Services

The purpose of analysis is to identify the key issues that the organization needs to address (Iles 1997). The analysis will provide an understanding of what is being delivered, how well it is being delivered, and whether it is meeting the expectations of the stakeholders.

There are a number of frameworks that can be used as tools to analyse the strategic environment; many of the frameworks within strategic management literature are geared towards analysing the competitive environment e.g. Porter's (1980) five forces. These frameworks provide useful insights into aspects of public health delivery and should not be dismissed, especially in the light of a more competitive environment emerging within health and social care. This chapter will present four frameworks for analysing the public health strategic environment:

- strengths, weaknesses, opportunities and threats (SWOT) analysis;
- political, economic, sociocultural, technological, environmental and legal (PESTEL) analysis;
- needs assessment;
- stakeholder analysis.

The frameworks can be used in any order. The approach to analysing the strategic environment should be iterative, with information from one framework being combined with the other frameworks so that an integrated view is developed.

9.2.1 SWOT analysis

An analysis of strengths, weaknesses, opportunities and threats is useful as it provides a simple framework to evaluate the current public health services. *Strengths* are aspects of public health which are delivered well and are meeting the needs of the local population, *weaknesses* are aspects which are not achieving targets or making a difference to public health. Strengths and weaknesses often relate directly to the internal organization in terms of how well current resources are being used in the delivery of public health. Box 9.1 provides some key questions to assist in analysing strengths and weaknesses.

Opportunities and *threats* relate to aspects within the external environment; these should also be evaluated against the strengths and weaknesses identified, e.g. opportunities can only be capitalised upon if there are sufficient and appropriate resources to meet the challenges posed. Threats are only threats if the capabilities to deal with them do not exist (Thompson 2001).

SWOT analysis is normally presented as a matrix (Table 9.1), and should be limited to those factors that have most impact so that attention can be concentrated upon these. Factors identified through the SWOT analysis may fit into more than one category, so something that is seen as a strength may also be identified as a threat. The SWOT analysis aims to identify internal strengths to take advantage of external opportunities and to avoid threats whilst addressing weaknesses (Dancar 2006).

An analysis of the external environment within which public health is being delivered is also important as there are many factors that impact upon public health and these should be taken into consideration when developing the strategy.

9.2.2 PESTEL analysis

Political, economic, sociocultural, technological, environmental and legal factors provide a framework to analyse and categorise environmental influences impacting upon public health. Sometimes the same topic may feature under two or more aspects of PESTEL analysis, e.g. government policies provide insights into priorities (political) but also may be a driver for technological advances. A PESTEL analysis enables the identification of public health opportunities provided by environmental conditions as well as current or emerging threats (Box 9.2).

The information from the PESTEL analysis can be used to further develop the SWOT analysis, e.g. local facilities for family planning may have been identified as a strength within the SWOT analysis. The PESTEL analysis may reveal the need to reduce the number of teenage pregnancies. There is therefore an opportunity to use one of the strengths identified (family planning facilities) to address the issue of reducing the number of teenage pregnancies. However, the SWOT analysis may have also identified a weakness in that the family planning services are not situated near any of the schools, so there is restricted access to these facilities (Table 9.2).

Future opportunities can be identified by reviewing current and emerging governmental and organizational policies related to public health and assessing how well these are or can be met within current constraints. Threats include anything that impacts upon the ability to deliver public health to the population, e.g. funding issues, legal constraints, etc.

The SWOT and PESTEL analyses provide a view of how well the current public health strategy is being achieved, and what the future challenges may be. In order to develop a meaningful public health strategy a needs assessment will also have to be undertaken.

9.2.3 Needs assessment

The first three chapters of this book provide details on the process of needs assessment. The data collected through needs assessment are used to present a case for health improvement. Jolly and George (cited in Rowe 2002) describe the following methods for identifying needs:

- comparing local provision with what is provided elsewhere;
- asking different stakeholders what they want and reaching a consensus;
- studying epidemiology and the cost-effectiveness of providing interventions to address the problems caused by disease.

BOX 9.1

A framework for analysing organizational strengths and weaknesses.

The following provides examples of the sort of aspects you may wish to consider when analysing your organizations' performance. *It is not an exhaustive list.*

Internal processes
1. Are the physical resources (buildings, etc.) suitable for the public health service being delivered?
2. Do the members of staff have the information they need to deliver public health?
3. Do you have the necessary human resources?
4. Would a different skill mix enable more effective delivery of services?
5. Are there sufficient support roles to enable staff to use their skills appropriately?
6. Are reports useful and accurate, e.g. population/health statistics for your local area?
7. Are there any problem areas within the process of delivering public health services?
8. Do you have appropriate technology to support the public health service?

Performance of staff
1. Do the team members work well together?
2. Do all members of the team share relevant information?
3. Do all staff members have an equal workload?
4. Do you regularly review achievement of standards by your team?
5. Has each member of your team received adequate training to perform the functions of their public health role?
6. Does each member of the team take appropriate responsibility for his or her work?
7. Do staff members have the knowledge and skills required to make the right decisions?
8. Are members of staff willing to make decisions?
9. Is there a high turnover of staff?
10. Are there mechanisms in place to encourage retention of staff?
11. Are the public health objectives/goals clear to all staff?
12. Do members of staff embrace or resist change?

Client satisfaction
1. Are the local population's public health needs clearly identified?
2. Are the clients involved in the development of ideas and service provision?
3. Do the public health services provided meet client needs?
4. Do the public health services provided meet the needs of clients from differing backgrounds/with complex needs?
5. What aspects of the public health service do your clients like/dislike?
6. What are the unmet needs of your clients?
7. Are the public health services provided in a timely fashion?
8. What are the 'value added' aspects of the public health services provided?
9. Is there an established process for reviewing public health services in relation to client needs?
10. Is client satisfaction monitored constantly?
11. How much are clients using the public health services provided?
12. How do clients access the public health services?
13. How do clients obtain information about the public health services?
14. What are the costs of providing these public health services?

Improving services
1. Do staff members make suggestions to improve the public health services provided?
2. What voice has the consumer?
3. Are suggestions for improvement followed up?
4. Is there a mechanism to identify new public health services?
5. How many staff/teams are developing new public health services?

Financial performance
1. Is the public health service provided within budget?
2. Are different ways of delivering public health services explored in terms of cost benefit?
3. Could productivity be increased within the current budget?
4. Are all assets utilised to the full?

Stakeholders
1. Who are your stakeholders?
2. What are the differing needs of your stakeholders?
3. How closely do your public health services meet those differing needs?
4. What are the tensions between the different stakeholders?
5. What are the unmet needs of your stakeholders?

Table 9.1   SWOT analysis: 'Prevention of fall in the home' initiative from a district nurses team.

Strengths	Weaknesses

A recognition and desire to improve the health of individuals through cooperation, collaboration and empowerment
Local knowledge of the community
Access to the vulnerable
Access to local data
Ongoing access to users and families
Established communication networks both formal and informal
Developed understanding of working patterns across traditional boundaries:
    primary care
    secondary care
    private sector
    voluntary and independent sector
Expertise in nursing in the home
Established risk assessment processes
	Current financial climate very restricted, limited funds for new initiatives
	Long-term care initiative thus difficult to present hard data re potential savings
	Existing staff and expertise already committed to existing work
	Data often stored on separate IT systems
	The initiative would cross established health and social care boundaries:
	    cultural
	    physical
	    economic

Opportunities	**Threats**
To manage for health – empower individuals to maintain their independence and wellbeing To reduce hospital admissions Potentially to reduce costs for the local health economy Opportunity to improve working relationships with other health and social care provider's e.g. occupational therapists Demonstrate a way of meeting PCT performance targets To develop and expand the nursing team's understanding of care Establish new networks and links in the community To validate and refine data and information collection tools To carry out relevant research in the care context IT, information technology, PCT, Primary Care Trust.	A dilution of existing service provision if no new recruitment took place No new money available Low on PCT priority list compared with other needs This represents a long term investment not a quick fix Incompatibility in IT systems External providers Limited evidence base for practice People may be change weary

Three main elements are assessed within the needs analysis:

1. Sociology, which provides the wider context for the study of public health, e.g. the impact of poverty on health.
2. Epidemiology.
3. Health economics.

Stakeholders can have a major impact on the emerging strategy; they can also influence the strategy when it is being implemented, so it is essential to be aware of the stakeholders and gain a view of their aspirations.

9.2.4   Stakeholder analysis

Stakeholders are defined as any individuals or groups who have a vested interest in public health, or those people on which the organization depends to deliver public health (Box 9.3). Stakeholder analysis is important in order to identify the expectations of different stakeholders, the degree of interest they may have in the strategic development, and the degree of power they have to influence the strategy. Figure 9.2 is an example related to healthy walks.

The concerns of stakeholders will differ depending on how interested they are in the emerging strategies (Johnson *et al.* 2005). Different stakeholders may hold distinct expectations of each element

BOX 9.2

PEST(EL) analysis. *Source*: Johnson *et al.* (2005).

Political factors
- Political agenda
- Current and emerging policies
- Government stability
- Political parties/alignment
- Taxation policy
- Social welfare policies
- Local health or social need
- Local health and social care infrastructure e.g Foundation Trust

Economic
- Gross domestic product (GDP) trends
- Interest rates
- Inflation
- Local commissioning priorities
- Consumer expenditure and disposable incomes
- Unemployment
- Investment by the state/private sector
- Costs of:
  - energy
  - transport
  - communication
  - raw materials
  - human resources
  - training and development

Sociocultural
- Social indicators of health
- Population demographics
- Social mobility

- Community resources
- Shifts in values/culture
- Changes in lifestyle
- Attitudes to work and leisure
- Distribution of income
- Education and health

Technological
- Improved screening for diseases e.g. cervical smear tests
- Government and European Union investment policy
- Research initiatives
- New discoveries/developments
- Speed of change and adoption of new technology
- Rates of obsolescence
- Access and compatibility of information technology systems – single assessment process
- Health registers, e.g. for diabetes

Environmental
- Transport systems
- Environmental protection laws
- Health hazards within the local area
- Waste disposal
- Energy consumption

Legal factors
- Monopolies legislation
- Employment law
- Health and safety
- Professional regulation

Table 9.2   Combining SWOT and PESTEL analyses in relation to teenage pregnancies

	Strengths	Weaknesses	Opportunities	Threats
Political	Existing policy framework	Socialcultural influences	Partnership and collaborative working practices	Lack of community engagement
Economic	Reduce overall costs/ health and social	Might need to come from new finances	Crossboundary commissioning	Reduced funding
Sociocultural	Building for the future, establishing and supporting positive lifestyle choices. Young people friendly	May perpetuate establish social boundaries and enforce negative beliefs	To positively influence healthy lifestyle choices. Potential to increase user involvement	Misunderstanding of the purpose of the facilitator
Technological	To utilise modern advancements in the field	New technologies increase costs and often require training packages to be financed	To operate a safer more efficient and effective service, and be able to collect local data. Meeting local need	Lack of operator knowledge and skills Obsolescence
Environmental	Dedicated facility that is accessible and equitable	High resource costs due to location, limiting interagency working	To be part of the community infrastructure Based on local need	Negative press
Legal	Meets Trusts performance targets	Parental objection	To promote a positive understanding of the law	Risk assessment could restrict the development

BOX 9.3

Type of stakeholders. Example of how stakeholders may differ at various stages of development of the public health strategy.

Review current public health services
- Director of Public Health
- Epidemiologists
- Primary Care Trust/Acute Boards
- Local authority leads
- Health Care Commission
- Researchers

Options for the public health strategy
- Director of Public Health Office
- Health Care Commission
- User groups/public forums and consultations
- Residents associations/community leaders
- Chamber of commerce
- Voluntary sector
- Primary Care Trust/Acute Boards
- Local authority leads

Plan the implementation
- User groups/association
- Practitioners from:
  - health
  - local authorities
  - statutory services
  - voluntary sector
  - independent sector
  - managers and commissioners
  - economists

Review progress
- Users
- Managers
- Commissioners
- Researchers

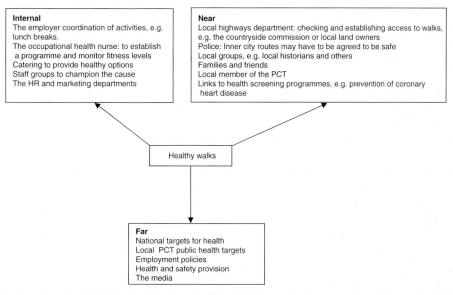

Figure 9.2   Examples of stakeholders involved in a health walks initiative for factory workers. Primary Care Trust (PCT).

of the public health strategy. The success or otherwise of the public health strategy will depend on the level of support from the stakeholders. Understanding the relative power of the different stakeholders is also important in order to analyse the extent to which they are able to influence or persuade others to follow a particular course of action.

Johnson *et al.* (2005) state that the power of the different stakeholders can be identified by analysing the sources of power:

1. *Status.* An individual or group status can be analysed by identifying the position within the hierarchy or other aspects such as reputation, grade or salary. In terms of external groups their status can be determined by the way in which they are referred to by staff, and how quickly demands are responded to.

2. *Claim on resources*. This includes such aspects as the size and number of staff within a department and the proportion of the budget that is allocated to public health. It may also include those groups of clients that make a large claim on public health resources.
3. *Representation in powerful positions*. If a group are represented on the management board they are likely to have more power than groups that are not represented. The degree to which client groups are involved in negotiating and agreeing the public health strategy will give an indication of their relative power.
4. *Symbols of power*. This may be indicated by such things as the size and position of a person's office, whether they have support staff, style of dress, etc. The level of attention paid to communicating with client groups differs, and so provides an indicator of their relative power.

Table 9.3   Stakeholder mapping. *Source*: Adapted from Eden and Ackermann (2004).

Degree of interest	Power	
	High	**Low**
High	Work closely alongside as they have the capacity to influence the emerging strategy	Keep informed they are interested enough to lobby more powerful stakeholders
Low	Often the most difficult. Keep informed and never underestimate their level of interest	Uninfluential bystanders

Eden and Ackermann (2004) advocate the use of a matrix in order to identify stakeholder interest and power (Table 9.3). This matrix identifies and categorises stakeholder according to:

- the level of interest a stakeholder group will have in the emerging strategy (and therefore the degree to which they will expect to influence the strategy);
- the degree of power each stakeholder group has (and therefore the level of influence they will have on the emerging strategy).

The matrix indicates the type of approach that needs to be taken with the stakeholders within each category. As the strategic options are identified it will be important to review the acceptability of these options with the most powerful and interested stakeholder group as clearly the strategy will fail if this influential group do not support it.

The stakeholders who are categorised as having high levels of power but low degree of interest are the most difficult group because they may suddenly become interested in the strategy, and actively wish to influence its development. It will be important to keep them informed and to try to raise their level of interest by provision of good information. Stakeholders who are interested, but have low power should be kept well informed as they can prove to be very useful allies and will lobby and influence the more powerful stakeholders.

The stakeholder analysis may also reveal the key blockers and facilitators of the strategy (Johnson *et al.* 2005), and appropriate plans can thus be made to manage the anticipated responses to the strategy.

Having undertaken an internal and external analysis of public health, the strategic direction which should be taken will be emerging.

9.3   Strategic Choice: Options for Developing the Public Health Strategy

The emerging strategy may require changes to the way things are currently done, and in turn this may necessitate a review of the public health mission statement.

9.3.1   Revising the public health mission statement

Mission statements are generalised statements of the purpose of an organization. The purpose of a mission statement is to present a focus for the strategy in terms of providing a broad direction to work towards (Johnson *et al.* 2005).

BOX 9.4

Example of a mission statement. *Source:* **Health Development Agency (2004, p. 2).**

The Health Development Agency is the national authority for England providing information on what works to improve people's health and reduce health inequalities. It gathers evidence and produces guidance for policy makers, professionals and practitioners at the national, regional and local level. Working in partnership across the public, private, voluntary and community sectors, the Agency supports informed decision making and the development of effective practice at all levels.

The Department of Health states that the role of public health professionals is to:

> monitor the health status of the community, identify health needs, develop programmes to reduce risk and screen for early disease, control communicable disease, foster policies which promote health, plan and evaluate the provision of health care, and manage and implement change. (DH 2006)

This provides a broad direction from which the mission statement can be developed.

The mission statement should reflect the essential purpose of public health in terms of:

- why public health is important;
- the nature of public health activities undertaken;
- the population it seeks to serve and satisfy;
- the beliefs and principles that guide the work.

Box 9.4 is an example of a mission statement provided by the Health Development Agency, which clearly addresses each of the elements above. The mission statement is important because it provides a clear vision of what public health aims to achieve and how it expects to achieve the vision. This clear strategic direction will guide the decisions that are made with regard to the options available to achieve the strategy.

9.3.2   Identifying strategic options for the public health strategy

Emerging strategic options and themes will be identified through the SWOT, PESTEL, needs and stakeholder analyses. The different options will also require differing strategies and investment to implement them, for example some aspects of current public health activity will be seen as meeting needs and should continue to be provided; this will not require any changes to current strategy or resources. However, the analysis may also have revealed that new public health activities are needed to support different needs or groups. To achieve this will require more investment in terms of recruiting/developing staff; producing different programmes to reduce risk, etc. It is useful to categorise the options in order to identify the different strategies and level of investment that will be required in order to implement them. Table 9.4 presents four developmental directions, and the options emerging from the strategic analysis can be arranged under these categories:

1. Maintain/improve the current public health activities that are meeting existing needs (do the same things better). This option includes withdrawing from public health activities which are not cost-effective, or where the necessary competencies to deliver public health are lacking.
2. Develop new ways to deliver public health to meet the existing need, e.g. explore partnership working.
3. Expand existing public health activities to deliver public health to different areas or groups identified as having needs which are currently not being addressed.
4. Diversify the public health activities so that new competencies are developed in order to satisfy needs in different ways.

It can clearly be seen that each of these four categories will require different strategies and levels of investment in order to implement them. A combination of these strategic directions may be pursued within the public health strategy.

Table 9.4   Options for developing a public health strategy for healthy eating in school.

	Existing public health activities	New public health activities
Existing needs	Maintain/strengthen current public health activities, e.g. do nothing	Develop existing competencies and look at new ways to deliver public health e.g. develop the infrastructure to support healthy eating including training staff; improving kitchen facilities and food supply chain
New needs	Expand existing public health activities into different areas/to different groups e.g. target education to parents	Diversify into new public health activities/build new competencies, e.g. include healthy eating in school curriculum

9.3.3   Evaluating and selecting the strategic options

Having identified the strategic options these should now be evaluated before a decision is made as to whether or not to pursue them within the strategy. Johnson *et al.* (2005) propose three criteria by which to evaluate the strategic options:

1. *Suitability*. This looks at the fit between the strategic options and future trends and changes (which will have been identified through the PESTEL analysis). It also looks at how the options will exploit the strengths (identified within the SWOT analysis).
2. *Acceptability*. To analyse acceptability it is necessary to identify the stakeholders' likely reaction to each of the strategic options and to identify whether the strategy is in line with their expectations.
3. *Feasibility*. This examines whether the strategy is likely to work in practice. Such issues as resources (financial as well as human and material) need to be examined. Clearly a strategy cannot be pursued if the skills needed to implement it are not available.

Table 9.5 provides a way of comparing the relative merits of the different strategic options in terms of the fit with key factors that the strategy must align with, e.g. government policies, resources, stakeholder expectations and the public health mission statement. This comparison will enable the selection of the most viable strategies. The example in Table 9.5 shows the ranking of possible strategies to improve healthy eating in schools. By comparing the merits of the proposed strategic options it is clear that it is not feasible to continue with the current strategy, and that there is a need to develop and expand the existing strategy.

Having identified the viable strategic options the next stage is to plan and implement the strategy.

9.4   Strategy Implementation

The changes which will need to be made in order to deliver new services or do things differently have to be identified (Thompson 2001). There are numerous books and articles on the subject of managing change that provide guidance and further information of relevance. This chapter will concentrate on those aspects that need to be considered when implementing public health strategy.

9.4.1   Communicating public health strategy

It is important not to underestimate the extent to which the various stakeholders will understand the need for change and what the strategy aims to achieve. The stakeholder analysis will have revealed the individuals and groups who have a vested interest in the public health strategy. A communication strategy will need to be formulated in order to keep these parties informed about the strategic plan and what is involved in implementing the strategy.

When considering the communication strategy the following points should be taken into consideration:

1. *Provide a vision*. The reasons for changing the public health strategy may be complex, and it is essential that it is communicated in such a way that a clear picture of the strategic direction is provided which encapsulates the significance and challenges of the strategy.

Table 9.5 Ranking strategic options for healthy eating in schools.

Strategic options	Key factors the strategy must be aligned with				
	Current strengths (suitability)	Political drivers (suitability)	Resources (feasibility)	Stakeholder expectations (acceptability)	Ranking
Maintain current activities (change nothing)	Y Existing weight and measurement programme	N Government drivers to improve healthy eating, e.g. 5 a day campaign	Y No extra resources needed	? School governors may be more concerned with budget	Low (abandon stategy)
Develop, e.g. develop infrastructure for meal provision	Y Localised data on obesity. Existing school nurse network Local farmers market	Y *National Healthy Schools Status* (DH 2005) *Choosing Health* (DH 2004) *Every Child Matters* (DFES 2003,2004)	N New kitchen facilities needed Staff development	Y Improves healthy eating of child	High (pursue strategy)
Expand activities, e.g. target parents	Y Existing health and social care networks – opportunity for partnership working	Y Extended schools *Every Child Matters* (DFES 2003,2004)	Y Existing and new health promotion and education resources	? Equality of access and freedom to make choices	High (pursue strategy)
Diversify, e.g. include healthy eating as part of curriculum	Y National curriculum therefore inclusive approach	? *National Healthy Schools Status* (DH 2005) *Choosing Health* (DH 2004) *Every Child Matters* (DFES 2003,2004)	? Dependent on human resources and flexibility of local education delivery	? Increase costs May not be seen as priority in curriculum development	Low (abandon strategy)

Y, fits with key factors; N, does not fit with key factors; ?, uncertain/irrelevant.

2. *Clarify and simplify priorities.* Rather than trying to impart all of the complexities of the strategy, provide a few key themes that sum up the whole strategy.
3. *Choose how the strategy will be communicated.* There are many different ways in which the strategy can be communicated, e.g. via face to face meetings, telephone/video conferencing, bulletins or circulars. The communication methods selected will have an impact on the success of the communication strategy. For instance, conveying complex information in an email is likely to be less successful than meeting face to face where others have the opportunity to ask questions and seek clarification.
4. *Ensure that there are opportunities for others to feedback.* The communication strategy should be seen as a two-way process. When formulating a strategy it is rare that all of the implications have been thought through, and others may be able to feedback on where they can foresee difficulties with the implementation.

9.4.2   Ensuring the organizational structure is in place to support the new strategy

Members of staff need to be empowered in order to implement the strategy, so when implementing the public health strategy it will be necessary to address structural issues such as:

1. *Division and allocation of work.* The implementation of the strategy will involve new and perhaps different activities being undertaken. Those responsible for delivering each aspect of the strategy will need to be identified, trained and prepared to undertake the role. Consideration will also need to be given to how the work will be coordinated. The more complex, interdependent or diverse the activities are, the more coordination is needed.
2. *Formal communication and reporting channels.* If new ways of working and new activities are being implemented, the staff involved will need to know who to report to and also what to report.
3. *Formal versus informal decision making.* Consideration needs to be given to the level at which decisions can be made about each aspect of the work. Members of staff need to know at what point they have to refer to a higher authority for a decision regarding the work.
4. *Policies and procedures.* Policies and procedures provide staff with guidelines on how to undertake the work and give a clear indication of the standards expected. Decisions will need to be made with regard to the extent to which policies and procedures need to be agreed and formalised.

When managing a strategic change it is also important to consider the culture of the organization and to ensure that the strategy and culture are aligned.

9.4.3   Ensuring the culture and strategy are aligned

The different values, interests and expectations of stakeholders will influence and change the strategy, especially during the implementation phase (see Figure 9.1). Culture is defined as the 'pattern of basic assumptions ... developed by [a group] that has worked well enough to be considered ... as the correct way to perceive, think and feel in relation to ... problems" (Schein 1985, p. 9). Hall (1995) describes three levels of culture:

1. *Surface level.* This level is characterised by aspects such as customs (language used) and visible objects such as clothing and the layout of the work space.
2. *Deeper level.* This level comprises behaviours and actions such as the way decisions are made, how teams work together or styles of problem solving.
3. *Deepest level.* At this level are the core morals, beliefs, values and judgements about right or wrong/ fair or unfair.

The deepest level of culture will influence the ability of the strategist to 'sell' the strategy to members of the organization because it will determine if people will give their support and commitment to the proposed strategy. If the strategy transgresses core beliefs or values then stakeholders are unlikely to embrace it.

The potential for being able to change an existing culture is affected by such things as the strength and history of the existing culture, how well the culture is understood, and the personality and beliefs of the strategic leader. There is, however, no empirical evidence to support the assumption that a culture can be changed. The ability for culture to change assumes that:

- there is a discernable culture that affects quality and performance;
- although cultures may be resistant to change, they are malleable and manageable;
- it is possible to identify aspects of the culture that facilitate or inhibit change, and therefore managers should be able to design strategies for cultural change.

Indeed, cultural change may be considered so difficult that it is considered better to select a strategy that fits with the existing culture – hence the importance of identifying stakeholder values and beliefs during the strategic analysis.

9.4.4 Reviewing progress and amending the strategy

The strategic management process should be viewed as cyclical and it is important to continuously review progress and monitor the realization of the strategy, making the necessary adjustments to the strategic plan.

Activity

Explore the website for childrens' workforce development on developing and implementing an integrated local children's service workforce strategy on www.cwdcouncil.org.uk/advice/index.htm.

Conclusion

The development of a public health strategy is a complex process and is influenced by numerous factors. Strategic analysis is essential in order to gain a view of current strengths that can be built upon, factors within the strategic environment which are influencing the strategic direction, and the public health needs of the local population. Stakeholder analysis is essential because the stakeholders can influence the development of the strategy at any phase of the development. This is especially important during the implementation phase, particularly if the proposed strategy does not fit with cultural values and beliefs.

Implementation of the public health strategy is the most challenging aspect. This chapter has not gone into detail on management of change as there are numerous texts on the subject. Successful strategy implementation is dependent to a large extent on how the strategy has been promoted to the stakeholders. Choosing the right method to communicate the strategy provides a means to success. When implementing strategic changes it is important to pay attention to structural aspects as this empowers those involved to work with the changes.

References

Clegg S., Kornberger M., Pitsis T. (2005) *Managing and Organisations: an introduction to theory and practice.* London: Sage Publications.

Dancar A.C. (2006) *SWOT Analysis.* University of St Framnces, IL. www.stfrancis.edu/ba/ghkickul/stuwebs/btopics/works/swot.htm.

DH (Department of Health) (2004) *Choosing Health: making healthier choices easier.* London: HM Stationery Office.

DH (Department of Health) (2005) *National Healthy Schools Status – a guide for schools.* http://www.wiredforhealth.gov.uk/doc.php?docid=7265 (accessed 22 Jan 2007).

DH (Department of Health) (2006) What is public health? http://www.dh.gov.uk/AboutUs/MinistersAndDepartmentLeaders/ChiefMedicalOfficer/Features/FeaturesBrowsableDocument/ (accessed 7 Aug 2006).

DfES (Department for Education and Skills) (2003) *Every Child Matters.* London: HM Stationery Office.

DfES (Department for Education and Skills) (2004) *Every Child Matters: next steps.* Nottingham: DfES Publications.

Eden C., Ackermann F. (2004) *Making Strategy: the journey of strategic management.* London: Sage Publications.

Hall W. (1995) *Managing Cultures.* Chichester: Wiley.

Section 3

Health Development Agency (2004) *Annual Report*. London: Health Development Agency.

Iles V. (1997) *Really Managing Health Care*. Maidenhead: Open University Press.

Johnson G., Scholes K., Whittington R. (2005) *Exploring Corporate Strategy*, 7th edn. Harlow: Prentice Hall.

Porter M.E. (1980) *Competitive Strategy: techniques for analysing industries and competitors*. New York: Free Press.

Rowe J. (2002) Planning public health strategies. In: *Public Health in Policy and Practice: a source book for Health Visitors and Community Nurses* (ed. Cowley S.). Edinburgh: Bailliere Tindall.

Schein E.H. (1985) *Organisational Culture and Leadership*. San Francisco: Jossey-Bass.

Thompson J.L. (2001) *Strategic Management*, 4th edn. Adelaide: University of South Australia.

CHAPTER 10

Health Protection and the Role of the Public Health Nurse

Janet McCulloch and Jacqui Prieto

Public Health Skills: Interpretation and application of policy legislation into practice

- Environmental health protection: health and safety in the wider community (occupational and private life)
- Infection control
- Interpreting codes of practice with regard to the environment and wider community

Introduction

Health protection is a branch of public health that seeks to protect the public from, or limit exposure to, hazards that may be harmful to health. More specifically, it is concerned with the prevention, investigation and control of infectious diseases as well as environmental hazards. These hazards relate to:

- food, water, air and environmental quality and safety;
- transmission of communicable diseases;
- outbreaks and other incidents that threaten public health (NHS Education for Scotland and Health Protection Scotland 2006).

Environmental hazards can be chemical, including poisons and pharmaceuticals, or radiological, including ionizing and non-ionizing radiation. Communicable hazards are infectious agents capable of causing disease in humans that are transmitted from one person to another. Today, health protection is also concerned with readiness for emergency situations that may impact on human health, including acts of terrorism and the deliberate release of hazardous agents.

Health protection has assumed a higher profile in recent years following disasters such as the attack on the World Trade Centre in New York in 2001, the London Underground bombings in July 2005, the oil depot fire at Buncefield in 2006 and the South Asian tsunami in 2005. More recent examples include the investigation into public health issues surrounding polonium-210 in January 2007 and the worldwide outbreak of H5N1 avian influenza (including poultry farms in Suffolk and Norfolk in 2007. However, most people's experience of hazards to health does not arise from major incidents, but from everyday exposure to hazards in their own communities and homes such as air pollution, household moulds, lead in dust and pipework, and occupational and other hazards.

Communicable diseases remain a significant threat to health. Whilst in the UK the major infectious diseases including diphtheria, typhus, cholera and tuberculosis affect only a small number of people compared to the past, infections such as meningococcal disease, gastrointestinal and respiratory infections are commonplace (DH 2002a). Added to this is the threat of new or previously unrecognised diseases, including high profile emerging infections that have a global impact such as human immuno-deficiency virus (HIV), severe acute respiratory syndrome (SARS), avian influenza and pandemic flu (DH 2002a).

Traditionally, public health approaches to the management of communicable disease have focused predominantly on the prevention of individual diseases, the emphasis being on biological processes and single causative agents (MacDonald 2004). However, there is growing recognition that a different approach is needed to take account of the many interactions, multifactorial and cumulative effects concerning health protection (HPA 2005a). This requires consideration of the biological, social, political and environmental conditions that impact on health protection (Susser 1998).

10.1 Impact on Health

The Health Protection Agency (HPA) report on the burden of disease used existing data to quantify the impact of infectious diseases, environmental, chemical and radiological hazards, poisons and injuries on health and health services in the UK (HPA 2005a). The report estimates that in the UK infections cause approximately 10 per cent of all deaths each year and the cost of treatment is about £6 billion per annum, with primary care having the greater share of the cost burden, i.e. £3.5billion (HPA 2005a). Yet the reported incidence of infection and infectious disease is underestimated for several reasons. Many communicable diseases remain undetected and some are subclinical or asymptomatic, e.g. some sexually transmissible infections. Others are self-limiting, e.g. many gastrointestinal infections. In the absence of a clinical diagnosis or positive laboratory result many cases never feature in national or international surveillance data.

Communicable diseases can have important consequences in the short or long term, such as time away from work or school, impaired fertility and other sequelae such as deafness and congenital abnormalities. In addition to this, their ability to spread from one person to another has added impact on others.

Environmental hazards, such as radiation, pollutants and chemicals may also adversely affect our health, although the HPA (2005a) report asserts that evidence for much of this is less strong, due to confounding factors, lack of surveillance systems to monitor health over the longer term following exposure, and the difficulty in proving cause and effect. Indeed, the report acknowledges the considerable amount of work still required in order to identify the real burden of disease. For example, data on the toxicity and maximum exposure limits of chemical and radiological hazards are limited. There are 30 000 chemicals in use today but toxicity has been assessed in less than 1 per cent of these (Royal Commission on Environmental Pollution 2005). The impact of radiological hazards that are naturally occurring, such as radon, background radiation and sunlight, are particularly difficult to assess since the risk to health may vary according to factors such as location, season, duration of exposure and age at exposure.

10.2 Inequalities

As mentioned above, health is affected by the interaction of physical, biological and social factors and is often associated with social inequalities. For example, a study of the relationship between hospital admissions for gastrointestinal infection and socioeconomic factors among residents in the West Midlands, UK found that gastrointestinal infection resulting in hospital admission was more common in areas of social deprivation than in affluent areas. This difference was most marked among young children aged 0–4 years in the most deprived areas, who were twice as likely to be admitted to hospital as those in the least deprived category (Olowokure *et al.* 1999).

Poor quality housing has adverse impacts on the health of children and adults and is frequently associated with some of the most disadvantaged groups in society: the poor, the elderly, immigrants and asylum seekers, travellers and the homeless. Overcrowding has been associated with a number of infectious diseases including meningococcal disease and tuberculosis; asthma and respiratory disease have been associated with damp and mouldy housing (Howden-Chapman 2004).

The public and media are concerned about the siting of telephone masts, landfill sites and incinerators near to heavily populated areas and the building of homes and schools on previously contaminated land. These developments often affect the most deprived communities and their impacts on health are difficult to quantify (HPA 2005a).

Children and infants in particular are vulnerable to exposures to biological and environmental hazards. They can be affected preconception or during developmental stages before or after birth due to childhood physiological factors and dietary factors (Bearer 1995). Children spend more of their time on the floor than adults and in this way may be exposed to chemical residues, lead, radon, soil or animal faeces from soiled footwear, or to discarded hazardous objects such as needles or sharps. Young children also have the habit of putting objects in their mouths and sucking their thumbs. These behaviours increase their risk of exposure to microorganisms and other hazards. For example, as long ago as 1914, lead was identified as a hazard to the health of children (Lockhart Gibson 2005). It has since been linked to developmental and behavioural problems (Lewendon *et al.* 2001). Many of the quantified risks to health from environmental hazards have been based on adult, rather than child, exposure.

10.3 Promotion of Health and Prevention of Ill Health

While governments and national agencies take the lead in ensuring that structures and processes are in place to prevent and manage health protection incidents, it is individual professionals and lay-people that practice health protection on a daily basis. Public health nurses have a key role in protecting the health of the public through their own engagement with the public and communities and are at the frontline of health protection.

Involvement in health protection and promotion programmes has been identified as one of the three core functions of public health nurses, who have an important role in the prevention of disease associated with biological and environmental hazards in the home, community and workplace (DH 2002b). This role requires public health nurses to know and understand the issues and policies, to support their local communities, translate information into language and messages suitable for their patients and clients, to undertake safe practice and educate others, to report unusual events, and to be aware of where further advice and guidance can be obtained. Some examples of the health protection role of public health nurses can be seen in Figure 10.1.

Public health nurses are involved in health protection through a variety of primary, secondary and tertiary interventions aimed at reducing the incidence of disease and its consequences and at promoting wellbeing in affected individuals and groups (DH 2002a; Horton & Parker 2002).

10.3.1 Primary prevention

Primary prevention is the active promotion of health and prevention of ill health. It includes the policy and legislative structures to support and promote a safe and healthy environment. A spectrum of structures extends from macro policy making at international, European or UK government level, through organizational policy and systems, to individual compliance.

One example of this relates to food safety in the UK. The Food Safety Act 1990 is regulated by the Food Standards Agency, enforced by local authority environmental health officers and implemented by individuals working in catering establishments, food outlets and in health and social care environments. The principles of food safety also have relevance within the home. Implementation at a local level involves an understanding of local policy and safe practice underpinned by the Food Safety Act.

Public health nurses can play a part in communicating the principles of food hygiene to groups and individuals, acting as a role model, educating and supporting clients and their families in making choices and decisions. For example, breast feeding contributes to reducing the risk of gastrointestinal

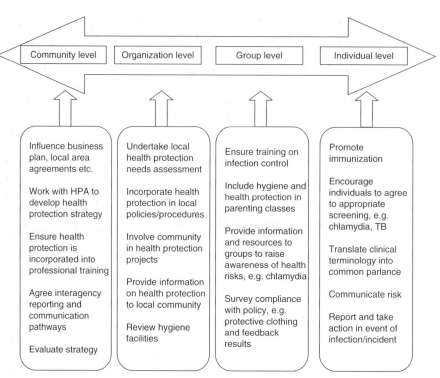

Figure 10.1   Examples of health protection roles for public health nurses. HPA, Health Protection Agency. *Source*: DH (2006b).

infections in babies (Kramer & Kakuma 2006). However, hygiene measures for breast and bottle feeding are also important in prevention of infection. Avoiding the consumption of certain high-risk foods (unpasteurised dairy products, undercooked eggs, pâtés and soft cheeses) by particularly vulnerable groups, such as children under 5 years old, pregnant women and older people, will reduce the risk of listeria and salmonellosis (Food Standards Agency 2006). Some public health nurses have an important direct role in promoting these choices, or indirectly by encouraging families and support groups.

Another example of primary prevention is the national childhood immunization programme. The schedule is health service policy rather than legislation and its aim is to protect health by preventing a range of diseases through 'herd immunity'. Herd immunity is a phenomenon that relates to the immunity of an entire population, such that enough people within that population have developed immunity to confer protection to the population as a whole. Many public health nurses are directly involved in the routine immunization of children and adults (DH 2006a, 2006b). They need a range of knowledge and skills to support them in this role, including knowledge of the role of immunization in protecting health, the interactions and contraindications and immunological responses. National standards for the training of immunisers have now been developed (HPA 2005b).

Childhood immunization can be a hotbed of controversy. A small number of parents have profound objections to immunizations of any kind; some others feel uncertain or fearful about subjecting their baby to a painful procedure or unknown risk; whilst the majority are supportive of immunization as a way of protecting the health of their own baby and others. Over 90 per cent of children are immunised with most of the available vaccines by the age of 2 years, although the level of coverage with the measles, mumps and rubella (MMR) vaccine is not quite so high (HPA 2005c). Public health nurses need negotiating and persuading skills and clinical credibility to counter emotive stories presented in the media. They are trusted sources of information and advice but they also need to demonstrate their own confidence in the system, as hesitation will be quickly communicated to uncertain parents and may undermine their support (DH 2002b).

It is also important that public health nurses know where to obtain additional information and expertise; this can include the local child health department, health protection team, the Department of Health website and professional journals and networks. The uptake of the MMR vaccination is now increasing, thanks to the excellent work of primary care teams and public health nurses in explaining the benefits and risks to parents (HPA 2005c).

The management of radon gas in certain parts of the UK, such as Cornwall, is another example of public health nurses' involvement in primary prevention. Exposure to radon gas increases the risk of lung cancer. It is a particular risk for children as it is a heavy gas and is found in larger concentrations nearer the floor at child height. Public health nurses can promote health and prevent ill health by supporting local policies and initiatives to control radon, as well as providing advice to individual families regarding ventilation, safer play areas and access to services and financial assistance.

Public health nurses working in occupational settings are also involved in primary prevention. By identifying hazards through risk assessment, incident review, health surveillance, immunization, etc. they can create healthier workplaces and introduce safer ways of working, preventing injuries or exposure to substances hazardous to health. Those working in schools, health care settings and communities can undertake similar activities.

10.3.2 Secondary prevention

Secondary prevention concerns the early detection and treatment of cases arising from exposure to infectious or environmental hazards, and is often associated with screening for disease.

One example of public health nurse involvement in a secondary prevention programme is chlamydia screening. Chlamydia is a sexually transmitted infection with increasing incidence in young people. The infection may be asymptomatic but can result in pelvic inflammatory disease and female infertility. The aim of the screening programme is to opportunistically offer screening, in the form of a vulval swab or urine sample, to young people aged 18–25 years who present to the health services so that cases can be detected and the infection treated before it can cause significant damage (DH 2004).

Public health nurses may be involved in this, or similar programmes such as prevention of pulmonary tuberculosis. They need to understand and describe the epidemiology of the infection, to persuade clients who are otherwise well to take part in the screening or contact-tracing programme and to accept appropriate treatment should the results be positive. This requires sensitivity, a non-judgemental attitude and good communication skills.

Health screening is also used in occupational settings, for example to monitor exposure to chemicals, radiation and other non-communicable hazards. Health screening must be supported by efforts to minimise risks to health by eliminating or controlling exposure to hazards. This may be achieved by changing work practices to avoid the hazard altogether, introducing safer techniques or using appropriate personal protective equipment. Health screening is also used to identify those who are at risk of occupationally acquired infections such as hepatitis B in health care and public sector workers, and measles, mumps or rubella in those working with children. Immunization is usually recommended for these vaccine-preventable diseases if employees are found to be susceptible (DH 2006b).

10.3.3 Tertiary prevention

Tertiary prevention is the prevention of deterioration, complications and relapse. A health protection example of this is the administration of antiviral drugs, such as aciclovir, to someone with shingles. Another example is the administration of antiretroviral therapy to people with HIV in order to slow down progression of disease.

10.4 Health Protection Structures

Following publication of the Chief Medical Officer's infectious disease report, *Getting Ahead of the Curve* (DH 2002a), the HPA was instituted to lead health protection and provide a coordinated and national centre to protect the population from infectious diseases and also chemical and

Section 3

radiological hazards. A number of existing organizations merged to form the HPA in 2003, as a non-departmental public body (Box 10.1).

The HPA can only fulfil its obligations by working in partnership with other stakeholders such as the NHS, local authority departments such as environmental health, transport and housing, the Health and Safety Executive, State Veterinary Services, the Drinking Water Inspectorate, water companies, waste disposal companies, occupational health services, emergency services (police, fire, ambulance) and other agencies such as the Food Standards Agency, Department for Environment, Food and Rural Affairs, and Environment Agency. Together these organizations prepare for and test plans to prevent and respond to incidents, outbreaks and emergencies and take action in the event of their occurrence.

Health protection is underpinned by numerous European legislations, regulations and acts of Parliament including the HPA Act 2004, Civil Contingencies Act, Health and Safety at Work Act 1974, Environmental Protection Act 1990, Clean Air Act 1993, Food and Environmental Protection Act 1995, Food Safety Act 1990 and the Control of Substances Hazardous to Health regulations 2002 (Irwin *et al.* 1999).

10.5   Notification of Infectious Diseases

Surveillance systems relating to chemical and radiological hazards are limited but becoming increasingly sophisticated (Health Protection Scotland 2006; HPA 2006a). However, there is a well-established and diverse system of surveillance in the UK (DH 2002a). This is used to monitor trends in communicable diseases and to identify clusters of cases and outbreaks, to measure the effectiveness of interventions (such as immunization programmes, legionella prevention, food safety and sexual health strategies) and to measure the burden of disease.

Certain infectious diseases are notifiable by law under the Public Health (Control of Disease) Act 1984 (Box 10.2) and the Public Health (Infectious Diseases) Regulations 1988 (Box 10.3). Medical practitioners who are aware of, or suspect, that a person is suffering from a notifiable disease or food

---

BOX 10.1

Organizations that combined to form the Health Protection Agency (HPA).

- Public Health Laboratory Service (PHLS)
- National Radiological Protection Board
- Centre for Microbiology and Research (CAMR)
- National Poisons Information Service
- National Focus for Chemical Incidents
- Health Emergency Planning Advisers
- Some former public health and reference laboratories
- Health authority communicable disease control teams

BOX 10.2

Diseases notifiable under the Public Health (Control of Disease) Act 1984.

- Cholera
- Food poisoning
- Plague
- Relapsing fever
- Smallpox
- Typhus

BOX 10.3

Diseases notifiable under the Public Health (Infectious Diseases) Regulations 1988.

- Acute encephalitis
- Acute poliomyelitis
- Diphtheria
- Dysentery (amoebic or bacillary)
- Leprosy
- Leptospirosis
- Malaria
- Meningitis
- Meningococcal septicaemia (without meningitis)
- Mumps
- Ophthalmia neonatorum
- Paratyphoid fever
- Rabies
- Rubella

- Scarlet fever
- Tetanus
- Tuberculosis
- Typhoid fever
- Viral haemorrhagic fevers (Lassa fever and Marburg disease)
- Viral hepatitis
- Whooping cough
- Yellow fever

---

poisoning is required to notify, in writing, the proper officer for the local authority who is usually a consultant in communicable disease control. These cases are reported to the HPA Centre for Infection, together with other cases identified via laboratory systems and outbreak investigations, etc. These data form the basis of national statistics on notifiable diseases published by the HPA in its *Health Protection Report* (formerly *Communicable Disease Report*) and on its website.

Other infections and infectious diseases that are not statutorily notifiable are also reported via national and international reporting systems, such as laboratory reports, mortality data, K60 forms for sexually transmissible diseases, reporting of occupationally acquired infections, case reporting by spotter GP practices, and reporting of symptoms by the public to NHS Direct.

10.5.1 Responding to cases and incidents

Where possible, exposure to hazardous substances should be prevented or controlled by following the principles described in the *Control of Substances Hazardous to Health Regulations* (HPA 2002):

- assess the risks;
- identify appropriate precautions;
- prevent or control exposure to the hazard;
- ensure controls are implemented and maintained;
- monitor exposure;
- carry out health surveillance;
- prepare incident, outbreak or emergency plans;
- ensure appropriate training or information is provided.

The response to an event such as an outbreak of infection is concerned primarily with disease prevention in a defined population rather than health improvement in an individual. The disease in question drives the investigation, the object being to identify the interventions required to manage individual cases and prevent further cases. Conversely, an alternative approach is required in response to an event involving exposure to a non-communicable hazard, since this may not be linked to a well-defined disease or, indeed, be one that manifests close to the time of exposure. Instead, assessment of the exposure drives the investigation in order to identify the population affected, control measures required and the likely health end point (Griffith & Aldrich 1993).

When investigating an occurrence or outbreak of infection, a common starting point is to use a specific cause model, based on the classic epidemiological triad of host–agent–environment (MacDonald 2004). Its purpose is to identify a causal chain linking the source, those at risk and the mechanism of exposure in order to identify the strategies required to prevent disease.

10.5.2   Chain of infection/exposure

One such model, known as the *chain of infection* is applied to the control of communicable disease. In this model, the 'agent' is the microorganism responsible for causing infection. The 'host' is the source of infection, which most commonly is a person or people, but may also be an environmental reservoir such as contaminated food, water or equipment. The 'environment' concerns the mechanisms by which the microorganism escapes from the person or reservoir and find its way to the new host.

The chain of infection model is depicted such that breaking any of the links in the chain prevents exposure of others to the infectious agent and thereby reduces the risk of infection. An understanding of the events leading to the spread of infection in a given situation enables identification of the necessary interventions. Figure 10.2 illustrates the model as applied in the event of an outbreak of meningococcal disease.

Importantly, for infection to occur, the new host must be susceptible to infection. The risk of acquiring infection is not uniform, but depends on the susceptibility of the given individual. Assessing a person's susceptibility, or indeed the susceptibility of a given population, is a key component of the chain of infection model and an important public health skill. Factors that affect a person's susceptibility to infection include age, immunity, physical wellbeing, psychological wellbeing, hygiene, underlying or chronic diseases or medical conditions (e.g. diabetes mellitus, cancer, chronic chest, heart problems), other existing infections, medical interventions (e.g. invasive procedure, indwelling medical device) and medical treatment (e.g. cancer chemotherapy).

The ways in which infection may spread varies from one microorganism to another. When these are well understood, specific measures can be directed towards interrupting spread. The provision of clear guidance on the actions required to minimise the risk of spread does much to allay people's fear and anxiety. The key modes of infection transmission are detailed in Box 10.4. Many microorganisms are spread by more than one route. Moreover, certain environments may augment the spread of infection, such as health care settings, schools, catering establishments and indeed any situation where large groups of people are gathered and where there are many opportunities for exposure, albeit unwittingly, to sources of infectious microorganisms.

In environmental public health the chain model is usually conceptualised as the triad of source–pathway–receptor, which is similar to the chain of infection and is described here as the

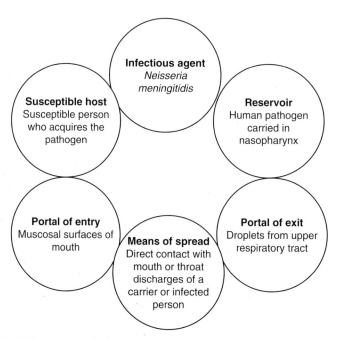

Figure 10.2   The chain of infection as applied to meningococcal disease.

chain of exposure. Environmental agents may be transmitted via similar routes to those listed in Box 10.4. Person to person transmission may occur via contact with contaminated skin, clothing or inhalation of exhaled gases. This is illustrated in Figure 10.3.

10.5.3   Breaking the chain of infection/exposure

An understanding of the chain model is essential to identify appropriate interventions to manage single cases and prevent further cases. Possible interventions include:

- improving the outcome for cases through early administration of appropriate treatments: antimicrobial, antitoxin, immunoglobulin, antidotes;
- identifying other exposed individuals and offering appropriate prophylaxis, treatment or advice;
- preventing further exposure of other individuals by decontamination of exposed individuals, environment and objects; sheltering populations from continuing sources of exposure such as plumes of smoke; isolating cases if necessary; closing implicated wards, food outlets or businesses; excluding cases or high-risk contacts from work or school;
- identifying and controlling sources, e.g. contaminated food, medical devices, cooling towers, showers, effluent, waste disposal sites, lead paint or pipework, radon, etc.

BOX 10.4

Key modes of infection transmission.

- Contact: direct or indirect. It includes: direct contact (person to person), indirect contact (food, water, inanimate objects, the environment) via faecal–oral route, sexual transmission, vertical transmission (mother to baby *in utero*, during delivery or via breastfeeding), inoculation such as exposure to contaminated sharps, blood and body fluids, and via insects and parasites
- Airborne (aerosol, droplet or vapour)

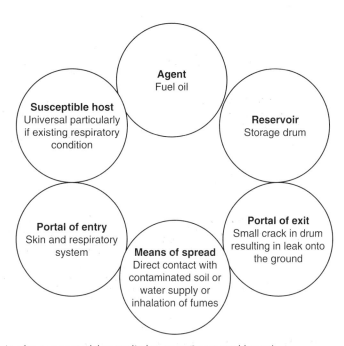

Figure 10.3   The chain of exposure model as applied to an environmental hazard.

Section 3

Standard precautions are required to interrupt exposure to infectious or environmental agents and these include:

- hand hygiene;
- appropriate use of personal protective equipment, e.g. disposable gloves, aprons/gowns, respirators/facemasks or eye protection;
- careful disposal of contaminated items, waste and sharps;
- appropriate decontamination of equipment and environment;
- safe preparation and storage of perishable items (e.g. food);
- aseptic techniques in a clinical environment;
- immunization against vaccine-preventable infection risks (e.g. hepatitis B).

Additional technical or engineering controls such as ventilation controls and containment measures (e.g. physical segregation or isolation) are required for specific hazards. More specific guidance and advice is available from local health protection units, infection control teams or environmental health departments.

Meningococcal disease

The example identified in Figure 10.2 illustrates the chain of events that may lead to the spread of infection in the case of meningococcal disease. *Neisseria meningitidis* is a bacterium that causes meningitis (infection of the brain linings) and can invade the bloodstream (septicaemia). This life-threatening disease has a rapid onset and requires emergency admission to hospital and prompt treatment with parenteral antibiotics. Its seriousness generates anxiety amongst the general public and health professionals alike.

Neisseria meningitidis is a normal inhabitant of the human nasopharynx (HPA Meningococcus Forum 2006). It is carried without harm by approximately 10 per cent of the population, with the highest carriage (approximately 25 per cent) among 15–19-year-olds (HPA 2006b). Only a small proportion of carried strains are responsible for most cases of invasive disease (HPA Meningococcus Forum 2006). It remains unknown why some individuals carry the bacteria harmlessly, while others go on to develop meningococcal disease, although the characteristics of the strain acquired as well as variations in environmental and host factors are important features (HPA Meningococcus Forum 2006).

All cases where a diagnosis of meningococcal disease is suspected should be reported promptly to the local health protection team (HPA Meningococcus Forum 2006). Comprehensive information on cases and their contacts is then gathered in order to minimise the risk of secondary spread. Those who have had prolonged, close contact with the case during the 7 days prior to onset of illness, including people living in the same household and kissing partners, are offered prophylactic antibiotics. In vaccine-preventable strains of *N. meningitidis*, these people are also offered the appropriate vaccine.

Given the heightened level of alarm caused by a single case or outbreak of infection, the provision of clear and consistent advice by health professionals, including public health nurses, is vital. UK guidelines (HPA Meningococcus Forum 2006) recommend that leaflets and other printed information about meningococcal disease should be widely available and quickly distributed after a case has occurred. Ideally information should be provided in advance at times when incidence is known to rise, such as the beginning of the autumn term, to raise awareness of the signs and symptoms.

When a case arises in an educational institution (i.e. pre-school groups, schools, colleges and universities), letters are usually sent to other parents/students to inform them of the situation and provide information about the disease, its signs and symptoms, and the action to be taken in the event of illness. Involvement of frontline staff such as school nurses as a key point of contact for students and their parents may do much to allay anxiety.

In relation to infectious disease epidemiology, the chain model has been used to illustrate how the response to an occurrence of infection or, indeed, increased incidence or an outbreak of infection may be conceptualised. By establishing a causal chain of events it is possible to identify the strategies required to prevent disease, including measures required to interrupt transmission and to enhance host resistance. This may be at an individual level or at a population level. Using the example of meningococcal disease, interventions at the level of the individual include provision of prophylactic antibiotics to close contacts to prevent further transmission of the organism to other susceptible hosts. A population-level intervention involves the addition of meningococcal C conjugate vaccine to the routine childhood immunization schedule to reduce the number of susceptible people in the community.

Salmonellosis

Interventions to break the causal chain of events can be illustrated using another example: *Salmonella* in eggs. At an individual level, by recognizing the risk that eggs may be contaminated with *Salmonella*, individuals can reduce their risk of infection by purchasing eggs with a quality mark, cooking eggs thoroughly and washing their hands after handling eggs. At a population level the risk is reduced by immunizing flocks, improving living conditions for flocks to reduce opportunities for transmission on farms, introducing and monitoring quality standards and public awareness campaigns, etc.

Environmental hazards

Using the example shown in Figure 10.3, exposure to an environmental hazard can be eliminated or controlled after a risk assessment by targeting one or more links in the chain. This involves eliminating the *source* (agent and/or reservoir), controlling or removing the *pathway* (portal of exit and/or means of spread), or protecting the *receptor* (susceptible host and/or portal of entry). In this example this may be achieved by:

- eliminating the source of the hazard by replacing fuel oil with an alternative such as gas or electricity;
- preventing leakage of the fuel oil by replacing or repairing the storage drum;
- wearing appropriate protective equipment when dealing with the fuel oil or decontaminating the area;
- keeping vulnerable people away from the area until it is made safe;
- maintaining and monitoring the condition of the storage drum and associated pipework to prevent further leaks.

Summary

In practice, the development of strategies to combat infectious diseases and indeed illness arising as a result of exposure to non-communicable hazards, requires consideration of the wider context, including the social and environmental factors that influence the distribution and causes of disease and the determinants of health-related states. In relation to the example of meningococcal disease, its increased incidence amongst infants, children and young adults, those living in overcrowded conditions, those exposed to passive smoke, and those with preceding influenza A infection (HPA Meningococcus Forum 2006) signifies the importance of a broader perspective.

10.6   The Role of Public Health Nursing in Outbreak/Incident Management

There are various definitions of outbreaks and incidents. The following are based on the definitions of the Scottish Executive (2003).

1. An *outbreak* is defined as one of the following:
   - two or more linked cases of the same illness (associated in person, place or time);
   - where the observed number of cases of an illness unaccountably exceeds the expected number.
2. An *incident* is defined as one of the following:
   - a single case of a rare or serious illness with major public health implications, such as polio, rabies or variant (v)CJD;
   - the exposure (or possible exposure) of a population to an infectious or environmental hazard (e.g. contaminated water, fire plume, failure of hospital autoclaves);
   - the exposure of a population to a natural disaster (e.g. flooding, heat wave);
   - two or more linked cases of an illness possibly associated with a common known or unknown agent.

Section 3

The scale of an outbreak or incident is related to:

- the public health impact, including morbidity and mortality, risk of transmission to or exposure of others, and effectiveness of control measures;
- the perception of risk by the public, media and professionals;
- its impact on services and resources.

For example, an outbreak of infection may be restricted to a few people, may be easily contained and have few adverse health impacts. One example of this may be an outbreak of *campylobacter* gastroenteritis in a school associated with the consumption of egg sandwiches on a school outing. Although outbreak investigations and control measures will be initiated, it is usually relatively easy to bring this type of outbreak under control once the source is identified. *Campylobacter* tend to be self-limiting and there is no person to person transmission. On the other hand, a single case of legionnaires' disease acquired in a health care setting will be considered to be more serious in that it has a mortality rate of up to 39 per cent (Chin 2000). Also, it has occurred in a vulnerable group and there is likely to be a continuing source with the potential for further transmission.

The HPA (2004) has identified the main objectives of outbreak and incident management.

1. To provide care for cases and others affected.
2. To control the source of the outbreak/incident.
3. To determine the extent of the outbreak/incident.
4. To prevent others being affected.
5. To monitor the effectiveness of control measures.
6. To prevent recurrence.
7. To consider whether the incident may be a result of deliberate release.

An outbreak/incident control team is usually convened to manage outbreaks and incidents. These are comprised of relevant specialists and managers who can coordinate the response and command resources to support this. Membership varies depending upon the nature, location and severity of the outbreak or incident. Typically an outbreak control team will include:

- a health protection consultant/specialist;
- an infection control consultant/specialist;
- the Director of Public Health (or their deputy);
- a laboratory manager;
- an environmental health officer;
- a communications manager;
- and others, depending upon the circumstances, e.g. senior managers (nursing, operations, catering, facilities, etc.) or specialists in toxicology, radiation, etc.

Public health nurses may be involved at various stages and in various roles depending upon their responsibility for the affected population. For example, in an outbreak of legionnaires' disease affecting workers in a factory, the occupational health nurse may support the outbreak control team in identifying potential sources of infection, providing information and counselling to workers who may have been exposed, or supporting cases who have returned to work.

In an outbreak of mumps in a secondary school, the school nurse may be involved in implementing the outbreak control plan to immunise non-immune school children with the MMR vaccine (DfES & DH 2006). This may require identifying susceptible children, assessing risks such as contraindications to the vaccine, providing information and counselling, obtaining consent, providing vaccination, identifying further cases, etc.

During influenza pandemics, public health nurses are likely to play a variety of roles, including triaging patients, mass vaccination, follow-up of cases at home and, in the event of staff shortages, supporting clinical teams. They may also be involved in the response to natural disasters such as flooding and heat waves – identifying vulnerable groups, supporting them during the crisis and remedial phases, liaising with emergency services, rest centres and local authorities, and many other activities.

Senior public health nurses may be members of the outbreak/incident control team and play their part in the coordination of the delivery of the control plan, supporting other members of the primary care team, approving the release of resources required to deliver the plan, prioritizing workloads, and organizing support services such as waste collection, delivery of supplies and provision of refreshments, etc. They should also have the opportunity to participate in the evaluation of the incident, known as 'wash-up meetings', and in developing and revising outbreak and incident plans.

Case Study Example

An outbreak of *Escherichia coli* O157 occurred in a large pre-school nursery in a market town. Over a 1-week period, five children developed clinical symptoms and positive stool samples. One child was admitted to hospital with haemolytic uraemic syndrome. *E. coli* O157 has a low infectious dose (about 100 organisms), is transmitted by the faecal–oral route and children under 5 years and people over 65 years old are at risk of serious infection.

An outbreak control team met and comprised of:

- a health protection consultant and nurse;
- an environmental health officer;
- a consultant microbiologist;
- the nursery manager;
- the health visitor attached to the nursery.

An action plan was agreed as indicated in Table 10.1. No common food source was identified; all food consumed at the nursery was low risk. A sandpit had been used for play, but the sand was discarded after one use. One of the cases had visited an animal petting centre in the days prior to becoming ill.

Seventeen asymptomatic individuals tested positive on screening. This included a parent who worked as a caterer for a large department store, who required exclusion and microbiological clearance before returning to catering duties. The 5-year-old sibling of a case also tested positive. This child attended the nearby primary school and it was agreed she could attend school if she could demonstrate a good knowledge of hand washing, used a good hand-washing technique and was supervised.

Due to excellent team working the nursery was only closed for three working days before staff and children who were microbiologically clear were permitted to return.

Table 10.1 Action plan for dealing with an outbreak of *Escherichia coil* O157

Action	Chain target
Close nursery immediately until environment is thoroughly cleaned	Eliminate source of infection
Individuals may only return to nursery when microbiologically clear two negative stool samples obtained at least 48 hours apart	Interrupt route of transmission
Administer *E. coli* O157 questionnaire to obtain histories of recent food intake and high-risk activity	Identify common source
Inspect catering and toilet facilities and practices	Identify common source
Screen high-risk household contacts of all cases. Exclude from work/school until microbiologically clear	Interrupt route of transmission
Ensure that facilities, knowledge and practice of hand hygiene is good amongst staff and children	Protect susceptible individuals at school and at home
Provide written and verbal information and support to parents and teachers	

Activity

As a public health nurse, what would your role be if a similar event to that in the case study occurred amongst your client group? Where could you obtain further information and guidance? What other agencies might be involved and do you know their contact details? Are there any health promotion activities you could initiate to prevent outbreaks such as this occurring? For further information, see Hawker *et al.* (2005).

Conclusion

This chapter has considered the structure and function of health protection as established in the UK setting. It has outlined the various ways in which public health nurses are engaged in health protection, the nature of these challenges and the key skills required. Inherently health protection is a multidisciplinary and multiagency sphere of public health in which public health nurses have key roles and will be increasingly important in the future. By engaging with health protection specialists, public health nurses can be involved in the management of incidents and outbreaks and influence local priorities and policies. By linking this engagement with their understanding of the local communities, public health nurses can reduce the risks of infection and disease associated with environmental hazards.

References

Bearer C.F. (1995) Environmental health hazards: how children are different from adults. *Critical Issues for Children and Youths* 5 (2), 11–26.

Chin J. (2000) *Control of Communicable Diseases Manual*, 17th edn. Washington, DC: American Public Health Association.

DfES (Department for Education and Skills), DH (Department of Health) (2006) *Looking for a School Nurse*. http://publications.teachernet.gov.uk/eOrderingDownload/0275-2006PDF-EN-01.pdf.

DH (Department of Health) (2002a) *Getting Ahead of the Curve. A strategy for infectious diseases (including other aspects of health protection)*. Report by the Chief Medical Officer. London: Department of Health.

DH (Department of Health) (2002b) *Liberating the Talents: helping Primary Care Trusts and nurses to deliver the NHS Plan*. London: Department of Health.

DH (Department of Health) (2004) *National Chlamydia Screening Programme (NCSP) in England: programme overview, core requirements, data collection*. http://www.dh.gov.uk/assetRoot/04/09/26/48/04092648.pdf.

DH (Department of Health) (2006a) *School Nurse Practice Development Resource Pack*. http://www.dh.gov.uk/assetRoot/04/13/20/70/04132070.pdf.

DH (Department of Health) (2006b) *Immunisation against Infectious Diseases*. http://www.dh.gov.uk/PolicyAndGuidance/HealthAndSocialCareTopics/GreenBook/fs/en.

Food Standards Agency (2006) *Health Diet: milk and dairy*. http://www.eatwell.gov.uk/healthydiet/nutritionessentials/milkanddairy/.

Griffith J., Aldrich T.E. (1993) Epidemiology: the environmental influence. In: *Environmental Epidemiology and Risk Assessment* (eds Aldrich T., Griffith J., Cooke C.). London: Chapman & Hall.

Hawker J., Begg N., Blair I., Reintjes R., Weinberg J. (2005) *Communicable Disease Control Handbook*, 2nd edn. Oxford: Blackwell Publishing.

Health Protection Scotland (2006) *Environmental Quality*. http://www.hps.scot.nhs.uk/enviro/surveillancesystems.aspx (accessed 15 Dec 2006).

Horton R., Parker L. (2002) *Informed Infection Control Practice*, 2nd edn. London: Churchill Livingstone.

Howden-Chapman P. (2004) Housing standards: a glossary of housing and health. *Journal of the Epidemiology of Community Health* 58, 162–8.

HPA (Health Protection Agency) (2002) *Control of Substances Hazardous to Health Regulations*. London: Health Protection Agency.

HPA (Health Protection Agency) (2004) *Initial Investigation and Management of Outbreaks and Incidents of Unusual Illnesses*. http://www.hpa.org.uk/infections/topics_az/deliberate_release/Unknown/Unusual_Illness_PH_Profs.pdf (accessed 20 Oct 2006).

HPA (Health Protection Agency) (2005a) *Health Protection in the 21st Century: understanding the burden of disease; preparing for the future*. London: Health Protection Agency.

HPA (Health Protection Agency) (2005b) *National Core Minimum Standards for Immunisation Training*. London: Health Protection Agency.

HPA (Health Protection Agency) (2005c) *Completed Primary Courses at Two Years of Age: England and Wales.* http://www.hpa.org.uk/infections/topics_az/vaccination/cover.htm.

HPA (Health Protection Agency) (2006a) *Chemical Incident Reports.* http://www.hpa.org.uk/chemicals/incident_reports.htm (accessed 15 Dec 2006).

HPA (Health Protection Agency) (2006b) *Vaccine to the UK Childhood Immunisation Programme and Changes to the Meningitis C and Hib.* http://www.hpa.org.uk/infections/topics_az/meningo/backgrd.htm (accessed 20 Nov 2006).

HPA (Health Protection Agency) Meningococcus Forum (2006) *Guidance for Public Health Management of Meningococcal Disease in the UK.* London: Health Protection Agency.

Irwin D.J., Cromie D.T., Murray V. (1999) *Chemical Incident Management.* London: HM Stationery Office.

Kramer M.S., Kakuma R. (2006) Optimal duration of exclusive breastfeeding (Cochrane Review). *The Cochrane Library* Issue 2. http://www.update-software.com/abstracts/AB003517.htm (accessed 21 Nov 2006).

Lewendon G., Kindra S., Nelder R., Cronin T. (2001) Should children with developmental and behavioural problems be routinely screened for lead? *Archives of Childhood Diseases* 85, 286–8.

Lockhart Gibson J. (2005) A plea for painted railings and painted walls of rooms as the source of lead poisoning amongst Queensland children. *Public Health Reports* 120, 301–20.

MacDonald M.A. (2004) From miasma to fractals: the epidemiology revolution and public health nursing. *Public Health Nursing* 21 (4), 380–91.

NHS Education for Scotland and Health Protection Scotland (2006) *Framework for Workforce Education Development for Health Protection in Scotland.* Glasgow: NHS Education for Scotland and Health Protection Scotland: Quality Assuring Continuing Professional Development.

Olowokure B., Hawker J., Weinberg J., Gill N., Sufi F. (1999) Deprivation and hospital admission for infectious intestinal diseases. *Lancet* 353, 807–8.

Royal Commission on Environmental Pollution (2005) Chemicals in Products: safeguarding the environment and human health. 24th report of the RCEP. In: *Health Protection in the 21st Century: understanding the burden of disease; preparing for the future* (Health Protection Agency). London: Health Protection Agency.

Scottish Executive (2003) *Managing Incidents Presenting Actual or Potential Risks to Public Health. Guidance on the roles and responsibilities of incident control teams.* http://www.scotland.gov.uk/Resource/Doc/47021/0013914.pdf.

Susser M. (1998) Does risk factor epidemiology put epidemiology at risk? Peering into the future. *Journal of Epidemiology and Community Health* 52, 608–11.

CHAPTER 11

Research and Development: Analysis and Interpretation of Evidence

Sheila Reading

Public Health Skills: Analysis and interpretation

- Evidence-based practice: critiquing evidence, implementing and evaluating practice
- Processes for evidence-based public health: recognizing an information need and asking questions
- Searching for evidence: critically appraising selective evidence and synthesizing the evidence
- Using evidence to inform public health practice: approaches to implementing evidence in public health practice and evaluating the impact of evidence on public health practice

Introduction

The aim of this chapter is to explore how evidence is used as part of research and development for nurses working in the field of public health. Evidence is important for public health practice because its purpose is to ensure that preventive care, treatment and services are of high quality and to improve health outcomes for client groups (Healthworks UK 2001).

The drive to encourage the implementation of evidence by practitioners (HDA 2004; Wanless 2004) requires public health nurses to develop a number of skills, including how to find, critically appraise, analyse and interpret existing evidence in order to make decisions about best practice for groups of people or populations. However, practitioners may not know how best to access evidence or possibly may suffer from information overload or a lack of confidence when trying to search for, and appraise, evidence that informs practice (Naidoo & Wills 2005).

The complexities of implementing evidence or using it to inform and alter practice are well recognised (Mulhall & le May 1999; Rycroft-Malone *et al.* 2004). In addition, the process of reaching a decision about how to use evidence to inform practice involves critical thinking that draws on the practitioner's experience, the patient's preference and knowledge of available resources (DiCenso *et al.* 1998).

Within this chapter, an overview of these issues will be explored and the topic of childhood obesity used as an example to illustrate how nurses can demonstrate the skills of public health activity in order to make use of a range of evidence to inform their practice.

11.1 Knowledge for Public Health Practice

While there are debates about the definition of public health (Heller *et al.* 2003) and at times confusion about the nature of public health practice (Craig 2000), it has become evident that public health nursing refers to the general contribution of *all* nurses to public health as well as to specific specialist practitioner roles such as health visiting, infection control and school nursing (Pearson 2002).

Public health nurses work in a variety of settings and have responsibility for the health and wellbeing of diverse populations. Furthermore, because health is determined by the wider social milieu within which populations live, factors such as the physical and social environment, lifestyles, housing, education and economic conditions have long been recognised as influencing health and the link between public health and social reform is well documented. It was Chadwick's (1965) report on the influence of poor working conditions, overcrowding and lack of sanitation on mortality and morbidity that led to the first Public Health Act of 1848. One hundred and fifty years later, Acheson (1998) referred to public health as 'the art and science of preventing disease, prolonging life and promoting health through organised efforts of society'. This definition recognises that the practice of public health involves more than scientific or epidemiological knowledge and that there is a need to view public health nursing as having a knowledge base influenced by the social, cultural and political context within which it is practised. The aim of public health practice is to improve the health of populations (Muir Gray 2001); the types of knowledge and information needed to achieve this can be developed and utilised by adopting an evidence-based approach to practice.

11.1.1 Types of evidence that inform public health

The drive for delivering effective health care brought about a focus on evidence derived from randomised controlled trials (Greenhalgh 2006). Clinical effectiveness focuses on the extent to which specific interventions improve health and deliver the best outcomes from available resources (NHS Executive 1996). In other words it is about providing evidence of what works. Randomised controlled trails (RCTs) and systematic reviews of RCTs provide evidence of the effectiveness of interventions. However, it is often not possible to carry out research using an RCT because of the ethical and practical difficulties of randomizing people to experimental or control groups. In an analysis of the limitations of evidence-based public health, Kemm (2006) argues that RCTs are often inappropriate for investigating public health interventions, because public health is concerned with interventions for communities that exist in specific social contexts for which there are unlikely to be matching controls. Instead, cohort studies, case controlled studies or case reports may be used to generate public health research knowledge. Where there is no research, other evidence should be considered, including theoretical knowledge, clinical guidelines, audit and performance data, expert knowledge and experiential knowledge. Data sources concerning lifestyle, housing, socioeconomic environment, education, leisure, culture and transport can also be used to inform public health practice in a specific local context (Heller 2005).

Significantly, Muir Gray (2001, p. 318) recognises that it is:

> necessary to draw evidence from a wide variety of disciplines if public health professionals are to continue to identify the causes of ill-health and to prevent disease and promote health.

What counts as evidence for public health embraces biological, psychological and sociological research and theories and includes descriptive and analytical literature on policy interventions (Kemm 2006). What research there is can inform public health practice in other ways. For example, needs assessments will give information which will help inform decisions on areas of priority. Official statistics on morbidity and mortality highlight social class and geographical differences in health. This can inform decisions about which populations need to be targeted and has been discussed in Chapters 1–3.

Also essential to making decisions in public health are clients' views. The NHS Plan (DH 2000) and the Nursing and Midwifery Council (NMC 2004) have indicated the importance to evidence-based practice of considering patient preferences, beliefs and values. There is therefore a need to generate evidence that takes account of client views and preferences, and values 'lay knowledge' (Kemm 2006). The tacit knowledge of an individual, group or population influences health behaviours and is also considered as offering data to inform practice:

> such data are usually inside the heads of those who have had the experience to provide the knowledge, and not available unless through the medium of discussions and presentations. (Heller 2005, p. 85)

Efforts to improve the health of populations involve accessing, interpreting and understanding this tacit knowledge.

Smith (2004) explores the issue of generating new modes of knowledge through participatory research involving diverse stakeholders, approaches and methods to investigate a number of health topics. She describes how autobiography and testimonies are 'other' legitimate sources of knowledge and argues that a range of flexible research methodologies and methods which capture different kinds of knowledge will increase dialogue between stakeholders and produce more user-friendly knowledge.

Debates about what evidence counts as knowledge often reflect the underlying concerns with upholding a scientific research approach and professional power that attaches lesser importance to lay perceptions (Popay & Williams 1996). They identify three aspects of lay expert knowledge relevant to public health research and practice:

- lay understanding of the relationship between individual behaviour and life circumstances;
- lay theories about causes of ill health;
- the predictive power of lay knowledge;

Schickler (2004) argues that an understanding of lay health beliefs is important in order to deliver effective health promotion programmes and in supporting professional–client interactions. However, Rycroft-Malone *et al.* (2004) indicate that in reality there is a lack of knowledge concerning the role of considering how client perspectives and preferences are incorporated into the practice of evidence-based health care.

As practitioners, nurses use various sources of knowledge and understanding gained from experience to become 'expert practitioners' or opinion leaders and this experiential knowledge is a further source of evidence that can be drawn on and shared with others. Table 11.1 identifies a pluralistic view of what constitutes evidence and how evidence is captured.

Activity

Think about what knowledge or evidence you use in your practice. Try and identify as many different sources as possible. What are the differences between research and evidence-based practice?

11.1.2   Hierarchy of evidence

The traditional hierarchy of evidence that places systematic reviews and RCTs at the top is problematic when considering evidence for public health (Petticrew & Roberts 2003). They argue that a hierarchy

Table 11.1   Evidence type and capture

Examples of types of evidence	Examples of methods available to capture evidence
Smoking in occupational groups	Randomised control trials
Attitudes to childcare	Social surveys, questionnaires
Multiagency assessment of need	Action research, participatory appraisal
Review of provision to improve quality and outcome	Clinical audit, risk assessment
Vignette to study role perception of public health nurses	Case study, ethnography

overlooks the importance of selecting the most appropriate research method to answer a specific research question. In public health, the policy makers and practitioners ask questions that are not merely to do with effectiveness.

> The possibility that the hierarchy may even be inverted, placing, for example, qualitative research methods on the top rung, is not widely appreciated. The hierarchy also obscures the synergistic relation between randomised control trials and qualitative research, and (particularly in the case of social and public health interventions) the fact that both sorts of research are often required in tandem. (Petticrew & Roberts 2003, p. 528)

Qualitative research methods provide an understanding of people's (and professionals') attitudes, beliefs and behaviours. The acceptance that health is socially determined has led to the use of qualitative research approaches which, among other things, can explore how social, political and financial factors affect people's behaviours. Qualitative research also provides an understanding of the meanings and experiences people have of health and illness (Green & Britten 1998). Jack (2006) notes that while public health has traditionally been informed by epidemiology and hence quantitative research methods, qualitative methods shed light on the important contextual influences that give an understanding of how successful public health programmes have been implemented.

Oakley (2001, p. 28) recommends that arguments about research paradigms should be left behind and that a combination of research approaches and methods be used to answer focused questions about how health promotion and other public health initiatives can 'enhance the quality and quantity of people's lives'.

The type of evidence to draw on will be driven by the specific practice question being asked. Because public health issues are complex, different sources of evidence may be used to provide an understanding of why individuals or populations behave in specific ways and how social and cultural factors have a bearing on public health programmes or interventions. Hunter (2003, p. 12) has argued that there is a need 'to widen the repertoire of what constitutes acceptable evidence if we are to embrace health as distinct from health care'.

11.1.3 Evidence for public health

Waters and Doyle (2002) have suggested that the focus needs to be not simply on the *kind* of evidence that can inform public health practice, but on ensuring that the *most relevant* questions are asked, answered and evaluated using the *most appropriate* research methods. They go on to indicate that the context of research on effectiveness of interventions (e.g. by schools or in geographical areas) as well as participants' perspectives and an understanding of the processes need to be explored through studies employing integrated methods.

Muir Gray (2001) identifies three key challenges to be confronted by those adopting an evidence-based approach:

1. To broaden the concept of effectiveness to take account of what people other than doctors and researchers mean by effectiveness and how they define 'effectiveness'.
2. To appraise evidence using extended criteria of equity, efficiency and affordability.
3. To supplement and complement evidence from quantitative research with other research methodologies including qualitative research. Behavioural research is also advocated.

Heller *et al.* (2003, p. 65) remind those in public health that central to adopting an evidence-based approach is the 'need to derive an evidence base relating to the effectiveness of methods for involving and being accountable to the public'. *Shifting the Balance of Power within the NHS* (DH 2001) also emphasises the idea that the users of health care must be at the centre of NHS services, participating in identifying public health priorities and evaluating services.

11.1.4 Evidence-based public health

Using research and development to improve health and wellbeing is one of the 10 key areas of practice identified in *National Occupational Standards for the Practice of Public Health Guide* (Skills for

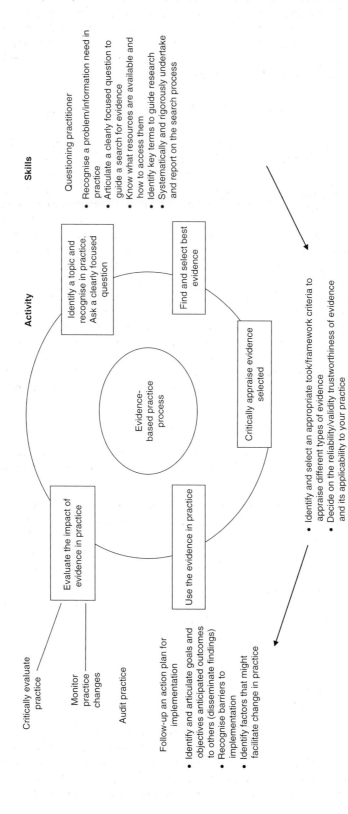

Figure 11.1 Evidence-based practice process.

Health 2004).This specifically requires practitioners to have the skills to interpret research findings and implement them in practice. There is an expectation of public health practice that nurses will have the knowledge and skills to lead and provide effective interprofessional evidence-based public health for individuals, communities and populations. To achieve this, nurses will have to demonstrate skills in searching for, selecting and critically evaluating a range of evidence in order to implement optimum public health practice underpinned by appropriate knowledge.

11.2 Using a Case Study Approach with Childhood Obesity

Although there are a number of major public health issues that are central to public health, for the purpose of this chapter the topic of childhood obesity has been selected to illustrate how evidence can be used in public health practice. A review of the literature will enable the practitioner to begin to have an understanding of key policy documents, research and other evidence informing the topic.

Childhood is a significant time when the foundations for good health are being put in place (Wright *et al.* 2001). Of particular concern currently is the continuing rise in childhood obesity and the link with lifestyle, diet and lack of physical activity. The past two decades has seen the prevalence of obesity, including childhood obesity, increase greatly worldwide (WHO 2000). The proportion of children with inappropriately high body weight has become a serious public health problem in Britain (DH 1994; Chinn & Rona 2001). The importance of having accurate estimates of obesity in children to assess preventive measures, monitor secular trends and identify high-risk groups has been emphasised (Prentice 1998). It is estimated that 50 per cent of children could be obese by 2020 (RCP 2004). Obesity in childhood causes a wide range of preventable health problems including heart disease, stroke, diabetes and osteoarthritis (National Audit Office 2001; DH 2002) and increases the risk of premature illness and death later in life, raising public health concerns (Ebbeling *et al.* 2002). Pearson (2005) identifies that managing obesity requires a focus on social, political, physical and environmental factors that influence the weight of populations with a focus on groups and individuals, such as children, who are particularly at risk of becoming obese.

11.2.1 The process of evidence-based public health

Evidence-based practice involves gathering all the best available evidence and critically appraising it to decide how it can best inform or be used in practice. The process according to Sackett *et al.* (2000) involves the following stages

1. Information needs or problems from practice are converted into clearly focused questions.
2. The questions are used as a basis for finding and selecting relevant 'best' evidence.
3. The selected evidence is critically appraised.
4. The evidence is used in practice alongside clinical expertise and people/clients' preferences.
5. The impact of the evidence is evaluated through a process of self-reflection, audit or peer review.

Figure 11.1 shows the key stages in the evidence-based process.

Using the example of childhood obesity, the skills required to undertake evidence-based public health are now addressed under the following headings:

- skill 1: recognise an information need and ask a clearly focused question;
- skill 2: search for evidence;
- skill 3: critically appraise the selected evidence;
- skill 4: use the evidence to inform and develop practice;
- skill 5: evaluate the impact of using evidence.

Skill 1: recognise an information need and ask a clearly focused question
Public health nurses need to constantly reflect on and ask questions about their practice. The starting point of the evidence-based process involves generating a practice-based question derived from an identified practice topic, problem or information need. This question will need to be defined and refined in terms of the context of practice and will drive the subsequent stages of the process, which are

to find evidence, critically appraise it and then act on the implications of the evidence that answers the question.

Questioning actions and practice is essential for good practice and provides the starting point for a search for information that will either support practice or lead to something being carried out in a different way. Many different questions arise from practice and may concern a group of patients or an aspect of public health nursing. For example, when exploring the subject of childhood obesity, a nurse might want an answer to questions about:

- the target group – what they want, their views, beliefs and attitudes;
- the environment in which the group live;
- the culture of the group – their norms, attitudes, behaviour and customs;
- what works – interventions;
- what is cost-effective;
- how public health nurses can best work with families and children who are obese;
- how to introduce interventions, and then monitor and support them.

Further examples of questions that might be asked about public health and child obesity include:

- Why do children become obese?
- What influence has the family on children's diets?
- To what extent is physical inactivity responsible for obesity?
- Does promoting healthy eating in schools make a difference to rates of obesity?
- Who specifically benefits from physical activity?
- What are the psychological needs of obese children?
- How can parents be involved in bringing about changes in children's lifestyles?
- What is the best intervention to reduce obesity in primary school children?

It is important to develop an idea into an explicit, well-phrased question. The PICO (population or problem, intervention, comparison and outcome) system devised by Sackett *et al.* (2000) can be used to structure a clearly focused question. While this framework is a helpful tool (Craig & Smyth 2002), clearly not all public health questions concern interventions; however, all questions need to be carefully defined and framed.

> Framing the question in a way which lends itself to searching while still reflecting the specific patient or service focus is an important stage to get right. That way, when you begin searching for evidence on the topic you have chosen, the volume of research will be manageable. (Flemming 1998, p. 36)

Activity

Reflect on your own practice and identify a topic about which you need more knowledge to inform your practice. Develop this into a clearly focused question.

Skill 2: search for evidence

It is important to be clear about the aim of the search – this will be driven by the practice question being asked. It is often necessary to undertake a review of relevant literature to help inform or focus the question being asked. Searching the literature can meet with different levels of success. In some cases a lack of evidence on a particular topic indicates where there is a deficit of knowledge and where specific research is needed. Sometimes there is a need to extend the scope of the search for evidence if there is little immediately available or, if there is a wealth of information, the focus needs to be narrowed. A search will reveal *how much* evidence there is and the *nature* of that evidence.

However, searching is a complex and sophisticated process and it is best to get help and support to learn the skills for accessing information from a professional librarian or informaticist (Greenhalgh 2006). Libraries often have guided self-help tutorials to assist and there are a range of sources which outline the stages of searching for evidence along with useful tips (Beaven 2002; Snowball 2005).

There are a range of different bibliographic databases which can be accessed, depending on the subject being explored such as CINAHL, PsychLit and Medline. In addition, databases of appraised and synthesised evidence include the Cochrane Database of Systematic Reviews, DARE (database of abstracts of reviews of effectiveness), Evidence Based Healthcare and Public Health and Evidence Based Nursing. Accessing such databases enables a systematic approach to searching for evidence that is rigorous and can be reported using a clear decision trail which others may replicate. Nevertheless, hand searching of journals and reference lists and personal contact with colleagues and expert professionals can help unearth 'grey literature' – that which is unpublished or produced only as a local report or as a student dissertation. This can provide further valuable sources of evidence.

When carrying out a search the question must be defined in terms that will guide the search. These are known as keywords or MeSH terms (medical subject headings) and are used to search the databases. It is important to develop inclusion and exclusion criteria in order to select the best, most relevant and current evidence for critical analysis and to avoid being overwhelmed by information that does not specifically address the question. This may involve setting limits on the dates of searches, e.g. 2001–2006, the specific population of patients, specific ages (e.g. children under 16) and identifying only evidence published in English.

Skill 3: critically appraise the selected evidence

Skills for Health (2004) focus on the need for the public health practitioner to be capable of evaluating and disseminating research about improving health and wellbeing. *Critical appraisal* is a systematic process by which the evidence that has been identified and selected following the search is assessed to judge its merits, weaknesses, relevance and applicability to practice. It requires the reader to think analytically and be objective and unbiased (McSherry *et al.* 2002). Waters and Doyle (2002) encourage public health practitioners who are evaluating and synthesizing evidence relevant to intervention studies to consider:

- whether the intervention/study was carried out as intended;
- what the geopolitical context/environment was, and where the intervention was carried out;
- whether the outcomes were appropriate to the intervention;
- whether the intervention was cost-effective.

Sackett *et al.* (1996) summarised the tasks of critical appraisal of evidence as:

- assessing if the information/results/conclusions are valid;
- coming to a decision about the clinical significance of the information for the investigator's own area of practice.

The process of appraisal can be aided by checklists or critical appraisal tools, which help provide a logical approach ensuring that potentially important information is not overlooked (Crombie 2002). Because practitioners have to appraise different kinds of evidence, depending on what is the 'best available' to answer a particular practice-based question (le May 1999), an ever-increasing number of tools are available and an appropriate framework is needed depending on the nature of the evidence available. No single tool can be applied when evidence is of a diverse nature.

Each critical appraisal tool or framework includes a series of questions to assist in assessing the validity and applicability of the evidence. Tools exist for the appraisal of quantitative and qualitative research studies, non-research papers, case studies, professional and patient biographies, consensus expert opinion, clinical guidelines and other sources of evidence (le May 1999; Crombie 2002; Greenhalgh 2006). There are also many websites that offer guidelines, such as the Critical Appraisal Tools Public Health Resource Unit Oxford (www.phru.nhs.uk/casp/casp.htm), and texts with worked examples to help guide the process, including Newman and Roberts (2002a, 2002b) and Cutcliffe and Ward (2003).

Activity

Visit the website www.phru.nhs.uk/casp/casp.htm and explore the critical appraisal tools available. Try one of the tools on a public health research article that you have read recently, or see if you can use the tool to help you with the last activity in this chapter.

11.2.2   Synthesis of evidence

Synthesis means bringing together all the evidence identified, possibly from a number of different sources as the evidence informing public health practice is diverse and complex. Mays *et al.* (2005) indicate that there is, as yet, no single framework that can enable decisions to be made using evidence from a range of sources. Instead, this process involves the practitioner identifying specific or common themes in a way that clarifies the current state of knowledge on a topic. Often the synthesis of findings begins with an overview of the evidence from each source, then narrative, along with tables, may be used to summarise central themes emerging from the evidence and synthesise key findings and indicate recommendations for practice. This is essentially describing, interpreting and summarizing the evidence, but it can be taken further and analysis can involve using the evidence to combine findings in order to provide new information or generate theories for future testing. It is likely that if the process is intended to inform clinical practice in a particular setting or community that more will be needed than just research evidence (Mays *et al.* 2005). Gomm and Davies (2000) give an overview of how practitioners can appraise diverse forms of evidence in order to decide the usefulness for their own practice.

Skill 4: use the evidence to inform and develop practice

Implementing evidence is complex and often recommendations for practice fail to be translated into practice. A significant problem in public health practice is that even when evidence does exist, it is often ignored (Wanless 2002). Public health is practised in a social and organizational context and there are known barriers to, and facilitators of, using evidence (Parahoo & McCaughan 2001). Organizational barriers and individual barriers to using evidence include problems in interpreting research, lack of organizational support (e.g. time to access evidence), lack of guidance from researchers on how to use evidence to inform practice, and lack of support for individuals to become involved in using research (McCaughan *et al.* 2002). Heller (2005) identified that organizational factors impacting on how knowledge generated from diverse sources is managed and used in practice include: leadership, access to and the use of information and communication technology, the culture of the organization, and the skills of the workforce. It is necessary to consider the structure of an organization and the sources of power and authority within it when translating evidence into action.

11.2.3   Dissemination of evidence

Communication and dissemination of evidence are important aspects for making colleagues, communities, groups and individuals aware of what can be changed or implemented in practice. Planning how to disseminate and present evidence to others is an important aspect of implementing evidence-based practice (Scullion 2002). Importantly, the nurse must consider the target audience and how to effectively communicate the message to them. Possibly the most important part of the evidence-based practice process is the careful consideration of how the evidence can be used with clients. Questions need to be asked about the match of evidence with the context of clients and the values and beliefs they hold in order to facilitate participatory decision making about the intervention (Box 11.1).

BOX 11.1

Chinese wisdom. *Source: Chabot (1976).*

Go to the people
Live among them
Love them
Start with what they know
Build on what they have
But for the best leaders
When their task is accomplished
Their work is done
The people all remark
We have done it ourselves

With communities, groups and individuals at the centre of public health practice, evidence has a place in ensuring that they get the best care. However, 'best care' must ultimately be defined by individuals as to what is good for them.

11.2.4 Approaches to implementation

There is a confusing array of theories and frameworks for implementing change in practice and a lack of evidence regarding the most effective approach to change management. Change operates at the level of individuals and also at organizational level. For both these there are constraints and barriers to achieving change. However, there are also factors that will promote change. Introducing any health promotion to improve the health of children, for example to reduce childhood obesity, typically seeks to facilitate change. If the advice cited in Box 11.1 is to be heeded, the process of facilitation must be unobtrusive and subtle and adopt a phased approach to its implementation over a period of time (Tones & Tilford 2001). Tones and Tilford (2001) suggest that change is a complex process and there are factors which facilitate and factors which resist change. It is important to plan to implement change and accept that the process requires time.

Kitson *et al.* (1998) argue that implementation of evidence into practice results from the interplay of the nature of the evidence, the environment into which the evidence is to be introduced and how the process is facilitated. They argue that a linear model of implementation fails to acknowledge the complexity which occurs when evidence confronts the reality of practice. Muir Gray (2001) suggests that the introduction of an intervention requires not only consideration of the evidence, but also the resources and the needs and values of the population.

In a study that described and analysed how multiagency 'communities of practice' processed and managed knowledge, Gabbay *et al.* (2003) concluded that a rationalist, linear model of implementing evidence-based practice was not evident. They suggested that the complexities encountered may be connected to the interaction between different types of evidence, how that evidence is used and the ways people work together to manage knowledge. Gabbay and le May (2004) found that primary care practitioners rarely use evidence from research or other sources explicitly in their everyday work, but instead rely on information from their own and others' (colleagues, opinion leaders, patients) experiences reconciled to the constraints and demands of the organization. They suggested that there may be

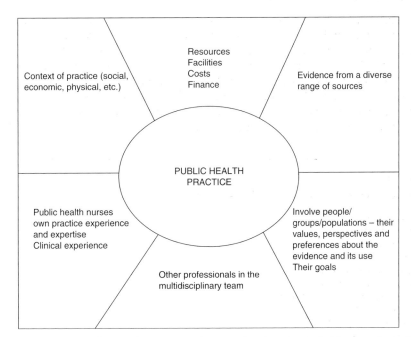

Figure 11.2 Factors to consider when implementing evidence. Rather than viewing evidence as the basis of practice, it is but one part of the total picture to be considered when using it to inform practice.

Section 3

a potential to make better use of existing networks to disseminate evidence to practitioners. Rather than evidence being viewed as the basis of practice, Figure 11.2 demonstrates that it is but one part of the total picture to be considered when using it to inform practice.

Activity

Reflect on what you can do to develop your own evidence-informed approach to public health practice.

- What *personal factors* will promote *your* skills and use of evidence?
- What *actions* are needed to support evidence-informed practice?
- Are there *people* who will work with you and support evidence-informed practice?

Skill 5: evaluate the impact of using evidence

Having decided to adapt practice as a consequence of finding new evidence or research information, it is important to monitor any changes and evaluate the outcomes. Using research to inform practice decisions should help to make explicit specific actions, and these may be used to develop an audit tool.

Activity

Reflect on any changes you have decided to introduce, the knowledge underpinning it and what you aim to achieve. Clearly identify and monitor the changes, processes and any associated outcomes (e.g. client satisfaction, health outcomes, costs, difficulties, achievements), and then feed this information back to others (dissemination). Finally, evaluate the impact of using evidence to underpin practice on you, clients, the organization and colleagues.

By recognizing the need to critically evaluate the impact of using evidence, the final stage of the evidence-based cycle is completed.

Case Study Example

As a nurse working in public health you may wish to implement a programme to reduce the obesity of school-aged children. You may be aware of different interventions but you want to know which is best or most effective or has the best outcome. Your question might be framed as:

What interventions are effective in reducing childhood obesity?

Using the PICO approach (Sackett *et al.* 2000):

- population or problem = children with obesity;
- intervention = any intervention;
- comparison = no intervention at all;
- outcome = reduction in obesity.

The question asked will indicate what type of evidence is likely to be accessed. The results from RCTs or a systematic review are likely to offer some answers.

To explore this question the Cochrane database was searched using the keywords 'childhood obesity'. This resulted in the discovery of a systematic review by Campbell *et al.* (2001) investigating the prevention of obesity and being overweight in children. The findings of the review indicated that there were limited quality data on the effectiveness of obesity prevention programmes. As a result no conclusions could be drawn.

A similar review carried out 5 years later and published on the Cochrane database (Summerbell *et al.* 2005) suggested that many diet and exercise interventions that aim to prevent obesity in children are not effective in preventing weight gain. Drawing on 22 studies from international locations with participants all under 18 years of age, the conclusion was that these was not enough evidence to prove that any single programme can prevent obesity in children.

(*Continued*)

Case Study Example (Continued)

Critical analysis and comment

Griffiths (2002) indicated that the problem of identifying effectiveness for public health interventions, such as childhood obesity, is that there are complex, multifaceted interventions, which have various outcomes and in practice are implemented in different ways. This may account for the fact that evidence of effectiveness for public health interventions dealing with childhood obesity is lacking. More than this, many initiatives introduced to tackle the problem of childhood obesity lack evidence to support their introduction and once introduced there are few rigorous attempts at evaluation beyond a description of how the programme was introduced. However, descriptions of the context and the process of any programme of implementation also need to be considered as this can give insight into the success, or failure, of any programme of implementation. Evaluations must be undertaken to determine if there has been any significant improvement in outcomes and to identify factors that will make the process more efficient (Sackett *et al.* 1996). RCTs are not the most appropriate method by which this can be achieved (Fulop *et al.* 2001). The focus needs to be on finding evidence of what works in 'real life' practice to advance health outcomes.

As well as asking if an intervention is effective, nurses may need to consider whether it can be used in their specific context or if it is acceptable to the population or target group with whom they work. As Kemm (2006) has argued, interventions that work in one context often do not transfer to other contexts. When critically appraising evidence there are also questions of differential impact; in other words does the intervention work for everyone or are there groups for whom it is more or less effective? Another question to bear in mind is the cost-effectiveness of any intervention. To answer these complex questions of practice related to childhood obesity inevitably demands that a wide variety of evidence is accessed.

But public health practice is about more than effectiveness. There is a wide range of evidence that will inform nurses in public health about childhood obesity. Asking a different question and searching for other evidence will reveal a wealth of diverse evidence that may inform specific aspects of practice. However, not all evidence is 'good' evidence and it is important to become a critical user of evidence and assess the potential contribution of various types for your own practice.

In one study, the strategies of mothers of overweight and obese children were explored using in-depth qualitative interviews (Jackson *et al.* 2004). This provides a very different kind of evidence that might inform public health nurses.

Activity

Having read through the case study example, consider whether it offers any evidence to inform your practice. Now think about critical appraisal:

- How will you go about this (critiquing tool)?
- What is the research question?
- What do you know about the method: its strengths and weaknesses?
- How would you comment on the sample size?
- How reliable/valid are the findings?
- How reliable/valid are the conclusions?
- What are the limitations, flaws, insights and benefits of the study?

Could you use the evidence to inform practice? Consider the following:

- Is the research generalizable to your context?
- What knowledge or evidence, if any, does it offer?
- Does it inform your practice?
- Is there anything you would alter about your practice having read it?

Finally, what have you learned from this exercise?

Conclusion

In conclusion, there is currently only limited evidence about what works in public health in terms of preventive interventions and how to most effectively implement them. Furthermore, there is little evidence of the impact of interventions on health inequalities (Wanless 2004). Nevertheless this is only one aspect of a complex picture, and so, while there is not a comprehensive evidence base for public health interventions, there is evidence that does exist and which must be accessed, analysed, synthesised and interpreted by practitioners in order to develop a knowledge base to inform and develop practice and identify gaps for future research.

Activity

As a final activity, review what you have learned about using research and evidence to develop public health practice. Now put into action those skills to develop you as an evidence-informed public health practitioner.

References

Acheson D. (1998) *Independent Inquiry into Inequalities in Health.* London: HM Stationery Office.

Beaven O. (2002) Searching the literature. In: *The Evidence Based Practice Manual for Nurses* (eds Craig J.V., Smyth R.L). Edinburgh: Churchill Livingstone.

Campbell K.J., Waters E., OMeara S., Summerbell C.D. (2001) Interventions for preventing obesity in children (Cochrane Review). *The Cochrane Library* Issue 2.

Chabot J.H.T. (1976) The Chinese system of health care. *Tropical Geographical Magazine* 2887, 134.

Chadwick E. (1965) *Report on the Sanitary Condition of the Labour Population of Great Britain* (reprint of Chadwick (1842). Edinburgh: Edinburgh University Press.

Chinn S., Rona R.J. (2001) Prevalence and trends in overweight and obesity in three cross sectional studies of British children, 1974–94. *British Medical Journal* 322, 24–6.

Craig J.V., Smyth R.L. (eds) (2002) *The Evidence Based Practice Manual for Nurses.* Edinburgh: Churchill Livingstone.

Craig P.M. (2000) The nursing contribution to public health. In: *Nursing for Public Health: population-based care* (eds Craig P.M., Lindsay, G.M.). Edinburgh: Churchill Livingstone.

Crombie I.K. (2002) *The Pocket Guide to Critical Appraisal.* London: BMJ Publishing Group.

Cutcliffe J.R., Ward M. (eds) (2003) *Critiquing Nursing Research.* London: Quay Books.

DH (Department of Health) (1994) *Nutritional Aspects of Cardiovascular Disease.* London: HM Stationery Office.

DH (Department of Health) (2000) *The NHS Plan: a plan for investment, a plan for reform.* London: Department of Health/HM Stationery Office.

DH (Department of Health) (2001) *Shifting the Balance of Power within the NHS: securing delivery.* London: HM Stationery Office.

DH (Department of Health) (2002) *Obesity: diffusing a time bomb.* Annual report of the Chief Medical Officer. London: HM Stationery Office.

DiCenso A., Cullum N., Ciliska D. (1998) Implementing evidence based nursing: some misconceptions (editorial). *Evidence Based Nursing* 1, 38–40.

Ebbeling C.B., Pawlak D.B., Ludwig D.S. (2002) Childhood obesity: public-health crisis, common sense cure. *Lancet* 360 (9331), 473–82.

Flemming K. (1998) Asking answerable questions. *Evidence Based Nursing* 1, 36–7.

Fulop N., Allen P., Clarke A., Black N. (eds) (2001) *Studying the Organisation and Delivery of Health Services: research methods.* London: Routledge.

Gabbay J., le May A. (2004) Evidence based guidelines or collectively constructed "mindlines?" Ethnographic study of knowledge management in primary care. *British Medical Journal* 329, 1013.

Gabbay J., le May A., Jefferson H., Webb D., Lovelock R., Powell J., Lathlean J. (2003) A case study of knowledge management in multi-agency consumer-informed "communities of practice": implications for evidence based policy development in health and social services. *Health: an Interdisciplinary Journal for the Social Study of Health, Illness and Medicine* 7 (3), 283–310.

Gomm R., Davies C. (2000) *Using Evidence in Health and Social Care.* London: Sage Publications/Open University Press.

Green J., Britten N. (1998) Qualitative research and evidence based medicine. *British Medical Journal* 316, 1230–2.

Greenhalgh T. (2006) *How to Read a Paper: the basics of evidence based medicine*, 3rd edn. London: BMJ Publishing Group.

Griffiths P. (2002) Understanding effectiveness for service planning. In: *Public Health in Policy and Practice. A sourcebook for health visitors and community nurses* (ed. Cowley S.). Edinburgh: Balliere Tindall.

HDA (Health Development Agency) (2004) *HDA Evidence Base: putting public health evidence into practice.* http://www.hda.nhs.uk/evidence/ (accessed September 2006).

Healthworks UK (2001) *National Standards for Specialist Practice in Public Health.* Public Health Register, London. http://www.riph.org/nationalstand.html (accessed September 2006).

Heller R. (2005) *Evidence for Population Health.* Oxford: Oxford University Press.

Heller R.F., Heller T.D., Pattison S. (2003) Putting the public back into public health. Part 1. A redefinition of public health. *Public Health* 117, 62–5.

Hunter D.J. (2003) *Public Health Policy.* Cambridge: Polity Press.

Jack S. (2006) Utility of qualitative research findings in evidence based public health practice. *Public Health Nursing* 23, 277–83.

Jackson D., Mannix J., Faga P., McDonald G. (2004) Overweight and obese children: mothers' strategies. *Journal of Advanced Nursing* 52 (1), 6–13.

Kemm J. (2006) The limitations of evidence-based public health. *Journal of Evaluation in Clinical Practice* 12 (3), 319–24.

Kitson A., Harvey G., McCormack B. (1998) Enabling the implantation of evidence based practice: a conceptual framework. *Quality in Health Care* 7, 149–58.

Le May A. (1999) *Evidence-based Practice.* Nursing Times Clinical Monographs No. 1. London: NT Books.

Mays N., Pope C., Popay J. (2005) Systematically reviewing qualitative and quantitative evidence to inform management and policy-making in the health field. *Journal of Health Service Research Policy* 10 (Suppl. 1), 6–20.

McCaughan D., Thompson C., Cullum N., Sheldon T.A., Thompson D.R. (2002) Acute care nurses' perceptions of barriers to using research information in clinical decision-making. *Journal of Advanced Nursing* 39, 46–60.

McSherry R., Simmons M., Abbott P. (eds) (2002) *Evidence Informed Nursing: a guide for clinical Nurses.* London: Routledge.

Muir Gray J.A. (2001) *Evidence based Health Care: how to make health policy and management decisions.* Edinburgh: Churchill Livingstone.

Mulhall A., le May, A. (eds) (1999) *Nursing Research: dissemination and implementation.* Edinburgh: Churchill Livingstone.

Naidoo J., Wills J. (2005) *Public Health and Health Promotion: developing practice*, 2nd edn. Edinburgh: Balliere Tindall.

National Audit Office (2001) *Tackling Obesity in England.* London: HM Stationery Office.

Newman M., Roberts T. (2002a) Critical appraisal 1: Is the quality of the study good enough for you to use the findings? In: *The Evidence Based Practice Manual for Nurses* (eds Craig J.V., Smyth R.L.). Edinburgh: Churchill Livingstone.

Newman M., Roberts T. (2002b) Critical appraisal 2: Can the evidence be applied in your context? In: *The Evidence Based Practice Manual for Nurses* (eds Craig J.V., Smyth R.L.). Edinburgh: Churchill Livingstone.

NHS Executive (1996) *Promoting Clinical Effectiveness: a framework for action in and through the NHS.* Leeds: HM Stationery Office.

NMC (Nursing and Midwifery Council) (2004) *Code of Professional Conduct: standards for conduct, performance and ethics.* London: Nursing and Midwifery Council.

Oakley A. (2001) Evaluating health promotion: methodological diversity. In: *Using Research for Effective Health Promotion* (eds Oliver S., Peersman G.). Buckingham: Open University Press.

Parahoo K., McCaughan E.M. (2001) Research utilization among medical and surgical nurses: a comparison of their self reports and perceptions of barriers and facilitators. *Journal of Nursing Management* 9, 21–30.

Pearson D. (2002) Public health and health promotion. In: *Public Health in Policy and Practice: a sourcebook for health visitors and community nurses* (ed. Cowley S.). Edinburgh: Balliere Tindall.

Pearson D. (2005) Obesity. In: *Key Topics in Public Health* (ed. Ewles L.). Edinburgh: Churchill Livingstone.

Petticrew M., Roberts H. (2003) Evidence, hierarchies, and typologies: horses for courses. *Journal of Epidemiology and Community Health* 57, 527–9.

Popay J., Williams G. (1996) Public health research and lay knowledge. *Social Science and Medicine* 42 (5), 759–68.

Prentice A.M. (1998) Body mass index standards for children. *British Medical Journal* 317, 1401–2.

RCP (Royal College of Physicians) (2004) *Storing Up Problems: the medical case for a slimmer nation.* London: RCP Publications.

Rycroft-Malone J., Harvey G., Seers K., Kitson A., McCormack B., Titchen A. (2004a) An exploration of the factors that influence the implementation of evidence into practice. *Journal of Clinical Nursing* 13 (8), 913–24.

Rycroft-Malone J., Seers K., Titchen A., Harvery G., Kitson A., McCormack B. (2004b) What counts as evidence in evidence based practice? *Journal of Advanced Nursing* 47, 125–32.

Sackett D.L., Richardson W.S., Rosenberg W., Haynes R.B. (2000) *Evidence-based Medicine: how to practice and teach EBM*, 2nd edn. Edinburgh: Churchill Livingstone.

Sackett D.L., Rosenberg W.C., Gray J.A.M. (1996) Evidence based medicine: what it is and what it is not. *British Medical Journal* 312, 71–2.

Schickler P. (2004) Lay perspectives and stories – whose health is it anyway? In: *Shaping the Facts: evidence based nursing and health care* (eds Smith P., James T., Lorentzon M., Pope R.). Edinburgh: Churchill Livingstone.

Scullion P.A. (2002) Effective dissemination strategies. *Nurse Researcher* 10 (1), 65–77.

Skills for Health (2004) *National Occupational Standards for the Practice of Public Health Guide*. Bristol: Skills for Health.

Smith P. (2004) Gathering evidence: the new production of knowledge. In: *Shaping the Facts: evidence based nursing and health care* (eds Smith P., James T., Lorentzon M., Pope R.). Edinburgh: Churchill Livingstone.

Snowball R. (2005) Finding the evidence: an information skills approach. In: *Evidence Based Practice: a primer for health care professionals*, 2nd edn (eds Dawes M., Davies P., Gray A., Mant J., Seers K., Snowball R.). Edinburgh: Elsevier.

Summerbell C.D., Waters E., Edmunds L.D., Kelly S., Brown T., Campbell, K.J. (2005) Interventions for preventing obesity in children. *Cochrane Database of Systematic Reviews* Issue 3.

Tones K., Tilford S. (2001) *Health Promotion: effectiveness, efficiency and equity*. London: Nelson Thornes.

Wanless D. (2002) *Securing Our Future Health: taking a long term view. Final report*. London: HM Treasury.

Wanless D. (2004) *Securing Good Health for the Whole Population*. London: HM Stationery Office.

Waters E., Doyle D. (2002) Evidence-based public health practice: improving the quality and quantity of the evidence. *Journal of Public Health Medicine* 24 (3), 227–9.

WHO (World Health Organization) (2000) *Obesity: preventing and managing the global epidemic*. Geneva: World Health Organization.

Wright C.M., Parker L., Lamont D. (2001) Implications of childhood obesity for adult health: findings from thousand families cohort study. *British Medical Journal* 323, 1280–4.

Section 4

Facilitation of Public Health Activities

Section 4 Introduction: Facilitation of Public Health Activities

Key Public Health Skills

- Developing quality and risk management within an evaluative culture
- Developing health programmes and services and reducing inequalities
- Ethically managing self, people and resources to improve health and wellbeing

The last section of this book examines some of the frameworks available for practitioners in facilitating health-enhancing activities. The chapters in this section provide a variety of examples from the field of public health practice and demonstrate how identified public health skills are applied to practice. Of particular relevance to this section is the evidence provided in acknowledging that public health practitioners are in a position to develop and sustain networks within local communities, organizations and agencies as well as within primary care and other local health economies. Such networks enable communities, groups, families and individuals to access public health activities and facilitate the referral between and across networks. By working in partnership to promote health and prevent disease, practitioners are acting as facilitators, innovators and change agents in the fostering of decision making for achieving optimum health and wellbeing.

Introduction to Chapter 12

Public Health Skills: quality frameworks and risk management in primary care settings

- Developing prescribing for nurses: extended and supplementary prescribing
- Prescribing and meeting the health needs of the population: patient group directives and prescribing for children
- Administration of medicines and risk management systems: principles, evaluation and strategies
- National Patient Safety Agency seven steps to patient safety: patient feedback, complaints and clinical governance

Chapter 12 covers one of the key aspects of the modernizing agenda for nurses – medicines management. In this context it considers risk management as part of the drive to improve quality in the NHS and the focus is on the role of the nurse in developing effective strategies to enable patient's safe and timely access to medicines in today's health care environment. The activities of the nurse as a prescriber are considered against the *Standards for Better Health* report and the author explores the principles for the administration of medicines and patient safety.

Introduction to Chapter 13

Public Health Skills: quality frameworks and risk management

- Quality and risk management: safeguarding children and working with vulnerable groups
- Assessment frameworks for quality: defining risk, risk assessment and management, managing risk to personal safety (lone worker) and working with vulnerable children and their families
- Frameworks for the assessment of need and risk: the assessment framework, common assessment framework, working in areas of deprivation and poverty as a practitioner (Sure Start, supporting families) and evaluation of public health initiatives

Chapter 13 explores the concept of risk and risk management in relation to vulnerable children, young people and their families. Consideration is given to the nature of risk within modern society and the responsibilities of the public health nurse in safeguarding vulnerable groups. The chapter examines the process of the identification, assessment and effective management of vulnerable groups and the impact of this on lone workers, in particular their personal safety. Finally, the chapter closes with discussion on frameworks and strategies within health and social care provision that aim to minimise risk to vulnerable children, young people and their families, and the evaluation of these strategies.

Introduction to Chapter 14

Public Health Skills: developing programmes and projects

- Programme and project planning: development, implementation, management, evaluation and review
- Developing existing skills and essential new skills: community development, project management and effective leadership
- Four steps to developing public health programmes and services

Chapter 14 takes a realistic and practical approach and serves to explain the skills needed to work with other professionals, agencies and lay people to make real differences to local people. A scenario is used to demonstrate the application of these skills to the planning, implementation, management, evaluation and review of a comprehensive multiagency public health project. The emphasis in this chapter is on skills and the application of these skills, rather than the theoretical and policy framework that underpins public health, which lies at the heart of Section 3 of this book:

Introduction to Chapter 15

Public Health Skills: programme planning

- Preparation for programme planning
- Delivery, management and evaluative skills in programme planning for health education: children and young people's health, public health and inequalities

- Ideology and strategy in the 'Healthy schools' initiative, accessing health services and planning framework for a health fair

Chapter 15 analyses and discusses the public health skills required to plan, deliver, manage and evaluate programmes designed to improve the health and wellbeing of children and young people. It contains a very practical case study example demonstrating the six key steps undertaken by a school nursing team in planning health education targeted at young people within a school environment. The example given is that of a multiagency venture resulting in the delivery of a health fair coordinated by a school nursing team together with their education partners.

Introduction to Chapter 16

Public Health Skills: managing self, people and resources ethically

- Ethical theories, ethical principles and their application
- Concepts of ethics: utilitarianism and deontology as applied to the client and practice
- Legal and professional frameworks and their application
- The role of advocacy and reflections on practice and dilemmas raised

Chapter 16 concludes the book by considering some of the ethical and legal issues that nurses working in the field of public health need to understand. The ethical and legal issues relate to the management of self and others as well as resources. The chapter is designed to enable the nurse to become aware of and apply legal and ethical frameworks that guide and inform practice. The chapter uses a scenario, in the form of a case study, to provide examples of ethical and legal issues and these are examined through an example assignment, written by a registered nurse undertaking a unit of learning on ethical and legal concepts at her local university. Learning is demonstrated through the case study, which raises ethical and legal issues around a patient who is being cared for in her own home by a multiagency team. Discussion points are raised during the chapter in order to explore some of the dilemmas faced within everyday practice.

CHAPTER 12

Quality and Risk Management in Primary Care Settings

Linda Childs

Public Health Skills: Quality frameworks and risk management in primary care settings

- Developing prescribing for nurses: extended and supplementary prescribing
- Prescribing and meeting the health needs of the population: patient group directives and prescribing for children
- Administration of medicines and risk management systems: principles, evaluation and strategies
- National Patient Safety Agency seven steps to patient safety: patient feedback, complaints and clinical governance

Introduction

This chapter will consider risk management as part of the drive to improve quality in the NHS. The focus will be on the role of the nurse in developing effective strategies to enable patients' safe and timely access to medicines in today's health care environment. The activities of the nurse prescriber will be considered against the *Standards for Better Health* (DH 2000a).

12.1 Development of New Roles for Nurses

The plans for modernization of the NHS proposed widespread changes in the roles of those employed in it and the shape of the services provided (DH 2000a). Further change was announced in *The NHS Improvement Plan* (DH 2004a, 2006a) for primary care trusts (PCTs) to place patient and service user needs at the heart of services, with decision making devolved to local level to provide health care nearer to home. As a consequence of this growing shift of provision from hospital to community, 70 per cent of patients' contact with the NHS now occurs in primary care settings. These changes, coupled with the crisis in medical manpower, and demand for health care, have prompted nurses to develop new roles to meet these needs. Plans to further transform services were compounded by the numbers of non-emergency cases presenting at emergency units, fewer GPs providing out of hours (OOH) services, and standards falling within traditional unsustainable systems (DH 2006b; National Audit Office 2006). The potential for nurses to extend their roles and influence the development of 'first contact' nurse-led services had already been established (DH 2000b, 2002). Walk in centres (WiCs) and minor injuries units (MIUs) were cited as areas in which nurses' practice might continue to build to provide alternative services to deliver the care traditionally delivered by doctors. The increasing flexibility and specialist skills of nurses remain central to developing primary care services. The nurse's extended role requires increased knowledge and skills to deliver complete episodes of care (DH 2006c). Nurse prescribing is identified as an essential skill, not only for specialist community public health nurses (SCPHNs), health visitors, school nurses, occupational health nurses, community health care nurses (CHCNs), district nurses, community children's nurses, community mental health nurses, community learning disability nurses and general practice nurses, but also for advanced nurse practitioners especially those in first contact care (DH 1999a, 2000a).

12.2   Introducing Prescribing for Nurses

Nurse prescribing is not new to health visiting or district nursing. The potential for nurse prescribing to improve patient care and enable efficient use of resources was identified by Dame Julia Cumberlege (DHSS 1986). The report was considered by the Crown Committee of the Department of Health (DH 1989), which proposed that those with health visitor or district nurse qualifications, working in the community, be given authority to prescribe from a limited formulary.

The Medicinal Product Prescribing by Nurses Act 1992, enacted in 1994, enabled the first health visitors and district nurses to be trained at pilot sites. In 1998, training was rolled out for district nurses and health visitors in England, allowing prescribing from a limited formulary known as the *District Nurse and Health Visitors Formulary*. This was revised periodically and renamed in 2006 the *Nurse Prescribers' Formulary for Community Practitioners* (Royal Pharmaceutical Society 2005). From 1995, the prescribing curriculum has been embedded in the initial post-qualifying training for all SCPHNs and CHCNs. Prescribing training may now be accessed by all nurses on these programmes.

The second Crown Report (DH 1999a) recommended prescriptive authority be extended to nurses with expertise in specialised areas and other groups of health professionals. Extended formulary nurse prescribing commenced from 2003. Nurses completing a training course (over 3–6 months) had access to an extended formulary known as the *Nurse Prescribers' Extended Formulary* (DH 2003g) to prescribe for certain conditions.

Supplementary prescribing for nurses and pharmacists was introduced in 2003. This enabled prescribers to manage any diagnosed medical condition by adjusting dosage or prescribing any medicine within the *British National Formulary* (BNF) (BMA 2006a) and some controlled drugs, providing that a clear clinical management plan was completed in advance and the patient agreed. The term 'non-medical prescribing' is used for all prescribing activities of nurses and allied heath professionals. Later courses for nurses enable qualification as both an independent and supplementary prescriber. However, the restrictions of extended formulary nurse prescibing limited, in some cases, the benefits of supplementary prescribing to patients (Latter *et al.* 2005), as it could not be used in all settings where patients would benefit (e.g. first contact and emergency care), as it required a clinical management plan signed by a doctor before the nurse could prescribe.

In March 2006, following further consultations, the *BNF* was opened to all extended formulary prescribing nurses, enabling the prescribing of any licensed product listed within the *BNF*, for any medical condition, and some controlled drugs (DH 2006c). More than 29 000 nurses in England have trained to prescribe from the *Nurse Prescribers' Formulary for Community Practitioners*, with a rapid growth from 2000 nurse independent/supplementary prescribers in 2004, to 7800 nurses today (Robinson & Potter 2006).

At the time of going to print a Department of Health consultation is considering further expansion by removing the restrictions on prescribing of controlled drugs.

12.3   Prescribing and Meeting the Health Needs of the Population

Prescribing has enabled nurses to meet the needs of the population to access their medications. Services for the homeless, outreach and OOH services deliver appropriate health care to disadvantaged groups and those who do not access traditional health care services. Public health is further promoted by nurses actively providing advice and medicines for sexually transmitted infections, preventing and treating coronary heart disease, smoke stop, hypertension, raised cholesterol, substance misuse, obesity and many more conditions. Prescribing also enables symptom relief and maintains health for those with chronic health and long-term conditions, and for those requiring emergency care and for minor ailments.

12.3.1   Patient group directions: the supply and administration of medicine

In addition to prescribing, nurses working in the field of public health may also be involved in the administration of medicines. The majority of prescriptions are supplied and administered by patient-specific directions, the traditional way for any nurse to administer medicines, via a written instruction on a patient's records or ward drug chart, from a doctor, dentist, nurse or other prescriber, to a named patient. Since August 2000, patient group directions (PGDs) have provided a legal framework to allow the supply and administration of medicines or vaccines directly to a patient, without the need for a prescription, subject to certain conditions being met. PGDs are for specified groups of patients and must be drawn up and signed by a doctor in advance of the treatment delivered by a qualified nurse or certain qualified health professionals (DH 2000c).

The supply of medicines under a PGD should be reserved for the limited number of cases where this offers an advantage to the patient without compromising safety (DH 2006c). Currently PGDs are widely used in primary care with, for example, 50 medicines being administered under this framework in one PCT (St Helen's PCT 2004). They are commonly used for delivery of the childhood immunization programme, flu vaccines and emergency contraception. Indeed some controlled drugs and antibiotics may now be issued under PGDs. The use of PGDs in walk in centres and minor injuries units supports the principle of reforming emergency care (DH 2001a). They have enabled timely access to treatment and a reduction in waiting times as nurses may 'see and treat'. Having made a thorough assessment and diagnosis, with agreement from the patient/client, nurses may select and implement the relevant PGD. The NHS Library for Health (2006) has 39 easily adaptable national PGD templates for emergency care and others for primary care/public health (see Appendix 12.1).

To comply with legislation, each PGD must state the clinical condition, patient inclusion and exclusion criteria, information on the medicine, instructions for use, warnings regards adverse reactions, arrangements for further advice, referral, follow-up and record keeping. Practitioners proposing to use the PGD must be named by the trust and a record kept (DH 2000c). The use of PGDs must also be consistent with appropriate professional relationships and accountability with practitioners working within their scope of competence. In practice, PGDs may replace protocols as they incorporate detailed instructions of best care and provide a means of auditing care. Where adjustments are required in the dosage of long-term medicines, PGDs are not considered suitable and supplementary prescribing by an appropriately qualified prescriber would provide a better option (DH 2006c).

Caution is required when prescribing or developing PGDs for antimicrobials, black triangle drugs, those used 'off label' or for children. For antimicrobials, consideration of the risks of increasing resistance within the general community is a priority (DH 2003a; BMA 2006b). Advice from a microbiologist and the drugs and therapeutics committee must be upheld. ('Off label' refers to drugs used outside their summary of product characteristics, their use should be the exception and justified by best practice. Black triangle drugs are newly licensed drugs for which special reporting arrangements for suspected adverse reactions are required.)

12.3.2   Advice on prescribing for children

The NMC guidelines (2006b) advise that prescribing for children be confined to nurses with relevant knowledge, competence and experience. This also applies to issuing medicines under a PGD for a child and is of particular importance for nurses employed in WiCs, MIUs, OOH services and nurses working in general practice who must work within their competence and refer to another prescriber when care falls beyond their expertise and competence. Attention to the child's weight, size and maturity when considering suitability of the medicine is imperative (BMA 2006c).

Activity

Why not visit the website for the National Service Framework for Children (DH & DfES 2004) and explore this further: http://www.dh.gov.uk/en/Policyandguidance/Healthandsocialcaretopics/ChildrenServices/Childrenservice sinformation/index.htm.

Since 2003, PGDs may be legally used in non-NHS organizations, independent hospital agencies and clinics registered under the Care Standards Act 2000, prison health care services, police services and defence medical services. Unlike prescribing, there is no specific training required before nurses may use PGDs; however employers normally initiate annual training and set and monitor standards for competence before nurses are sanctioned to supply and administer medicines by this method. The National Prescribing Centre (NPC 2004) has issued a competency framework for staff using PGDs. This includes the ability to: complete a holistic assessment; make a diagnosis as well as differential diagnoses; consider non-pharmaceutical approaches, and public health and health promotion issues; consider concordance issues and patients' perception; and possess knowledge of the condition presenting, the medication (its actions and interactions) and how mechanisms may be altered, for example the influence of age on renal conditions, etc. Nurses are best advised to adhere to local and professional guidelines at all times (NMC 2004a, 2006a) when administering medicines.

12.3.3   Principles for the administration of medicines

Medicines Management (NMC 2006a) lists the principles for the administration of medicines and states that nurses must:

- possess knowledge of the therapeutic use of the product, normal dosage, precautions, contraindications and side effects;
- establish the identity of the patient to receive the medicine;
- establish the clarity of the prescription and/or the label on the medication to be dispensed;
- check the expiry date;
- consider the dosage, method, route and timing of the administration in the context of the patient's condition, diagnoses and coexisting therapies;
- check that the patient is not allergic to the medication nor that it is contraindicated;
- contact the prescriber (or if unavailable, another doctor or authorised prescriber) immediately if there are any contraindications or reactions, or where assessment of the patient indicates that the medicine is no longer suitable;
- make a clear, accurate, legible and immediate record of all medicine administered, or intentionally withheld, or refused by the patient with a signature (follow any additional local guidelines). It is the nurse's responsibility to ensure a record is made when delegating the administration of a medicine;
- clearly countersign the signature of any student whom you have supervised in the administration of medicines (NMC 2005a).

12.3.4   Errors with the use of medicines

Mistakes made with the administration of medicines are the most common threat to patient safety (Neale *et al.* 2001) and pose concern worldwide. Each day over one million people visit their GPs and many more are treated by nurses in a variety of settings, with 1.5 million prescriptions issued and dispensed in primary care (NPSA 2006a). Amongst all this activity the potential for risk, which is inherent in all aspects of health care delivery, is high, with the consequence that some patients are harmed as a result.

The Nursing and Midwifery Council *Code of Professional Conduct* (NMC 2004b) clauses 1.4, 8.1, 8.2 and 8.3 place a duty on nurses to minimise risk and deliver safe and competent care to their patients or clients. An understanding of risk and the risk management process is therefore required.

12.4   Risk and Risk Management in Primary Care Settings

Risk may be defined as the potential for unwanted outcome (Wilson 1994). The NPSA (2006a) define potential risk as the chance of something occurring that will have an impact on individuals or organizations. Risk management is therefore the systematic identification, assessment and reduction of risk to patients and staff through a means of modifying systems and behaviours to reduce the potential for health care risk (DH 2000d). It involves all the processes in identifying, assessing and measuring risks, attributing ownership, taking actions to mitigate or anticipate risk, and monitoring and reviewing progress (NPSA 2004). Consequently, risk is an element of day to day practice and the aim of PCTs and nurses is to minimise its effect by managing it.

Wilson (1999) states that avoidable risk may be a consequence of the following:

1. Systems failure, where there are inadequate or non-existing policies, guidelines or protocols for procedures.
2. Poor communication, either with service users and carers or amongst professionals and agencies.
3. Staff taking short cuts, which may be precipitated by heavy workloads or staff shortages, etc.
4. Poorly defined role responsibilities so staff may work beyond their scope of competence.
5. Inadequate training so staff are not fit for purpose.
6. Poor team coordination, within the organization and with other agencies.
7. Deliberate damage to patients by staff (although this is the exception).

12.4.1   Risk management systems

Risk management systems are concerned with risk identified within the organization. They are concerned with patient dissatisfaction; they consider complaints, near misses, clinical incidents and clinical negligence. Wilson (1999) stated that risk management consists of identifying risk, risk analysis, risk treatment and evaluation. However, this author also proposed to add two further dimensions to this: (i) following evaluation it is necessary to revisit practice to reinforce the activity or implement changes to maintain safe practice; and (ii) then audit to measure how far the recommendations have been implemented or embedded in practice (Figure 12.1).

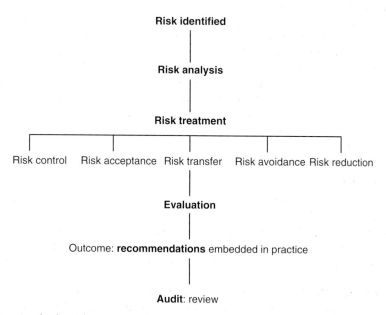

Figure 12.1   Steps involved in risk management.

12.4.2 Risk identification

Risk identification involves awareness by the organization of the actual or potential risk posed. Practitioner involvement in the early reporting of incidents, near misses and mistakes will influence effective risk management. Organizations are required to compile a risk register listing all identified risks.

12.4.3 Risk treatment

Risk treatment involves one of the following:

1. *Risk analysis.* This is an estimation of the potential severity of loss re the risk and the probability of recurrence. The process of risk analysis seeks to answer the questions, 'What can go wrong? How often? How bad? Is there need for action?' (NPSA 2006a).
2. *Risk control.* Risk can be controlled by containing the risk and reducing the outcome of adverse occurrences by following clinical guidelines, education and training for avoidance, and contingency or disaster plans. An example of this is organizational activity to educate and train staff, and set local policies that adhere to the national immunization guidelines (DH 2006d) including treating anaphylaxis.
3. *Risk acceptance.* This involves managing a risk that cannot be reduced, avoided or transferred. Estimates of the potential losses of the risk are made with plans to cover financial losses.
4. *Risk avoidance.* Risk avoidance employs alternative ways of providing care which reduce the greater risk posed by the original method. An example is providing medicine in liquid form for patients who have dysphagia.
5. *Risk reduction.* This is a common activity within PCT risk management programmes. It includes: staff education and training policies, safety and induction training, policy and procedure review, and health and safety updates. It may also include annual updates on using PGDs, and an annual medicines management and drugs calculations test.
6. *Risk transfer.* This involves shifting the loss to others. Arrangements with the Clinical Negligence Scheme for Trusts protects the organization from financial loss in cases of claims. Similarly, nurses may obtain indemnity insurance from a professional body.

12.4.4 Risk evaluation and outcome

This may be performed by various activities including clinical audit, benchmarking against national and local standards, and audit of compliance with mandatory training. *Essence of Care* (DH 2003b) provides benchmarks to measure quality of care. Following risk evaluation, recommendations for best practice should be made.

Outcome recommendations may entail changing practice and policy, and setting new guidelines for practice. Outcome activity should be revisited after a period of time to measure how far the recommendations and action have been embedded in practice by auditing.

12.5 Development of Risk Management Strategies

The development of risk management strategies within the NHS is associated with the annual increase in claims for clinical negligence. The NHS Litigation Agency (2006a) report spiralling legal costs incurred for litigation, reaching £579.3 million in 2006/7 for all clinical negligence claims for incidents sustained after 1995. A consequence of this is the drain on financial resources away from patient care to settle these claims. Although the focus of adverse events, risk assessment and monitoring has been on the care delivered in the acute sector, little research is available to quantify risks in primary care, although it is certain that similar challenges apply (NPSA 2006a). Earlier reports (DH 2000d) identified 850 000 adverse events each year in the NHS hospital sector, estimated at an annual cost exceeding two billion pounds, and recommended that a systematic approach be developed, similar to that used in aviation and other industries to analyse mistakes and failures in order to learn lessons and prevent recurrence. The proposals given in the government's implementation document *Building a Safer NHS for Patients* (DH 2001b) included:

- a mandatory reporting scheme;
- strategies to improve understanding of why things go wrong through initiating research into patient safety incidents;
- a new system for handling investigations and inquiries;
- setting up the new National Patient Safety Agency (NPSA).

Four specific areas of risk were targeted, two of which related to medicines safety – to reduce to zero the number of serious errors relating to spinal injections, and to reduce by 40 per cent the number of serious errors in the use of prescribed drugs across provision, which accounted for 20 per cent of all clinical negligence litigation (DH 2001b).

The NPSA was established in 2001 to improve patient safety by promoting a culture of reporting and learning from adverse incidents and near misses. The National Reporting and Learning System was developed by the agency to analyse information on adverse events and near misses, to publish statistics, to identify trends, and to deliver effective, practical and timely solutions. The development of the single, mandatory reporting system for all adverse events and near misses, with the encouragement of a reporting and questioning culture throughout the NHS, to identify underlying causes of failures and to learn from experiences were strategies proposed to improve national safety. Staff may anonymously report incidents in which they are involved or are witness to, directly to the NPSA (www.npsa.nhs.uk/stafform/). Organizations are required to inform the NPSA of locally reported patient safety issues. This enables national collation of all incidents and the sharing of outcomes and alerts via the NPSA distribution system. NHS organizations are informed of recommendations from national inquiries in order to take steps to prevent similar safety incidents. An example is the safer practice notice issued in 2005 after 93 school children were wrongly vaccinated with Repevax – a whooping cough vaccine. Similar names and packaging of the two vaccines, Repevax and Revaxis, were identified as contributory factors (National Audit Office 2005; NPSA 2005a). The NPSA continues to monitor events and influence the pharmaceutical industry to make changes in labelling and packaging to avoid recurrence.

The yellow card scheme enables staff and the public to notify the Medicines and Healthcare Products Regulatory Agency and the Commission of Human Medicines of suspected adverse drug reactions by completing a yellow card available in the *BNF* or electronically at www.yellowcard.gov.uk. Reporting is required for all severe reactions and any suspected adverse reactions to newly licensed medicines under intensive monitoring (identified with a black triangle in the *BNF*) so that risk may be investigated.

Patient safety forms part of the remit of board-level managers; usually the medical or nursing director takes the lead. In addition to this strategic lead, an operational risk manager is required to work with practitioners to monitor and coordinate patient safety and to manage risk. Risk managers take a lead in identifying and managing risk, collating evidence and establishing mechanisms for the distribution of patient safety alerts and notices. Trusts are required to compile a risk register that lists all the risks within the organization. Plans to address and reduce identified risks are required along with regular reviews of progress. This activity links with work required for assessment for the Clinical Negligence Scheme for Trusts. Those achieving the highest standards pay lower contributions. The NHS Litigation Agency risk management standards for PCTs measure performance against set risk standards, which include incident reporting, complaints and investigation, infection control, health records, and the validation and monitoring of professional registration, clinical care and training. New standards are being developed for 2007 to be piloted in 2008 (NHS Litigation Agency 2006b). Although risk managers take an overall responsibility for risk management, nurses and the multidisciplinary team are required to lead in situations where they possess the knowledge and expertise to address risk in their practice area, and to share responsibility for patient safety (NMC 2004a).

12.6   The NPSA's Seven Steps to Patient Safety

This was launched as a manual for all staff to improve patient safety (NPSA 2004). Although aimed at all health care settings, it was considered more relevant to the acute sector. Within NHS-funded primary care, advances in technology and knowledge have enabled more than one million people to be treated safely and successfully each day. This, however, has resulted in a complicated health care system which, coupled with the speed of change, is acknowledged by the NPSA as bringing its own set of risks. Subsequently a patient safety manual was published for all primary care staff (NPSA 2006a). This document presents seven key areas of activity for members of primary care organizations to work through to develop strategies to improve patient safety over the next 3–5 years (Box 12.1). It postulates that patient safety can only be improved with systems whereby all staff learn from mistakes. For this to happen, a change is required in both the culture and systems in the workplace (DH 2000d) – to become an effective learning organization which treats staff fairly, where staff challenge poor practice and report any errors or practice that may cause harm. Comparisons of the health care environment with that of the aviation industry (Sexton *et al.* 2000) identified that a move was necessary, away from the ethos of infallibility to one where mistakes and near misses are acknowledged and learnt from.

Changes in medical training (Sharpe & Faden 1998) and the closer working relationships between doctors and nurses to enable partnerships and joint decision making (Fisher & Burn 2003) were found to be essential for this shift. Dean *et al.* (2002) noted that junior doctors and nurses were reluctant to question senior staff, especially consultants, even if they suspected errors in clinical practice, including medicines errors.

The recommendations were for a shift in culture to an open, questioning and learning environment. Similar observations were noted in the recommendations following the Bristol Royal Infirmary Inquiry (2001) and, more recently, after the Shipman Inquiry (Smith 2004). The new training for health professionals has embraced this concept and it is hoped that by openly reporting and learning from events, and developing frameworks for scrutiny, safety will be enhanced.

12.7   Errors Involving the Use of Medicines

A study by Bates *et al.* (1993) found that errors involving the use of medicines pose the most common threat to patient safety. Bates *et al.* (1993) defined medication error as any error in the process of

---

BOX 12.1

The steps to patient safety for primary care. *Source*: NPSA (2006a).

Step 1   Build a safety culture
Create a culture that is open and fair

Step 2   Lead and support your staff
Establish a clear and strong focus on patient safety throughout

Step 3   Integrate your risk management activity
Develop systems and processes to manage your risks and identify and assess things that may go wrong

Step 4   Promote reporting
Ensure that staff can easily report incidents both locally and nationally

Step 5   Involve and communicate with patients and the public
Design ways to communicate openly with and listen to patients

Step 6   Learn safety lessons
Encourage staff to use root cause analysis to learn how and why incidents happen

Step 7   Implement solutions to prevent harm
Embed lessons through changes to practice, processes or systems

prescribing, dispensing, preparing, administering or monitoring of drug therapy, regardless of whether injury occurs or potential for harm exists. To date only a small percentage of safety incidents in primary care have been reported (NPSA 2005b), with documentation errors most commonly reported (23 per cent of total reports), followed by medication errors (20 per cent). Many patients receive care from both the acute and primary care sector and it is following discharge from acute care that patients are most at risk of medication errors. The Royal Pharmaceutical Society (2006) found 20 per cent of patients experience an adverse event following discharge from acute care or between care providers, and have published guidelines for the multidisciplinary team in their discharge and transfer planning workbook. Further issues identified were that 25 per cent of discharge letters were lost in the post and that 80 per cent of consultant's letters took more than a month to reach the GP. Emphasis on the importance of developing and maintaining processes for timely information sharing to avoid patient harm is required.

The importance of recording treatment and medications prescribed, ensuring that systems are in place and adhered to, in order to inform the patient's physician of new or changed medication is paramount. Guidance and frameworks are provided by the National Prescribing Centre (2003), the Nursing and Midwifery Council (NMC 2004a, 2006a) and the Department of Health (DH 2006c). One of the advantages of the imminent introduction of the electronic patient medical record is that it has the potential to improve the situation as a summary of the individual's medical information will be available, whenever and wherever they present for treatment. If a man living in Carlisle presents at a WiC in Cornwall, whilst on holiday, his records may be accessed. The NHS Care Record Service is scheduled to be introduced in 2007 and rolled out nationally in 2008. Electronic prescriptions have the potential to increase safety by timely recording of prescribing information and medicines dispensed. The potential to receive alerts specific to a patient's episode of care and information such as possible risks, reactions and interactions, all contribute to safer prescribing decision making (NHS Connecting for Health 2006).

In a survey of older people, Barat *et al.* (2001) identified that, of all reported medicine errors, 71 per cent were taking a different dose than prescribed and a further 66 per cent were varying the doses. The importance of communication, providing information and developing a partnership approach with patients is apparent. The reasons for non-compliance are complicated and include issues related to patients' health beliefs and intentional actions, as well as misunderstanding (Marinker & Shaw 2003). No single intervention has been found to be effective in promoting adherence. However, multiple interventions – which include further follow-up, written information, compliance aids, dosage boxes, simplified regimes, better communication and education strategies – are recommended (Haynes *et al.* 1997; Vermiere *et al.* 2001). The National Prescribing Centre (NPC 2001, 2003) competency frameworks identify the communication competencies required by the prescriber to negotiate concordance. The *Essence of Care* (DH 2003b) provides benchmarks to measure communication performance across all nursing provision.

Roberts *et al.* (2002) identified that for all errors with dispensed medicines, nurses detected 45 per cent of the total errors reported. Categories of error were: 23 per cent wrong strength, 23 per cent wrong medicine, 10 per cent wrong directions, 10 per cent wrong quantity issued and 44 per cent 'other'. Barat *et al.* (2001) identified that, of the total errors identified, 22 per cent of patients were taking drugs that were different to those recorded on their medical record. There is scope for professional interventions to check medication and regimes on a regular basis, to empower those who are able to take an active role in agreeing and managing their treatment, and to enable a concordant approach to empower patients to actively monitor their medicines. However, there remains concern about the errors in the prescribing, dispensing and administering processes.

Two approaches to human error are described by Reason (2000): the person approach and the systems approach (Figure 12.2). The *person approach* attributes the error to the individual and the action tends to be 'name and blame'. Although practitioners must take responsibility for their actions, blaming individuals does not encourage reporting or learning.

The *systems approach* accepts that staff are fallible and that errors occur despite the competence of the practitioner. An 'error' is described as a planned action that fails to achieve the desired outcome. Focus is given to the conditions under which practitioners work and how these may predispose to

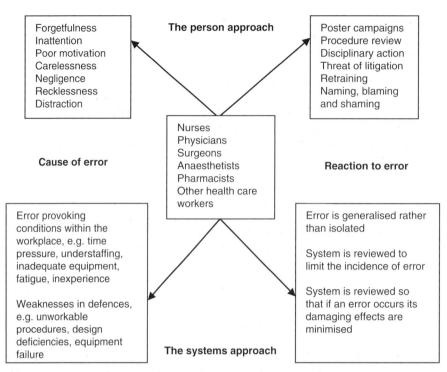

Figure 12.2 The person and systems approaches to medication error. *Source*: DH (2004a).

errors. It is only by acknowledging these predisposing conditions that system defences may be developed to avoid recurrence. Incidents reported, either directly or through the organization, enable the NPSA to map events and causal factors. It is more important to identify why and how a safety incident occurred, and to learn from this to prevent recurrence, than to attribute blame to one person (NPSA 2006a).

To enhance learning from a patient safety incident, *root cause analysis* (RCA) may be used. This is a technique for undertaking a systematic investigation that looks beyond individual actions (Woodward 2006). The root causes of an event may be sited in various factors such as poor documentation, lack of resources, skill mix, omissions, failure to diagnose or equipment error. RCA is a model based on the chronological chain of events. It is worked in reverse chronology. The level of analysis depends on the severity and complexity of the problem. A review of all factors that contribute to a patient safety incident is required, not merely those related to a staff member, as system failure is often a major factor (NPSA 2004). Recommendations are for patient safety leaders to oversee training and provide support for staff.

All causes of harm and potential harm, including drug prescribing and administration errors, must be reported. So must near misses or 'no harm' events. A drug error that was noticed before the drug was administered is an example of a near miss. There is evidence that near misses are underreported (NPSA 2006a). Guidelines and training on RCA and appropriate interventions are provided on the NPSA website (www.npsa.nhs.uk). The multidisciplinary team should analyse the patient safety event and consider all documentation and records when conducting the incident analysis. The NPSA (2004) provides a choice of 11 tools with which to consider contributory factors, such as the 'five whys', asking why five times (Ross 1994), and the fishbone tool (NPSA 2004). These are available online for NHS use. The use of online tools enables prompt RCA. This may then be used to collate safety information to provide advice and to enable learning to promote safety and improve the quality of care.

For risk management to be effective it requires the following:

1. A detailed consideration of the:
   - patient's needs and experiences;
   - use of appropriate supporting data;

- workforce capacity/capability requirements;
- available infrastructure;
- integrated services used;
- care professional's contribution.

2. The service to be comprehensively mapped.
3. The provider to identify all things that may go wrong – the 'what if' question.
4. The likely causes and consequences and failures to be identified and recorded.
5. Production of a risk matrix to assess the frequency, likelihood and impact of the identified failure.
6. Targeted recommendations and implementation strategies to reduce risk without introducing new risks (NPSA 2006a).

Activity

An example of the risk assessment process described above may be accessed from the NPSA website (NPSA 2006b), www.npsa.nhs.uk. Exploring incidents-improving safety demonstrates the key components of effective risk assessment whilst investigating a case study involving one patient in the community who had 24 contacts with seven health care agencies in 36 hours. It provides a working example of the effective risk management as described above.

12.8   Patient Feedback and Complaints

Patient feedback and complaints are one means of identifying risks. NHS organizations are responsible for improving performance and supporting those making complaints and engaging the Healthcare Commission in cases where speedy resolution has not been met. Practitioners remain accountable for complaints made against them and are required to take action to build quality improvements. Complaints should be handled efficiently, effectively and promptly in accordance with national guidelines and local policy. A single system to deal with complaints across health and social care (DH 2006e) is scheduled for 2009; this will build on existing procedures but will place more emphasis on supporting patients and relatives, rather than on process and procedure. Poor communication was found to be a factor in the majority of complaints.

Following patient safety incidents. Gallagher *et al.* (2003) identified that whilst doctors were reluctant to discuss errors or to apologise for fear of litigation, patients valued an explanation of events and wanted an apology. Both doctors and patients wished for support to deal with the emotional consequences of the incident. A survey involving 8000 people (DH 2003c) found that not only was an apology and explanation required but also an in-depth investigation. Being open decreases the trauma felt by patients following a patient safety incident (Vincent & Coulter 2002). The NPSA (2005a) provides guidance for developing a consistent approach to handling communications following a patient safety incident resulting in harm. The NPSA (2005b) recommends that a senior practitioner with good communication skills empathetically leads an open and honest discussion with the patient and their significant others, with support from either the risk manager or clinical lead. Focus should centre on clear explanations and the patient's or significant other's agenda, whist seeking resolution.

Complaints form part of the risk identification and risk management process. Risk management is an integral part of the clinical governance framework (DH 1999b) – a systematic approach through which NHS organizations manage quality assurance and quality control to ensure that patients receive the best quality of care that the NHS can provide. Nurses have a responsibility to deliver safe and high quality care at all times (NMC 2004b).

Clinical guidelines or protocols have been used in practice by nurses for some time as a tool to promote clinical effectiveness by identifying and implementing best practice and to standardise care to meet best outcomes. The drive for quality in the NHS has influenced the systematic development of many guidelines, which were adapted locally in order to assist practitioners and patients in best decision making (NHS Executive 1996). However, despite their usefulness, limitations arose from the fact that protocols tend to be specific to the care delivered by a single discipline of staff (e.g. nurses), while the complexities of modern health care delivery requires a multidisciplinary or multiagency approach, across acute and primary care, to provide seamless care and to prevent unnecessary delay or duplication. Consequently it is essential to have a tool that provides a map of care to be delivered by each discipline, which apportions accountability and states proposed outcomes. Integrated care pathways (ICPs) fit this remit.

12.9   Integrated Care Pathways

An ICP determines locally agreed, multidisciplinary practice based on guidelines and evidence for a specific patient/client group. It forms all or part of the clinical record, it documents the care given and facilitates the evaluation of outcomes for continuous quality improvement. ICPs were originally developed in America in the 1980s as a one-page tool to identify multidisciplinary interventions as a timeline to enable effective monitoring of patient care to allow outcome measurement and to assist with costing (Swage 2004). They were selected as part of a resource management initiative, adapted and developed for NHS settings. The NHS has developed a 'protocols and care pathways knowledge service' that provides access to a range of protocols and care pathways for professionals, which may be accessed electronically (National Library for Health 2004). Protocols can provide best evidence and may be used to set standards against which to audit the quality of care. As a strategy to raise quality standards, the Department of Health (DH 1998) announced the role of the National Institute of Clinical Excellence (NICE) to evaluate treatments and health care interventions in order to establish the most cost-effective options to guide national practice. The work of NICE in determining standards for quality care delivery may also reduce inequalities by specifying what treatments will be available nationally, and thus end the postcode lottery (where a patient living in one area was able to access the care or treatment that a patient in a neighbouring area was denied) (DH 2005). NICE has three functions:

1. To set clinical guidelines identifying treatment and care for patients with specific diseases within England and Wales.
2. To perform technology appraisals on the use of new and existing medicines and treatment including public health interventions.
3. To report on the interventional safety of procedures for diagnostics and treatment.

12.10   National Service Frameworks

National Service Frameworks (NSFs) set national standards for quality within the NHS and play a key part in NHS modernization. They present an entire systems approach to the prevention and management of health conditions, across primary and acute care (Pearce 2005), and identify long-term strategies for improving standards of care by setting measurable goals within set timeframes. There are currently eight NSFs, with others in the developmental stage. PCTs have a central role to play in implementing NSFs, which link directly with the three core functions of PCTs: to improve the health of the community, to develop primary care services and to secure secondary services. Subsequently, ICPs have incorporated best evidence, NSF and NICE recommendations. Evidence-based practice is expressed as actions for required outcomes (e.g. treatments, investigations). This in turn helps identify the skills required by the team and contributes to skills and workforce planning, and assists in identifying risk and developing policies for managing risk. It provides a systematic approach to clinical governance by providing a standard and a structure against which current and retrospective data may be audited.

12.11   Clinical Governance

Clinical governance is defined as:

> a system through which NHS organisations are accountable for continuously improving the quality of their services and safeguarding high standards of care, by creating an environment in which clinical excellence will flourish. (DH 1998, p. 17)

Table 12.1 *Standards for Better Health* for PCTs. *Source*: DH (2006f)

Seven domains	National targets
1. Safety	Improve the population's health
2. Clinical and cost-effective	Support long-term conditions
3. Governance	Access to services
4. Patient focus	Patient/user experience
5. Accessible and responsive care	
6. Care environment and amenities	
7. Public health	

Clinical governance was introduced to the NHS in 1997 as a comprehensive framework to improve the quality of health care (DH 1997a) following a series of highly publicised failures that resulted in a loss of confidence in the NHS and spiralling costs of health care litigation claims. A focus on failures included the Bristol Royal Infirmary Inquiry (2001) into the deaths of 23 children following cardiac surgery, the trials of nurse Beverley Allitt (DH 1994) and Harold Shipman (Smith 2004). This prompted the government's proposal for a quality assurance framework to consolidate the quality agenda within health care organizations to deliver safe, cost-effective care (Sale 2005). This was to be done through the monitoring of standards by national organizations which include the Healthcare Commission, the NPSA and the NHS Performance Framework. Locally, PCT governance leads set the agenda to implement national quality initiatives and local strategies to monitor and improve quality. Performance assessment in health care remains on the government's agenda, with new core and developmental standards replacing the previous star ratings. *Standards for Better Health* (DH 2006f) present 24 core and developmental standards within seven domains and the national standards against which a trust's performance is measured (Table 12.1). The effectiveness of this method has yet to be tested.

NSFs are central to the government's plan in driving quality improvements and have been used with the NICE guidance in the assessment framework *Standards for Better Health* (DH 2006f) by the Healthcare Commission since 2005 to measure health care achievements and build on quality performance year on year. PCTs are required to produce evidence of the quality of their services. User perspectives and audit are methods commonly employed. Audit is the continuous review or measurement by health professionals of their practice and care delivered against agreed standards. Review of the NSFs enables measurement of the entire patient journey through acute and primary care provision. The first NSF review was in 2005 using the *National Service Framework for Coronary Heart Disease* (DH 2000e) to map the patient journey, within one region, through primary care preventive services, emergency ambulance, secondary and tertiary care, and discharge back to primary care (Pearce 2005).

Professional standards provide guidelines for all nursing behaviour; further standards and targets for care may be set locally and nationally to provide frameworks for quality heath care against which practice may be measured. The Department of Health (DH 2006a) recommends that trusts provide a clinical governance framework for non-medical prescribing and provides examples of such. However, *Standards for Better Health* (DH 2006f) provides a framework against which all health care provision is measured annually to determine the level of quality attained and to enable targets to be set to improve quality year on year. Trusts are required to provide evidence of meeting core and developmental standards in their annual health check (DH 2006f).

In the following example, nurse prescribing will be considered against the standards in Table 12.1 and will be referred to as non-medical prescribing (NMP) as in the Department of Health guidance (DH 2006c).

Patient safety

- Organizations have in place an integrated policy for the management of non-medical prescribing nurses (NMPs) in line with monitoring all prescribing, and in consultation with the drugs and therapeutics committee, to minimise potential and associated risk.

- NMPs demonstrate evidence of integrating risk management into working practice (as previously discussed in this chapter).
- NMPs adhere to professional standards for prescribing practice (NMC 2006a) and current legislation, Medicinal Products: Prescription by Nurses and Others Act 1992, enacted in 1994. NMPs adhere to the Medicines and Human Use Prescribing, Amendments Order May 2006 and the associated medicines regulations (Statutory Instrument 2006/1015) when prescribing any licensed medicine in the UK and permitted controlled drugs.
- All NMPs have access to organizational systems for information pertaining to relevant clinical therapeutic and prescribing information, including patient safety notices and alerts from the Medicines and Healthcare Products Regulatory Agency and safety alerts broadcasts.
- NMPs are able to report suspected adverse drug reactions via the yellow card system.
- Systems exist to transfer information between other provider services.
- The organization follows NICE intervention processes and guidance in accordance with the national and international procedures programme, which includes clinical guidelines.
- Risk with medical devices is minimised and reusable devices are decontaminated.
- Infection control policy is implemented, maintaining high standards of hygiene and cleanliness to reduce the risk of health care infection and the safe disposal of sharps and waste (NICE 2003).
- Safe handling of medicines in accordance with statutory requirements of the Medicines Act 1986 and the Misuse of Drugs Act 1971, with guidance from the National Treatment Agency for Substance Misuse (for basic drugs training, prescribing options and models of care where indicated) in accordance with Department of Health guidelines and the Misuse of Drugs Regulations Amendments 2005 (Statutory Instrument 2005/271; Home Office Circular 48/2005).
- Controlled drugs – core activities, monitoring and inspection (Gerada 2006) – and controlled drugs record keeping (DH 2006h).
- Child Protection policy is understood and acted upon.
- Regular review/audit is evident.

Clinical and cost-effective considerations

- NMP leads oversee the systems and quality of NMPs.
- NICE guidance is followed by organizational policies and by NMPs in managing care, through health promotion, therapeutic use of medicines and investigations.
- Guidelines re the use of antimicrobials and prescribing of antibiotics are understood and implemented in prescribing decision making.
- National guidelines and targets for treatments are adhered to.
- National reporting systems are in place and alerts are acted upon.
- NMPs operate within local guidelines and take into consideration local formularies and the cost-effectiveness of medicines and treatments.
- Clinical care and treatment is carried out under supervision and leadership. NMPs have access to preceptorship immediately after qualifying and have clinical peer review support and mentoring arrangements are established. Models of clinical supervision agreed locally enable reflection on practice including prescribing activity (NMC 2006b).
- Annual performance appraisal and continuing professional development plans are acted upon to access activities to update and develop practice.
- NMPs participate in regular audit of practice and reviews of service.
- NMPs have access to prescription analysis and cost (PACT) data available from the NHS Business Service Authority (formerly known as the Prescription Pricing Agency) in electronic format from ePACT.net (details available from their website, www.nhsbsa.nhs.uk). For those prescribing on behalf of a GP practice, data are obtainable from ePFIP (electronic prescribing and financial information for practices) from the Business Service Authority. PACT data provide an account of an individual's prescribing activity and makes comparisons against local and national trends. It provides useful information for the audit of products prescribed and prescribing activity.
- NMPs work with other provider organizations so that patients may access appropriate care. Records of referrals are kept.
- Job description defines the NMP's prescribing role and leadership and management responsibility.

Governance

- Organizations demonstrate sound clinical and corporate governance to actively support and risk manage non-medical prescribing within the trust.
- Organizations demonstrate equity and an equal opportunities policy for staff and users.
- Staff induction programmes are accessed by all new staff, and retention and support strategies are in place.
- A nominated NMP lead ensures a consistent approach to managing prescribing, arranges access to the prescribing budget, and orders prescriptions for newly qualified staff.
- Workforce planning identifies the number of nurses required to have prescribing skills, and funding streams are identified.
- There are selection criteria in place for identifying nurses to train as NMPs in an area where they have specialist knowledge and where there is an identified need to prescribe (DH 2006c; NMC 2006b).
- Programmes for training are within higher education institutions (HEI), whose provision meets the outcome quality measures for education standards (DH 2003f). These are determined through the partnership and consensus of higher education institutions, strategic health authority commissioners for education, regulators (Nursing and Midwifery Council) and individual placement providers.
- Practice training and assessment for prescribing competency is provided by a community practice teacher for those prescribing from the community formulary, and by a designated medical practitioner for independent/supplementary prescribers.
- Personal development programmes and mandatory and in-service training enables staff development.
- NMPs work within their competencies and refer to others when care is beyond their expertise and competence (NMC 2004a, 2006b).
- A record of all prescribers and their prescribing status is maintained by the trust and may be confirmed electronically www.nmc-uk.org.
- NMPs maintain contemporaneous records of all treatment and contacts in keeping with local and national guidelines. Records of any medicines prescribed or administered by PGD entered in the patient's medical record contemporaneously (NMC 2004a) and according to local policy.
- NMPs adhere to policy on safe storage of prescriptions.
- Appraisal and audit of practice to make sure that NMPs meet safe practice requirements.
- The parameters of the individual's prescribing are agreed with their manager, local professional lead and employer.
- The drug and therapeutic committees are aware of the medicines to be prescribed by the nurse prescriber.
- NMPs comply with the continuing professional development standards for practice and prescribing (NMC 2005b, 2006a). NMPs keep up to date with evidence and best practice for the management of conditions for which they prescribe and update their knowledge of prescribing and therapeutics (NPC 2001; DH 2006c; NMC 2006b). NMPs collate evidence to support PREP (post-registration education and practice) requirements to renew registration with the Nursing and Midwifery Council.
- Staff are aware of reporting systems and the whistle blowing policy.
- Monitoring arrangements by the prescription pricing division of the NHS Business Services Authority check that community practitioner nurse prescribers adhere to prescribing from the community practitioners' formulary. For independent/supplementary prescribers this is executed by the employing trust.

Patient focus

- NMPs treat patients with dignity and respect (NMC 2004a).
- NMPs give patients information that is clear and accurate to meet patients' individual needs (NPC 2003; NMC 2004a).
- Prescribing and treatment decisions involve patients and their carers, ensuring consent (DH 2003e), and consider consent when working with children (DH 2001c).

- Patients and professionals seek concordance (Medicines Partnership 2003) and reach agreement on the course of treatment.
- Patient information about the service is available and questions invited.
- Patient information about their treatment plan and medication is available.
- NMPs honour patients' confidentiality (except where legislated to the contrary) and patients are made aware of confidentiality policy.
- Staff comply with policy relating to access to health records, the Data Protection Act 1998 and the Caldicott report (DH 1997b).
- Health care information is recorded and shared when necessary by all involved in care.
- NMPs are aware of, and act upon, the complaints procedure and support the patient's right to complain (DH 2006e). Patients have access to information about making a complaint and procedures, and about support services, e.g. Patient Advisory Liaison Services (PALS).
- NMPs access patient support, chaperone or advocacy services where required and act in accordance with policy when receiving complaints and feedback and take the necessary action following complaints, and seek to improve services accordingly (DH 2004a, 2006e).
- Patient feedback, surveys, user groups, etc. are used to gain information about the quality of the service and steps taken to make constant improvements. *Essence of Care* (DH 2003b) may be used to benchmark practice.

Accessible and responsive care

- Organizations involve users and carers in designing, planning and delivering services. National patient survey information, local patient surveys, PALS information, user group feedback and expert patient evidence is acted upon to shape services. Nurses are responsive to feedback and recommendations are acted upon.
- Health care organizations provide responsive care to meet the needs of patients equally (DH 2004b). This includes access to OOHs, WiCs, MIUs, NHS Direct, outreach and homeless health care teams, substance misuse services, school health services, family planning, emergency contraception, health promotion, smoke stop, mental health and counselling services, etc. (DH 2004c, 2004d).
- Patients with emergency health care needs are able to access services promptly within nationally agreed timescales (DH 2006g) and receive care commensurate with national expectations. The 4-hour target for see and treat is met, and patients have timely access to medicines.

Care environment and amenities

- A safe secure environment provided.
- NMPs uphold health and safety policy to protect patients and their property, equipment, themselves and the environment.
- The consultation areas are arranged to maintain patient privacy and allow confidentiality.
- NMPs support the organizations zero tolerance of violence to staff and patients.
- Records are stored securely.
- The health care environment is clean and well maintained.

Public health

- Health care organizations promote, protect and demonstrate improvements in the health of the community served and narrow health inequalities (DH 2003d).
- NMPs work in partnership with other services to meet the needs of the local population in meeting the needs of groups.
- Provide services to meet local targets for public health campaigns.
- Provide information, medicines and health advice and health promotion, e.g. teenage pregnancy, sexually transmitted infections, smoke stop, weight management, flu vaccine and childhood immunizations.
- Act on recommendations from the annual *Public Health Report* and support local campaigns.

- NMPs implement care according to national plans such as NSFs (e.g. coronary heart disease, diabetes, physical activity and smoking cessation), NICE guidance and locally agreed guidance on public health intervention.
- NMPs refer to others within the multidisciplinary team and work closely with social services.
- NMPs are aware of plans and actions required to meet emergency situations and incidents that affect the provision of normal services.

Activity

Read the risk management case study example and apply the information and guidelines given within this chapter to conduct an incident analysis. You may access the NPSA (2004) tools available from the website, www.npsa.nhs. uk, to aid your analysis. Then answer the questions posed and determine the best course of action.

Case Study Example

Nurse Mary Jones has worked as a staff nurse for 15 years. Today Mary is delivering the immunization programme to pupils in a local school with the school nursing sister, Sue Smith. It has been a busy morning and Mary has complained of a headache for which she had taken a simple analgesic before leaving home. The traffic is heavy on the way to the school and Mary arrives a few minutes late.

Mary checks the paperwork, the consent form for John Brown is in order, Mary checks his identity and that he is well and that the immunization is not contraindicated and proceeds to give him his immunization. She then tells John that his arm may feel a little sore for a few days. John replies that he knows all about this because he has recently changed schools and received the same immunization at his last school 3 months ago. Mary immediately tells Sue what has happened.

Now consider what actions should be taken:

- What should Mary Jones do?
- What are the responsibilities of Sue Smith?
- How may this be investigated?
- What were the contributory factors?
- What tools may be used for analysis?
- What would be the likely outcome and recommended actions?

Remember your actions should be the same in a near miss. That is, if Mary is in a position to give the immunization, with John's arm presented, when he discloses that he has had it before so Mary does not give the immunization.

Conclusion

This chapter has identified the role of the nurse in meeting the needs of the population by enabling timely access to medicines in order to prevent illness, and to promote and maintain health and wellbeing. Policy, professional guidelines, quality frameworks and strategies to manage risk have been identified as tools to enable best practice in primary care settings. Activities and practical examples have been provided to demonstrate application to practice.

References

Barat I., Andreasen F., Damsgaard E.M. (2001) Drug therapy in the elderly: what doctors believe and patients actually do. *Journal of Clinical Pharmacology* 51, 615–22.

Bates D.W., Leape L.L., Petrycki S.J. (1993) Incidence and preventability of adverse drugs events in hospitalised adults. *Journal of General Internal Medicine* 8, 289–94.

BMA (British Medical Association) (2006a) *British National Formulary*. London: RSPGB, BMA Publishing Group. www.bnfc.org.

BMA (British Medical Association) (2006b) *Healthcare Associated Infections: strategies for improvement. Improving health*. wwww.bma.org.optimaluseofantimicrobials.

BMA (British Medical Association) (2006c) *British National Formulary for Children*. London: RPSGB, BMA Publishing Group. www.bnfc.org.

Bristol Royal Infirmary Inquiry (2001) *Learning from the Bristol Royal Infirmary Inquiry. The report into the Public Inquiry into Children's Heart Surgery at Bristol Royal Infirmary 1884–1995*. London: HM Stationery Office.

Dean B., Schlatter M., Vincent C., Barber M. (2002) Causes of prescribing error: a prospective study. *Lancet*. 359, 1373–8.

DH (Department of Health) (1989) *Report of the Advisory Group on Nurse Prescribing*. London: Department of Health.

DH (Department of Health) (1994) *The Allitt Inquiry* (Clothier C. chair). London: HM Stationery Office.

DH (Department of Health) (1997a) *The New NHS: Modern, dependable*. London: HM Stationery Office.

DH (Department of Health) (1997b) *The Caldicott Committee Report*. London: HM Stationery Office.

DH (Department of Health) (1998) *A First Class Service Quality in the New NHS*. London: HM Stationery Office.

DH (Department of Health) (1999a) *Review of Prescribing Supply and Administration of Medicines*. London: Department of Health.

DH (Department of Health) (1999b) *Clinical Governance: Quality in the New NHS*. London. HMSO.

DH (Department of Health) (2000a) *The NHS Plan: a plan for investment, a plan for reform*. London: HM Stationery Office.

DH (Department of Health) (2000b) *Raising Standards for Patients. New partnerships in out of hours care departments (Carson Review)*. London: Department of Health. www.dh.gov.uk/en/Publicationsandstatistics/Publications/PublicationsPolicy andGuidance/dh_4007133 (accessed 30 Aug 2006).

DH (Department of Health) (2000c) *HSC Patient Group Directions in England*. London: Department of Health. www.dh.gov.uk/assetRoot/04/01/22/60/04012260.pdf.

DH (Department of Health) (2000d) *An Organisation with Memory: learning from an expert group from adverse events*. London: HM Stationery Office.

DH (Department of Health) (2000e) *National Service Framework for Coronary Heart Disease*. London: Department of Health.

DH (Department of Health) (2001a) *Reforming Emergency Services: first steps*. London: Department of Health.

DH (Department of Health) (2001b) *Building a Safer NHS for Patients*. London: HM Stationery Office.

DH (Department of Health) (2001c) *Seeking Consent Working with Children*. London: HM Stationery Office.

DH (Department of Health) (2002) *Liberating the Talents. Helping PCTs and nurses deliver the NHS Plan*. London: HM Stationery Office.

DH (Department of Health) (2003a) *Winning Ways: working together to reduce health care associated infections in England: report for the Chief Medical Officer*. London: Department of Health.

DH (Department of Health) (2003b) *Essence of Care: benchmarks for communication between patients, carers and health care personnel*. London: NHS Litigation Agency. http://www.cgsupport.nhs.uk/downloads/Essence_of_Care/Communication.doc.

DH (Department of Health) (2003c) *Making Amends: a consultation paper setting out proposals for reforming the approach to clinical negligence in the NHS*. London: HM Stationery Office.

DH (Department of Health) (2003d) *Tackling Inequalities: a programme for action*. London: Department of Health.

DH (Department of Health) (2003e) *Good Practice in Consent Implementation Guide: consent to examination or treatment*. London: Department of Health.

DH (Department of Health) (2003f) *Assurance Framework for Healthcare Education in England*. London: Department of Health.

DH (Department of Health) (2003g) *Nurse Prescribers' Extended Formulary*. London: Department of Health.

DH (Department of Health) (2004a) *The NHS Improvement Plan: putting people at the heart of public services*. London: HM Stationery Office.

DH (Department of Health) (2004b) *Equity and Diversity Strategy and Delivery Plan to Support the NHS*. London: Department of Health.

DH (Department of Health) (2004c) *Delivering Out-of-Hours Review. Securing proper access to medicines in the out-of-hours period*. http://www.out-of-hours.info/downloads/short_medicines_guidance.pdf.

DH (Department of Health) (2004d) *Building a Safer NHS for Patients: improving medication safety*. London: Department of Health. wwww.doh.gov.uk/buildsafenhs/medicationsafety.

DH (Department of Health) (2005) *NHS Continuing Care*. House of Commons Health Committee 6th Report. London: HM Stationery Office.

DH (Department of Health) (2006a) *Our Health, Our Care, Our Say: a new direction for community services.* London: Department of Health.

DH (Department of Health) (2006b) *New Steps to Further Improve GP Out of Hours Services.* Press release 5 May 2006, www.dh.gov.uk/publications.

DH (Department of Health) (2006c) *Improving Patients Access to Medicines. A guide to implementing nurse and pharmacist prescribing within the NHS in England.* London: Department of Health.

DH (Department of Health) (2006d) *Immunisation Against Infectious Disease: the Green Book.* London: Department of Health.

DH (Department of Health) (2006e) *Supporting Staff: improving services: guidance and support of the NHS Complaints Amendment Regulations.* London: Department of Health.

DH (Department of Health) (2006f) *Standards for Better Health. Annual Health Check 2006/7.* London: Healthcare Commission.

DH (Department of Health) (2006g) *Analysing A&E, MIU and WiC data.* London: Department of Health.

DH (Department of Health) (2006h) *Safer Management of Controlled Drugs: changes to record keeping requirements.* London: Department of Health.

DH (Department of Health), DfES (Department for Education and Skills) (2004) *National Service Framework for Children, Young People and Maternity Services. Standard 10.* London: Department of Health. www.doh.uk.

DHSS (Department of Health and Social Security) (1986) *Neighbourhood Nursing: a focus for care.* London: HM Stationery Office.

Fisher D., Burn M. (2003) Nurse diagnosed myocardial infarction: hidden nurse work and iatrogenic risk. In: *Limiting Harm in Health Care: a nursing perspective* (eds Milligan F.J., Robinson K.). Oxford: Blackwell Publishing.

Gallagher T.H., Waterman A.D., Ebers A.G., Fraser V.J., Levison W. (2003) Patients and physicians attitudes regarding disclosure of medical errors. *Journal of the American Medical Association* 289 (8), 1001–7.

Gerada C. (2006) *Guidance on Changes in the management of Controlled Drugs.* London: NHS Clinical Governance Support Team. http://www.cgsupport.nhs.uk/downloads/Primary_Care/Controlled_Drugs_Management_Changes.pdf.

Haynes R.B., McKibbon K.A., Kanani R., Brouwers M.C., Oliver T. (1997) Interventions to assist patients to follow prescriptions for medications. *The Cochrane Library* Issue 2. http://www3.interscience.wiley.com/cgi-bin/mrwhome/106568753/HOME?CRETRY=1&SRETRY=0.

Latter S., Maben J., Myall M., Courteney M., Young A., Dunn N. (2005) *An Evaluation of Extended Formulary Independent Nurse Prescribing.* Southampton: University of Southampton, Department of Health.

Marinker M., Shaw J. (2003) Not to be taken as directed: putting concordance for taking medicines into practice. *British Medical Journal* 326, 348–9.

Medicines Partnership (2003) *Project Evaluation Toolkit.* London: Medicines Partnership.

National Audit Office (2005) *A Safer Place for Patients: learning to improve patient safety.* London: HM Stationery Office.

National Audit Office (2006) *The provision of out of hours care in England: Mori out of hours patient survey.* NAO report HC1041 (2005–6) London. TSO.

National Library for Health (2004) *Protocols and Care Pathways.* http://www.library.nhs.uk/pathways/page.aspx?pagename=Icps.

Neale G., Woloshynowych M., Vincent C. (2001) Exploring the causes of adverse events in NHS hospital practice. *Journal of Research in Social Medicine* 94, 322–30.

NHS Electronic Library for Health (2006) *Patient Group Directions for Emergency Care.* http://www.library.nhs.uk/Pathways/searchResults.aspx?searchText=Patient&Group&Directions&emergency&care&pgIndex=0&.

NHS Executive (1996) *Clinical Guidelines: using guidelines to improve patient care within the NHS.* London: NHS Executive.

NHS Connecting for Health (2006) Electronic care records and prescribing. *Connecting for Health Clinical Collection* Issue 2. http://www.connectingforhealth.nhs.uk/delivery/serviceimplementation/engagement/clinical_connections_part2.pdf.

NHS Litigation Agency (2006a) *Factsheet.* http://www.nhsla.com/NR/rdonlyres/465D7ABD-239F-4273-A01E-C0CED557453D/0/NHSLAFactsheet20607.doc.

NHS Litigation Agency (2006b) *Risk Management Standard for PCTs 2006/7.* London: NHS Litigation Agency.

NICE (National Institute for Clinical Excellence) (2003) *Infection Control: prevention of healthcare associated infection in primary and community care.* http://www.nice.org.uk/page.aspx?o=CG002.

NMC (Nursing and Midwifery Council) (2004a) *Guidelines for the Administration of Medicines.* www.nmc-uk.org (accessed 16 Aug 2006).

NMC (Nursing and Midwifery Council) (2004b) *Code of Professional Conduct: standards for conduct, performance and ethics.* London: Nursing and Midwifery Council.

NMC (Nursing and Midwifery Council) (2005a) *Guidelines for Records and Record Keeping.* www.nmc-uk.org (accessed 16 Aug 2006).

NMC (Nursing and Midwifery Council) (2005b) *The Prep Handbook.* www.nmc-uk.org (accessed 16 Aug 2006).

NMC (Nursing and Midwifery Council) (2006a) *Medicines Management: advice sheet*. www.nmc-uk.org (accessed 16 Aug 2006).

NMC (Nursing and Midwifery Council) (2006b) *Standards of Proficiency for Nurse and Midwife Prescribers*. www.nmc-uk.org (accessed 16 Aug 2006).

NPC (National Prescribing Centre) (2001) *Maintaining Competency in Prescribing; an outline framework to help nurse prescribers*. Liverpool: NHS National Prescribing Centre.

NPC (National Prescribing Centre) (2003) *An Outline Framework for Supplementary Prescribers*. Liverpool: NHS, National Prescribing Centre.

NPC (National Prescribing Centre) (2004) *Patient Group Directions. A practical guide and framework of competencies for all professionals using PGDs*. Liverpool: NHS, National Prescribing Centre. npcetc.co.uk/publications/pgd/outline-framework.doc.

NPSA (National Patient Safety Agency) (2004) *Seven Steps to Patient Safety*. London: National Patient Safety Agency.

NPSA (National Patient Safety Agency) (2005a) *Ensuring Safer Practice with Repevax and Revaxis. MHRA Safer Practice Notice (07) 29 April 2005*. London: National Patient Safety Agency. www.npsa.nhs.uk

NPSA (National Patient Safety Agency) (2005b) *Being Open: communicating patient safety incidents with patients and their carers*. London: National Patient Safety Agency.

NPSA (National Patient Safety Agency) (2006a) *Seven Steps to Patient Safety for Primary Care*. London: National Patient Safety Agency.

NPSA (National Patient Safety Agency) (2006b) *Assuring Patient Safety through Risk Assessment: a guide to assist commissioners of out of hours service*. London: National Patient Safety Agency. http://www.saferhealthcare.org.uk/NR/rdonlyres/639CB556-2888-4515-BCF7-241195BE1111/0/PatientSafetyForOOHThroughRiskAssessment.pdf.

Pearce P. (2005) Review of the National Service Framework for coronary heart disease: a whole systems approach. *Clinical Governance Bulletin* 6 (1), 11–12.

Reason J. (2000*)* Human error: models and management. *British Medical Journal* 320, 768–70.

Roberts D.E., Spencer M.G., Burfield R., Bowden S. (2002) An analysis of dispensing errors in UK hospitals. *International Journal of Pharmacology Practice* 10 (Suppl. R6).

Robinson P., Potter C. (2006) The national perspective from the Department of Health. *Connecting Prescribers: National Prescribing Centre* 4, 3.

Ross R. (1994) The five whys perspective. In: *The Fifth Discipline Fieldbook: strategies and tools for building a learning organization* (eds Senge P., Kleiner A., Roberts C.). New York: Doubleday.

Royal Pharmaceutical Society (2005) *Nurse Prescribers' Formulary for Community Practioners (2005–2007)*. London: Royal Pharmaceutical Society.

Royal Pharmaceutical Society (2006) *Moving Patients' Medicines Safely: discharge and transfer planning book*. London: Royal Pharmaceutical Society.

Sale D. (2005) *Understanding Clinical Governance and Quality Assurance. Making it happen*. London: Palgrave.

Sexton J.B., Thomas E.J., Helmreich R.L. (2000) Error stress and teamwork in medicine and aviation. *British Medical Journal* 320 (7237), 745–9.

Sharpe V.A., Faden A.I. (1998) *Medical Harm: historic, conceptual, ethical dimensions of iatrogenic illness*. Cambridge: Cambridge University Press.

Smith J. (2004) *The Shipman Inquiry 4th Report, Regulations of Controlled Drugs*. Norwich: HM Stationery Office.

St Helens PCT (2004) *St Helens Patient Group Directions*. www.portal.nelm.nhs.uk-NELM-PGD.

Swage T. (2004) Quality initiatives the process of clinical effectiveness. In: *Clinical Governance in Healthcare Practice* (ed. Swage T.). London: Butterworth Heinmann.

Vermiere E., Hearnshaw H., Van Royen P., Denekens J. (2001) Patient adherence to treatment: three decades of research. A comprehensive review. *Journal of Clinical Pharmacy and Therapeutics* 26, 331–42.

Vincent C.A., Coulter A. (2002) Patient safety: what about the patient? *Quality and Safety in Health Care* 11 (1), 76–80.

Wilson J.H. (1994) Quality in clinical care: healthcare risk modification. *Health Business Summary* April.

Wilson J.H. (1999) Risk review and using a clinical risk strategy. In: *Clinical Risk Modification: a route to clinical governance?* (eds Wilson J., Tingle J.). Oxford: Butterworth Heinemann.

Woodward S. (2006) Learning and sharing safety lessons to improve patient care. *Nursing Standard* 20 (18), 49–53.

Appendix 12.1 Patient Group Direction (PGD) for the Supply and Administration of Pneumococcal Conjugate Vaccine (PCV) by Registered Nurses

Direction no:

Developed and produced by:	Name	Signature	Date
Senior Pharmacist			
Senior Nurse			
Doctor			

Adopted on........................

Review date.......................

To be reviewed by...............

Authorised by	Name	Signature	Date
Director of Clinical Development			
Chair, Executive Committee			
Pharmaceutical Adviser			

This PGD has been approved for use within.......................................Practice

Signed: Senior Partner (on behalf of the employer) ....

1. Clinical condition or situation to which the direction applies

Indication	For active immunization against invasive disease (including sepsis, meningitis, bacteraemic pneumonia, bacteraemia) caused by *Streptococcus pneumoniae* serotype 4, 6B, 9V, 14, 18C, 19F and 23F
Criteria for inclusion	Previously unvaccinated children aged from 2 months and under 2 years of age where: • parent/guardian consent has been given to receive the vaccine • as a primary course of PCV at 2 and 4 months of age with a booster dose at 13 months of age • as a catch-up programme for children born between: 04.02.06 and 03.07.06: two doses separated by 2 months with a booster at 13 months of age • 04.08.05 and 03.02.06: a single dose at 13 months of age • 05.09.04 and 03.08.05: a single dose
Criteria for exclusion	The vaccine should not be given to: • those who have had a confirmed anaphylactic reaction to a previous dose of PCV • those who have had a confirmed anaphylactic reaction to any component • those who have had a confirmed anaphylactic reaction to diphtheria toxoid • no valid consent has been given
Action if excluded	Specialist advice must be sought on the vaccine and circumstances under which the vaccine could be given. The risk to the individual of not being immunised must be taken into account
Action if patient declines treatment	Advise about the protective effects of the vaccine and the risks of infection, diseases and complications. Document advice given and decision reached. Inform or refer to GP as appropriate
Reference to national/local policies or guidelines	Department of Health (2006): *Immunisation against Infectious Disease* Current edition of *British National Formulary* Manufacturer's Summary of Product Characteristics (SPC) NMC (2006) *Medicines management* NMC (2004) *Code of Professional Conduct: standards for conduct, performance and ethics*

2. Description of treatment

Name, strength and formulation of drug	Adsorbed pneumococcal conjugate vaccine (PCV – Prevenar) suspension for injection in pre-filled syringe
Legal status	POM (prescription only medicine)
Dose/dose range	0.5 ml
Method/route	Prevenar is routinely administered by intramuscular injection

Vaccination by deep subcutaneous route should be reserved **only** for individuals with a bleeding disorder.

NB. Shake the vaccine well immediately before administration |
| **Frequency of administration** | A primary course of three doses to be administered at 2 months 4 months and 13 months

Infants aged 7–11 months: two doses separated by 2 months with a booster dose at 13 months of age

Children aged 8–13 months: a single dose at 13 months of age

Children aged 13 months to 2 years of age: a single dose |
| **Patient advice and follow-up treatment** | Inform of possible side effects and their management. Give advice on temperature control

Provide a patient information leaflet (supplied with the pack) |
| **Identification and management of adverse reactions** | Local reactions (pain, erythema, induration and oedema) following vaccination |
| **Reporting procedure of adverse reactions** | Any serious adverse reaction to the vaccine should be documented in a child's health records and on their medical records. GP should also be informed

Vaccines: any adverse events that may be attributable to PCV should be reported to the CHM using the yellow card system (www.yellowcard.gov.uk) |
| **Additional facilities** | Immediate access to epinephrine (adrenaline) 1 in 1000 injection |
| **Special considerations/ additional information** | Vaccine should be stored in the original packaging at a temperature of 2–8 °C. If the vaccine has been frozen, it should be discarded. Disposal should be by incineration. PCV should only be used as a primary immunization course in children from 2 months and under 2 years of age. Although PCV conjugate can be given at the same time as other vaccines, including MMR vaccination, it cannot be |

	given at the same time as Hib/MenC. If administered at the same time as other vaccines, it should be at a different injection site, preferably different limbs. If given in the same limb, they should be given at least 2.5 cm apart. PCV conjugate vaccine should be administered via the intramuscular route except where there is a bleeding disorder, when the deep subcutaneous route should be used
Records	Manual records including the personal held child record (PHCR – red book), computerised records and data collection for Child Health Information Services (CHIS) should include: patient's name and date of birth; dose, site and route of injection; brand, batch number and expiry date of vaccine; date given and by whom A computer or manual record of all individuals receiving immunization with combined diphtheria/tetanus/pertussis/polio vaccine under this PGD should be kept for audit purposes within each practice

3. Characteristics of staff

Qualifications required	Registered Nurse
Additional requirements	Competent to undertake immunizations Resuscitation skills and anaphylaxis training
Continued training requirements	Annual attendance at the PCT/ practice update on resuscitation skills and the management of anaphylaxis within the community Maintenance of own level of updating with evidence of continued professional development (PREP requirements)

*** The part below to be used for a single authorised nurse

This PGD is to be read, agreed to and signed by all registered nurses it applies to.

One copy will be retained by the nurse. The original signed copy will be retained by the nominated GP with responsibility for PGDs within the practice.

I confirm that I have read and understood the content of this PGD and that I am willing and competent to work under it within my professional code of conduct **Name of authorised nurse**.. **Signature of authorised nurse**..

Date signed ....

Name of GP responsible for

PGD..

Signature of GP..

Date signed ....

**Final page to be used where multiple staff are authorised within the practice area, e.g. walk in centre

PGDs DO NOT REMOVE INHERENT PROFESSIONAL OBLIGATIONS OR ACCOUNTABILITY.

It is the responsibility of each professional to practice only within the bounds of their own competence and in accordance with the NMC code of professional conduct.

Note to Authorising Managers: authorised staff should be provided with an individual copy of the clinical content of the PGD and a photocopy of the document showing their authorization.

I have read and understood the PGD and agree to supply/administer this medicine only in accordance with this PGD.

Name of professional	Signature	Authorising manager	Date

CHM, Commission on Human Medicines; MMR, measles, mumps and rubella;
NMC, Nursing and midwifery council;
PCT, Primary care trust;
PREP, Post-registration education and practice.

CHAPTER 13

Quality and Risk Management: Safeguarding Children and Vulnerable Groups

Wendy Wigley

Public Health Skill: Quality frameworks and risk management

- Quality and risk management: safeguarding children and working with vulneralble groups
- Assessment frameworks for quality: defining risk, risk assessment and management, managing risk to personal safety (lone worker) and working with vulnerable children and their families
- Frameworks for the assessment of need and risk: the assessment framework (DH *et al.* 2000), common assessment framework, working in areas of deprivation and poverty as a practitioner (Sure Start, supporting families) and evaluation of public health initiatives

Introduction

This chapter will explore the concept of risk and risk management in relation to vulnerable children, young people and their families. Consideration will be given to the nature of risk within modern society and the responsibilities of the public health nurse in safeguarding vulnerable groups. The chapter will examine the process of the identification, assessment and effective management of vulnerable groups and the impact of this on lone workers, in particular their personal safety. Finally, the chapter will discuss frameworks and strategies within health and social care provision that aim to minimise risk to vulnerable children, young people and their families and the evaluation of these strategies.

13.1 Defining Risk

What is *risk* and where does it come from? Plough and Krimsky (1987) suggested that the profession-alization of risk is a relatively new concept, which is born out of medical concerns for the health and social welfare of populations in the 18th century. The notion of risk was aimed at communicating formal health and safety interventions, such as the dangers of drinking unclean water and the need for a reduction in infectious diseases. They also suggested that a further formalization of risk emerged during World War II (1939–1945) when governments required scientifically based decision methodologies in order to understand chance processes and inform strategic military decisions (Plough & Krimsky 1987). The emergence of the assessment of risk can therefore be viewed as having roots in 18th century public health and the decision methodologies of war. In today's society these concepts relate more to

'A systematic way of dealing with hazards and insecurities induced by modernisation itself' (Beck 2002, p. 19). It could be argued that risk is intrinsic to the human condition and that throughout evolution the human race has had to adapt to, and assess, risk in order to survive (Plough & Krimsky 1987).

Risk in modern health and social care is a complex concept to define. The *Concise Oxford English Dictionary* (2006) describes the noun 'risk' as a situation involving exposure to danger; the possibility that something unpleasant will happen. Yet the *Collins Reference Thesaurus* (1993) suggests that the terminology of risk might also include 'chance'. Chance denotes an unpredictable course of events (*Concise Oxford English Dictionary* 2006), so for public health nurses the question is how to manage risk and chance? The nature of exposure to danger with risk-taking behaviours indicates there is no set pattern to behaviours and as a consequence risk is difficult to manage, as the notion of risk means different things to different people (Lucas & Lloyd 2005).

Case Study Example

Mark chooses to engage in action sports; he is at his happiest and most fulfilled when he is hurtling down a muddy precipice on his mountain bike into the unknown, yet has never contemplated smoking a cigarette because of the risks to his health. George, on the other hand, is terrified by the thought of dangerous off-road mountain biking and yet in his youth chose to smoke the occasional cigarette despite being professionally aware of the consequences to his health. What is the difference between these two behaviours?

The answer is that for Mark, participating in such dangerous activities, 'the risk is the actual point!' (Lucas & Lloyd 2005, p. 112).

A lifestyle and behaviour change model of health promotion (Naidoo & Wills 2000) would encourage people to take responsibility for there own health behaviour by choosing not to participate in risk-taking behaviour. For many people, they smoke because their peers smoke; it is 'the social norm' for the group of people they associate with and part of their group identity and desired image (Lucas & Lloyd 2005). They participate in this behaviour despite being informed and aware of the risks to their health.

Activity

Think about how risk can be managed effectively if, as Lucas and Lloyd (2005, p. 111) advise, 'To assume that individuals can be motivated to change their behaviour is naïve and simplistic, particularly if the chance of risk taking behaviours is indeed driven by personal choice.'

13.2   Risk/Need Assessment versus Risk Management

The writing of Ruckelshaus (1985) is largely focused upon the environmental risks of hazardous and toxic pollutants in the USA. He makes a distinction between *risk assessment* and *risk management* which when applied to the context of risk within the practice of public health nursing provides a useful parallel of risk assessment and risk management with clients. Ruckelshaus (1985, p. 28) suggests that:

> Risk assessment is an exercise that combines available data on a substance's potency [read: poor housing, substance misuse, or domestic abuse] in causing adverse health affects, with information about likely human exposure; and through the use of plausible assumptions, it generates an estimate of human health risk. Risk management is the process by which a protective agency [read: public health nurse] decides what action to take in the face of such estimates.

Therefore, for the public health nurse, risk assessment and risk management are key aspects of their protective role. Considering situations from which risk may evolve will help to set the context for the public health activity. The assessment and management of risk is key to ensuring protection of the vulnerable client or group.

The traditional bureaucratic mechanisms of the internal market of the early 1990s, based upon the needs of individuals, were challenged by the Labour administration in 1997 as they attempted to develop a 'Third way' of reform, different from both the internal market of past Conservative governments and the application of centralised planning by previous Labour governments. This heralded a shift from a needs-led welfare society to a risk-led society where the political philosophy of the 'Third way' is a mixture of social democracy and new right neo-liberalism. Kemshall (2002, p. 133) identifies five key strands in the 'Third way' as:

> social responsibility and obligations, the use of the labour market to achieve social justice, emphasis upon meritocracy [personal ability], residual welfare and targeting, and modernization.

The reason these political ideologies are so important to the public health nurse, is in how people are encouraged to view their health. These political ideologies view individuals as socially obliged and socially responsible, and, as such, are encouraged to take responsibility for 'risk management' within their own lives. Any deficit or 'need' is met by state provision; welfare is provided but is targeted by policy, thus state responsibility for risk management is reduced (Kemshall 2002).

Within this context risk management is clearly influenced by political thinking as identified by Ruckelshaus (1985). Risk management can be viewed as:

> the distribution of current resources to shape some desirable state; risk management at its broadest sense means adjusting our environmental policies to obtain an array of social goods – environmental, health related, economic, and psychological – that forms our vision of how we want the world to be. (Ruckelshaus 1985, p. 31)

What Ruckelshaus is saying is that risk management touches all areas of modern Western society; for risk management to be practical and effective it needs to be flexible, grounded in evidence (factual data determining that a negative outcome will occur if the risk is not addressed), supported by realistic governmental policy, and accepted by the public and those individuals who are identified as subject to risk.

Securing Good Health for the Whole Population (Wanless 2004), written 19 years later, would seem to reflect the Ruckelshaus (1985) definition and ideology, recognizing that although ultimately individuals are responsible for their own health and that of their children, it is the shared responsibility of the society in which we live (private sector, employers, media, voluntary and community sectors) to ensure that risks to individuals and the wider population are identified and minimised.

The publication of the Wanless (2004) report was followed by the governmental White Paper *Choosing Health: making healthier choices easier* (DH 2004). This paper describes an abundance of governmental reforms that aim to improve the long-term health of the population by increasing 'individual choice'. The paper outlines initiatives that are aimed at all of us and are designed to reflect the recommendations made by Wanless (2004) to 'fully engage' the public in their health. Both the Wanless (2004) report and *Choosing Health* (DH 2004) acknowledge that some vulnerable individuals in society – such as young children, those with severe mental health issues or suffering from certain learning disabilities – may lack the 'capacity' to make good decisions and choices regarding their health. Wanless (2004) recognised that individuals who experience high levels of stress and social inequality may struggle to access adequate resources and information to make healthy choices. *Choosing Health* (DH 2004) further recognises that vulnerable groups and individuals within our society have little or no 'choice' as to how to improve their health and social wellbeing, or that the 'choices' made by some individuals in society can have serious consequences for others, especially children.

Activity

Ask yourself what does the difference between need and risk mean for the public health nurse?

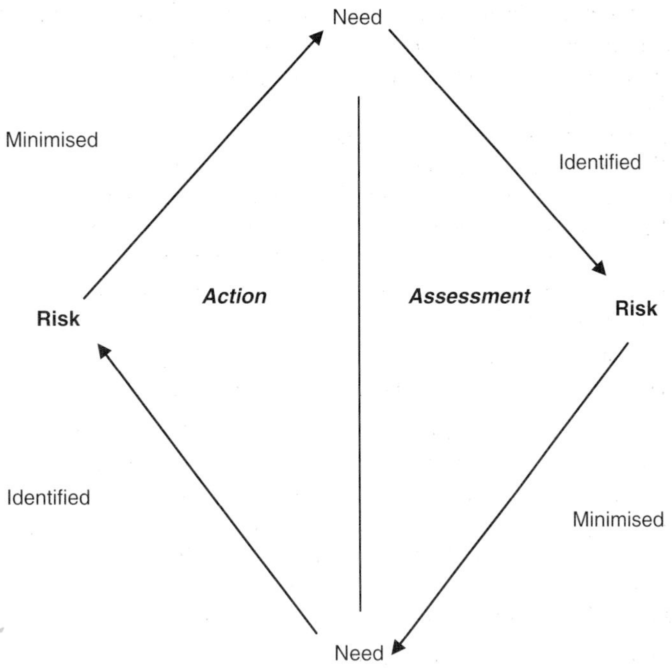

Figure 13.1   The need–risk cycle.

As public health nurses, we need to ask whether we are assessing need or risk and what the difference is between these two concepts. Section 8 of the NMC's *Code of Professional Conduct: standards for conduct, performance and ethics* (NMC 2004, p. 9) states that: 'As a registered nurse, midwife or specialist community public health nurse, you must act to identify and minimise the risks to patients and clients'. Vulnerable individuals who are unable to effectively manage risks to their own health are the ones who may require the public health nurse to act as an advocate on their behalf and, in doing so, take on the accountability of risk management.

Although not as far reaching as the Ruckelshaus (1985) definition, this type of risk management of vulnerable groups and individuals within a population is a cyclical process (Figure 13.1) and involves the assessment of negative and protective factors within an individual's health, behavioural, social and environmental culture. The public health nurse should then decide upon a course of action that ensures equity and access to services that offer environmental, health-related, economic, psychological and social support in order that need is identified and the risks from danger, abuse and harm to vulnerable groups and individuals can be minimised.

13.3   Vulnerability and the Vulnerable Child

Children are especially vulnerable to risk within many life experiences. Vulnerable children are identified by Hall and Elliman (2003, p. 346) as:

> Children with disabilities and children whose physical safety or emotional, cognitive and language development is being adversely affected by their environmental circumstances.

Such groups would include those clients identified in Box 13.1.

In addition to being included in one or more of the above, these vulnerable children may live with vulnerable parents or carers who are themselves considered vulnerable due to their own complex needs (Box 13.2). Identifying and then building a relationship with such families can be problematic and requires time, professional competency, patience and skill.

BOX 13.1

Vulnerable children as identified by Hall and Elliman (2003).

- Children with disabilities
- Children with special learning needs
- Children who are homeless, refugees, asylum seekers or members of a travelling community
- Children who live in poverty or on the edge of poverty and because of this have limited access to health care
- Children who are carers for sick parent(s) or other siblings
- Abused or neglected children
- Children looked after by a local authority
- Children being fostered or awaiting adoption

BOX 13.2

Examples of complex needs affecting vulnerable parents and carers.

- Parents/carers involved with prostitution
- Parents/carers who misuse drugs and alcohol
- Parents/carers who experience or are perpetrators of domestic violence or abuse
- Parents/carers who are socially isolated, with a limited supportive network of family and friends
- Parents/carers who experience mental health problems and have altered life perspectives
- Parents/carers who have learning difficulties
- Parents/carers who are disabled or experience poor health
- Parents/carers who withdraw from engagement with professionals

---

13.4   Managing Risks to Personal Safety: The Lone Worker

Because of the nature of their work, public health nurses often work and visit clients alone and are in a position of being accepted into the clients' home. However, working and visiting alone increases the vulnerability of the practitioner (Mayhew & Chappell 2001). In engaging with vulnerable families it is important to undertake what has been described as *entry work* (Luker & Chalmers 1990). Entry work is key to building a professional relationship and should aim to be objective and perceptive of the family's circumstances and should aim to inform and raise awareness of the services available to support vulnerable clients and their families.

In the initial stages of building a professional relationship with vulnerable families, it may be necessary to undertake what are commonly described as 'joint visits' with another colleague. This is especially important if the family is known to be potentially violent and/or abusive; ideally, no nurse should undertake any visit alone unless they have some information regarding the family's history or background. Many vulnerable families have had negative experiences involving health, social care and legislative systems and will be deeply suspicious of anyone perceived to be in 'authority' (Marcellus 2005).

The dangers of being subject to violence or attack when working alone have been well documented (Lamplugh *et al.* 1993; Lamplugh 1999). For example, in July 1986, during lunchtime, Suzy Lamplugh – an estate agent – was seen with a client leaving a property she was trying to sell. She was never seen again. Much evidence exists to suggest that experienced nurses have traditionally relied upon intuitive knowledge, particularly when making decisions about patient care and the needs of their client group (Neligan *et al.* 1974; Benner 1982; Chalmers 1993). However, as far as personal safety is concerned, practitioners may not use intuition as effectively. Diana Lamplugh (1999) suspected that her daughter Suzy had numerous different intuitive warning signals that the situation in to which she was entering might be dangerous but that she chose to ignore them – possibly because she was determined to prove that she could cope with her workload and as a result became less vigilant about her own safety.

Lamplugh *et al.* (1993) suggest that this is a common feature of the lone worker. They found that lone workers appear to be less concerned with the dangers of serious incidents to themselves than to their colleagues, often recalling reports of colleagues who have experienced dangerous incidents while at work. All employers within health and social care agencies should adopt a 'zero tolerance' policy with regard to violence and must provide clear procedures and guidance, education and training for all employees with regard to personal safety (National Audit Office 2003; Health and Safety Executive 2006). In addition, the *Code of Professional Conduct* (NMC 2004) places a responsibility on registrants to practice competently and safely, within the limitations of their practice (clause 6, NMC 2004). Therefore it is the responsibility of public health nurses to ensure that they are fully aware of the risks to their own and their colleagues' personal safety when visiting alone.

Clarke (1999) suggests that it is the responsibility of the employer to provide all reasonable protection, such as two-way radios or mobile phones. Ideally, practitioners should always carry a mobile phone so that they can either be text messaged or phoned by colleagues at the time the visit was expected to end, or to enable the practitioner to text or phone their colleagues when they have safely left the visit. However, some agencies for reasons of cost and funding do not provide mobile phones to their staff; in such situations the practitioner should leave clear information as to the address they are visiting, the purpose of their visit, the time of the visit, the estimated duration of the visit, and the expected time of return to office or base so that should they not return, colleagues can take appropriate action.

13.5   Vulnerable Children and their Families: The Work of the Public Health Nurse

It is not the role of the public health nurse to 'police' children, young people and their families in the identification of risk or vulnerability. However, the public health nurse has a 'duty of care' (clause 1.4, NMC 2004) and must also 'promote the interest of patients and clients' (clause 2.4, NMC 2004). This places a duty on the practitioner to safeguard vulnerable groups, which includes the protection of children 'in accordance with national and local policies' (clause 5.4, NMC 2004). In addition, section 175 of the Education Act 2002 and section 11 of the Children Act 2004 place duties on organizations and the individual to include the need to safeguard and protect the welfare of children.

Nurses working within a public health context will encounter vulnerable children and their families. Identification of the vulnerable child and their family is a complex process and to some extent may involve professional intuition (Benner 1982). However, the needs of such children and their families are far better served if this identification is based upon a sound professional judgement that is formulated through open and thorough assessment, undertaken in partnership with the client and that considers the client's previous history, the health and social care needs of the particular client group, and the prevailing needs of the community in which they live (DH *et al.* 2000).

The importance of comprehensive needs assessment is to minimise the risk to vulnerable children by ensuring the child, young person and their family have their health and social needs addressed by accessing appropriate services and professionals (DH *et al.* 2000). Some circumstances or events within the day to day lives of children and their families will necessitate a referral to local authority Children and Families Services (Social Services). Examples of such circumstances are shown in Box 13.3. Such circumstances are occasionally, but unlikely to be, an isolated event or crisis and are usually associated with other long-term issues and historical, familiar risk-taking behavioural patterns. Therefore, a comprehensive quality assessment process that enables the identification and communication of need is essential in the identification of such risks. All agencies (statutory and voluntary) and professionals involved with children, young people and their families are required to share information when risk is identified, and this commitment overrules any duty of confidentiality (Beckett 2005).

Section 4

BOX 13.3

Examples of circumstances or events within the day to day lives of children and their families that could necessitate a referral to Social Services.

- Domestic abuse or violence
- Frequent unexplained injury and/or accidents
- Persistent non-attendance for health appointments
- Persistent non-attendance at school
- A slowing or failure in growth and developmental progress in the absence of diagnosed disability
- Persistently inappropriately clothed and/or unclean child
- Persistent failure of the designated parent/carer to respond to the needs of a growing child
- Persistently left unsupervised or to care for other siblings
- Exposure, association and engagement with criminality, e.g. drugs and prostitution
- Unstable and unsupported mental health of parents or carers

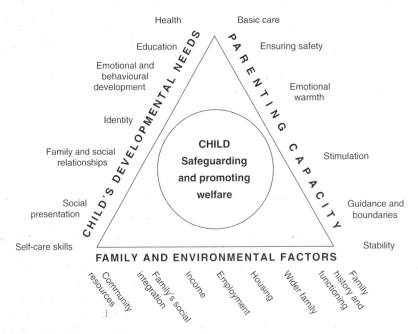

Figure 13.2   The assessment framework. *Source*: DH *et al.* (2000).

13.6   Frameworks for the Assessment of Need and Risk

The assessment processes used by health and social care professionals working with children, young people and their families are in general based upon the *Framework for the Assessment of Children and their Families* (DH *et al.* 2000) (Figure 13.2). This framework,

> provides a systematic way of analysing, understanding and recording what is happening to children and young people within the their families and the wider context of the community in which they live. (DH *et al.* 2000, p. viii)

Although frequently utilised by social workers in order to carry out a comprehensive and holistic assessment of a child's needs (Beckett 2005), the framework is also intended as guidance for professionals and other staff who will work in partnership with social workers, general practitioners and teachers in the assessment process of children in need and their families (DH *et al.* 2000). However, the framework should not be used as a 'checklist' approach to needs assessment. Several studies (Saunders 2001; Houston & Cowley 2002) acknowledge that any needs assessment should incorporate a client-centred, open and listening empowerment approach. It is essential that the public health nurse is aware that the use of such an approach is fundamental to establishing a trusting professional relationship with clients, even if the use of such an approach results in an initial assessment being carried out over several client contacts. It is also crucial that the assessment involves professional judgement and does not focus solely on the negative aspects of a family's circumstance, but rather seeks to identify the protective aspects of the family and the positive health-related practices that are 'embedded' in their everyday life and/or culture. A view supported by Christensen (2004) suggests that in promoting child and family health the professional should move away from labelling the 'problem family' – which serves no useful or constructive purpose for service provision, the professional or, indeed, the family.

In order to overcome any client perception of paternalism, the framework has been successfully adapted, implemented and integrated within the personal child health record (PCHR) by some children and families services throughout the country. It is used by public health nurses in partnership with the client alongside locally devised complementary tools that may contain 'trigger questions' (Saunders 2001) or 'a field of words' (Houston & Cowley 2002). Such tools allow the client, not the professional, to consider the client's own needs and as such are objective in nature and can facilitate client under-standing of, and contribution to, the assessment process. The inclusion of the assessment framework and supportive tools within the PHCR enables public health practitioners to assess, in *partnership* with their client, the health and social needs of the child and family and to ensure that clients are aware of, are offered, and have access to interventions and services that will be beneficial, supportive and promote their health and social wellbeing.

Activity

Revisit Chapter 6 and read a more detailed discussion on this aspect of work.

The principles underpinning the assessment framework (DH *et al.* 2000) can be used to inform the assessment process (Box 13.4). Within the context of public health these can also be used to consider the provision of coordinated and locally determined supportive public health services and interventions available within a community for vulnerable children and their families. It is important for public health nurses to remember that for a variety of reasons, including disruption in their lives, some vulnerable children and their families may have been reluctant or unable to access such services. Therefore, the role of the public health nurse is to work in partnership with such children, their families and other statutory and voluntary agencies in the identification, assessment, planning and subsequent engagement of families with the services and interventions, examples of which are illustrated in Table 13.1.

BOX 13.4

Principles underpinning the assessment process. *Source*: DH *et al.* (2000, p. 10)

- Child centred
- Rooted in child development
- Ecological in their approach
- Ensure quality and opportunity
- Involve working with children and families
- Build on strengths as well as identifing difficulties
- Interagency in their approach to assessment and the provision of services
- A continuing processes, not a single event
- Carried out in parallel with other actions and providing services are grounded in evidence-based knowledge

Table 13.1   Working in partnership.

Child's developmental needs	Illustrative public health supportive services/interventions
Health includes: • Growth and development • Physical and mental wellbeing • Receiving appropriate health care • Adequate nutritious diet • Exercise, immunization, developmental screening, optical care • Advice and information on sexual health and substance misuse	• Child health/well child clinics • Home visiting • Parenting groups • Parent and baby groups • Immunizations clinics/well child clinics • Connexions • Personal and social education (school) • Oral health educators • Speech and language therapy
Education includes: • Play and interaction with peers • Access to books • Acquiring a range of skills and interests • Experiencing success and achievement • An adult interested in the above • Recognition of special needs	• Child health clinics • Home visiting • Parenting groups • Parent and baby groups • Library initiatives: rhyme time, family literacy • Parent and toddler groups • Youth groups • Connexions
Emotional and behavioural development includes: • Appropriateness of response to parents and caregivers • Nature and quality of attachments • Temperament • Adaptation to change • Response to stress • Appropriate self-control	• Child health clinics • Home visiting • Parenting groups • Behaviour specialists • Parent and baby groups
Identity includes: • Sense of self and valued person • Abilities • Self-image and esteem • Individuality • Race • Religion • Gender • Sexuality • Disability • Belonging and acceptance	• Child health clinics • Home visiting • Parenting groups • Parent and baby groups • Connexions • Personal and social education (school)
Family and social relationships include: • Capacity for empathy • Stable and affectionate relationship with caregivers/parents/siblings • Age-appropriate friendships with peers • Appropriate parental response to above	• Child health clinics • Home visiting • Parenting groups • Parent and baby/toddler groups • Connexions • Breakfast clubs • After-school clubs

(Continued)

Table 13.1 **(Continued)**

Child's developmental needs	Illustrative public health supportive services/interventions
Social presentation includes: • Appropriateness of dress for age, gender, culture and religion • Cleanliness and personal hygiene • Availability of advice from parents/caregivers	• Child health clinics • Home visiting • Parenting groups • Personal and social education (school)
Self-care skills includes: • Acquisition of competences: practical, emotional, and communication for independence • Dressing and feeding • Independent living skills • Social problem solving	• Child health clinics • Home visiting • Parenting groups • Personal and social education (school) • Speech and language therapy

The assessment framework (DH *et al.* 2000), however, has not been without criticism. Morrison (2000, p. 365) expressed concern that the framework did not provide 'any formal multi-disciplinary framework for the management of complex and high risk "children in need" cases which are on the cusp or being diverted away from, the child protection process …'. Morrison's opinion was that the policy document did not consider children in 'true' need in any depth or provide good guidance as to how to achieve a needs-led family support approach to protecting children by any method other than a formal child protection process. Morrison's further concern was that the bureaucracy and complexities within individual agencies would impact on the internal management of staff and consequently the collaboration of staff across agencies.

It would seem that Morrison's concerns were justified; in February 2000 Victoria Climbie, aged 8, died. Her death was the result of systematic abuse by her carers, who were later convicted of murder in 2001. The subsequent inquiry into the circumstances of Victoria's death, led by Lord Laming in 2003 identified that there had been a complete lack of interagency communication and sharing of information by the numerous agencies – including health, social care, police and housing – that had all come into contact with Victoria and her family in the months prior to her death (Lord Laming 2003). The inquiry made many recommendations, most of which centred on the need for improved interagency training, communication, collaboration and integration.

As a result of the Climbie Inquiry (Lord Laming 2003), the policy approach by the government could be described as one of 'social change' (Naidoo & Wills 2000), a top-down process, targeted towards children, young people and their families and requiring commitment at the upper management level with the aim of addressing the inequalities experienced by vulnerable groups within this section of the population. This approach involved the publication of a plethora of documents, all aimed at streamlining children's services in order to improve the outcomes for children and young people. The key document that was to transform service provision in response to the Climbie Inquiry (Lord Laming 2003) was the Green Paper *Every Child Matters* (DfES 2003). In 2004 the Children Act was introduced by the government to provide the legislative underpinning foundation that has enabled the implementation of the policy document *Every Child Matters: change for children* (DfES 2004). This policy document is the key to a 'whole systems reform' of children's services and the provision of children's health and social care. Wellbeing is the term used in the Children Act 2004 to define the five 'Every child matters' outcomes, which were based on consultation with children and young people to determine 'what children want' and in turn form the basis of the 'Every child matters' programme. These five outcomes are listed in Box 13.5.

Section 10 of the Children Act 2004 provides statutory guidance on the 'duty to cooperate' by interagency collaboration that will bring together public, private and voluntary services working with children, young people and their families to improve the wellbeing of children. The Children Act 2004

BOX 13.5

Every Child Matters **(DfES 2003): the five outcomes.**

- *Being healthy*: enjoying good physical and mental health and living a healthy lifestyle
- *Staying safe*: being protected from harm and abuse
- *Enjoying and achieving*: getting the most out of life and developing the skills for adulthood
- *Making a positive contribution*: being involved with the community and society and not engaging in antisocial or offending behaviour
- *Economic wellbeing*: not being prevented by economic disadvantage from achieving one's full potential

---

provides the reinforcing framework for Children's Trusts, to be in place nationally by 2008 and will transform the way in which services for children and their families are delivered. The integration of services, systems and processes in the identification and subsequent effective meeting of the needs of children and their families is the key principle of *Every Child Matters*. As a result of these policy reforms, many local services across the country have begun to consider the introduction of a new tool and process for the assessment of children in need, known as the *common assessment framework* (CAF).

Activity

Revisit Chapter 1 and read about the introduction of the common assessment framework as a tool in the assessment of children.

13.7   Common Assessment Framework

The CAF is a standardised assessment process designed to be implemented and used across public, private and voluntary sectors by anyone working with children, as soon as any concern is identified. The CAF recognises that the identified needs of children and young people lie along a continuum that will range from children with no additional needs, through to children identified as having additional needs and, in some identified cases, children with complex needs. The 'Every child matters' programme recognises that children and their families should be supported by flexible and responsive health, social care and educational service provision, which will become increasingly targeted and specialised as the identified needs become more complex (DfES 2006a).

The CAF will enable practitioners to make an assessment and act upon the outcome of the assessment using a standardised format to record the assessment process, and where appropriate share information with others. This process will also involve the completion of a pre-assessment checklist in order to establish if the child would benefit from a more detailed assessment using the assessment framework (DH *et al.* 2000) (see Figure 13.2), which will still be applicable and utilised to inform in-depth and complex child safeguarding and child protection assessment and processes.

It is hoped that the benefits of the CAF will be that children, young people and their families need not be subjected to the potentially distressing and time-consuming process of providing the same information to a variety of workers from various agencies (DfES 2006a). Once a CAF has been completed and identifies that a child may need integrated support from a variety of agencies, a lead professional will be nominated. This decision will usually be made as part of an initial multiagency team meeting. Any individual who works with the child and family can be nominated as lead professional, regardless of role title or seniority, and may not necessarily be the person who carried out the CAF. The lead professional's role is to coordinate and create partnerships, not only with colleagues and other professionals but also with the child, young person and their family, to ensure that effective support is actioned, properly planned and reviewed and to prevent any overlap and inconsistency of service provision. Most importantly, the lead professional will be a single point of contact providing children, young people and their families with a trusted individual with whom they can communicate and share information (DfES 2006a).

In September 2006 *Working Together to Safeguard Children* (DH *et al*. 1999) was revisited (HM Government 2006) and updated by the government in the light of the Children Act 2004 and *Every Child Matters* (DfES 2003). This updated guide to interagency working to safeguard and promote the welfare of children, is more far reaching and comprehensive than its 1999 predecessor and recognises the need for a truly integrated approach in supporting children, young people and their families with the many complexities and risks of living in the 21st century.

As previously stated, an *integrated service* is the gold standard, best practice method of multiagency working. An integrated service involves different providers, such as health and education, working together from a central building that is highly visible to the community – such as schools, nurseries, community centres and, in some areas, places of worship. Integrated services are funded and managed by partner organizations such as local government, local authorities and health to ensure the effective joining of children's services. Examples of such provision are Sure Start Children's Centres and Extended Schools (DfES 2006a), which are situated in areas and communities traditionally associated with deprivation and poverty.

13.8 Working in Areas of Deprivation and Poverty as a Practitioner

The term *deprivation* is used to describe the ecological aspects of a given area and is usually measured by indices or scales. One such scale is the ACORN (a classification of residential neighbourhood) scale. This geodemographic tool is used to identify and understand the UK population and also the demand for products and services. Businesses also use this information to improve their understanding of customers and target markets and to determine where to locate operations.

Activity

You may be interested in accessing the website www.upmystreet.com to discover the indices/ACORN scale for the postcoded area in which you live. Now try putting in another postcode from another area within your community. How do the two areas compare? Are you surprised by the information you find?

In contrast, the term *poverty* is a difficult concept to define; the *Concise Oxford English Dictionary* (2006) describes poverty as 'a state of being extremely poor'. But what does it mean to be poor? To be poor in Africa is not the same as being poor within today's Western culture. Haralambos and Heald (1985, p. 140) describes absolute poverty as 'a judgement of basic human needs and is measured in terms of resources required to maintain health and basic human needs'. Without adequate fresh water, nutritious food and clean air, one might be described as being very poor, but few people within Western cultures experience such absolute poverty. In 21st century Western society one might conclude that a television and even a personal computer are a necessity to which all people should have access if wanted. Such an expectation would reflect Kemp *et al*.'s (2004, p. 3) definition of poverty as being a 'disadvantage that results from inequality in income, wealth and opportunity'.

From these two definitions we can see that a definitive description of poverty is impossible. Poverty is therefore a 'relative' concept; a concept that not only describes expected human needs but also the provisions, commodities and opportunities available and expected as 'the norm' by most people within a given society.

Many families live in poverty in areas that are considered deprived. When considering the term 'family', it is important to recognise that in the 21st century many families are not necessarily made up of mother, father and children. A family may include single or lone parents, same sex couples or a wider extended group of relations, and as such are described by Christensen (2004, p. 380) as 'a complex historical, social and cultural phenomenon'.

The public health nurse should recognise that the concept of 'family' is a private reality until the conception and subsequent birth of a child, which acts as the precursor for the intervention of a very 'public' health and social care system (Orr 1992). Christensen (2004, p. 377) suggests that, 'societal factors provide the material base for the family and will therefore to a large degree shape the resources available to the family'.

Families that live in areas of deprivation may not have their own transport, there might be a lone parent, or the family may be unable to find employment and consequently may rely on the benefit system for financial provision. The private sales of local government (council) house stock in the 1980s and early 1990s has left adequate and affordable housing in short supply. It might be necessary for some families to live with relatives or friends causing the accommodation to be overcrowded. Accommodation may be local council property; however, increasingly, families in areas of deprivation are housed in privately rented accommodation or temporary accommodation where rent is often charged at a premium. A consequences of this practice is that any housing benefit to which the family might be entitled may be insufficient to cover the full cost of the rent, and as a result a family may have to contribute from other necessary social welfare benefits that might have been granted to cover the cost of food and heating. The housing and homelessness charity Shelter undertook a postal questionnaire survey in 2003 of homeless households living in temporary accommodation and the responses are indicated in Box 13.6. In addition, Shelter (2006) suggests government figures show a number of other important statistics (Box 13.7).

From this discussion it is clear that housing need is inextricably linked to poverty, deprivation and poor health (Sandel & Wright 2006) and that some children and their families have little choice as to the environment in which they live. Despite this, the child's family may lack the capacity, have no desire or see no reason to change their living environment or their circumstances. Several studies have suggested that not only are nutrition and physical development compromised by poverty and deprivation, but those children and their families living in poverty and deprivation may experience problems with attachment (Utting 1995; Wilkinson & Marmot 2006). Others suggest that poverty can also have a profound effect on childhood behaviour and relationships (Rutter *et al.* 1998; Stuart-Brown 2005).

BOX 13.6

Main findings of the Shelter survey undertaken in 2003. *Source*: Shelter (2006).

- Over three-quarters of respondents (78 per cent) said that they had a specific health problem and half said that they were suffering from depression
- Over half of people said that their health or their family's health had suffered due to living in temporary accommodation
- Children had missed an average of 55 school days due to the disruption of moves into and between temporary accommodation
- Two-thirds of respondents said their children had problems at school, and nearly half described their children as 'often unhappy or depressed'

BOX 13.7

Government statistics on homeless families. *Source*: Shelter (2006).

- More than 100 000 children currently become homeless each year
- Over 300 000 families with children live in overcrowded housing
- More than 900 000 families with children live in poor housing
- 3.8 million children are in poverty after housing costs are deducted from the family income, compared to just under 2.7 million before housing costs
- 22 per cent (almost 28 000) of homeless households lost their home following relationship breakdown. Of these, 70 per cent were due to violent relationship breakdown – the main cause of the increased figures

Poverty and deprivation are therefore considered one of the greatest risk factors affecting children, young people and their families – not only impacting on many areas of their lives but also potentially on the parent or carer's ability to successfully acquire the skills necessary to parent their children successfully (Lucas & Lloyd 2005). Despite these findings, many parents living in social deprivation continue to do the best they can for their children; an in-depth qualitative analysis by Gilles (2006) found that parents struggling in difficult and demanding circumstances often took pride in their parenting abilities and did their utmost to parent well and provide for their children.

The terms poverty and deprivation therefore carry with them a stigma that suggests being poor and living in a deprived area is somehow demeaning. These terms should be considered and used with sensitivity by those practising in all public health and social care systems, failure to do so can discredit an individual, their family, community and the wider population. Public health nurses should be mindful that middle class values and attitudes to education, child development and parenting are often institutionalised by professionals (Gilles 2006) and in some circumstances may contribute to an unratified historical myth in relation to a specific geographical area or community.

13.9   Sure Start: Supporting Families

The concept for Sure Start was born out of the government Green Paper *Supporting Families* (Great Britain Home Office 1998), a document that aimed to improve social inequality and address social exclusion and which outlined the plans for the Sure Start initiative. This programme was to be the driver in the promotion of social inclusion and family support. Initially £540 million was set aside by the government for the funding of Sure Start local programmes (SSLPs) over 3 years. By February 1999, 60 'trailblazer' SSLPs were established in areas nationwide. In contrast to the social change approach of *Every Child Matters* (DfES 2006a) to supporting children, young people and their families, Sure Start has its roots in an empowerment approach to improving health and social wellbeing (Naidoo & Wills 2000), an ethos to initiate change by working with clients and communities in order to improve long-term health and social outcomes.

Activity

Revisit Chapter 4 and refresh your understanding of working towards empowering communities.

The Sure Start programme is not without its critics. The Sure Start concept was largely based on controversial research of a similar USA initiative, Headstart. Evaluation of the Headstart programme of the effect and outcomes for the children and families involved in the programme established ambiguous results, demonstrating either a positive effect, negative effect or no effect (Cook & Campbell 1979, cited by Griffiths 2002). Later studies showed an early positive effect on school performance, but that this tailed off over time (Barnes McGuire *et al*. 1997, cited by Griffiths 2002). As no long-term benefits were demonstrated the US programme was scaled down. (As an aside, readers may be interested to know that the one success that has continued in the USA from this programme is the children's educational television programme *Sesame Street*.)

However, the conclusion of a longitudinal study by Lazar and Darlington in 1982 demonstrated that those children who received the Headstart package completed their education and went on to full employment (Lazar & Darlington 1982, cited by Griffiths 2002). This finding is additionally supported by Hall and Elliman (2003) who suggest that there is substantial evidence that early intervention with children and their families can maximise and maintain socially supportive networks in order to improve health and wellbeing.

At its initial conception, SSLPs were only expected to benefit 5 per cent of children, but such was the response of applications from various areas to become a SSLP, that by July 2000 the government set aside funds of a further £315 million. The focus of SSLPs was the reconfiguration of services for

---

BOX 13.8

Sure Start local programme aims and objectives. *Source*: **DEE (1999).**

- Improving health and emotional development for children
- Supporting parents/carers as parents /carers and their aspirations towards employment
- Increasing the availability of childcare for all children
- Helping services develop in disadvantaged areas alongside financial help for parents to afford childcare
- Rolling out the principles driving the Sure Start approach to all services for children and parents

---

BOX 13.9

Sure Start local programme principles. *Source*: **DEE (1999).**

- Support for families from pregnancy until the child is 14 years, including those with special educational needs; for those with disabilities support up to the age of 16 years
- Working with parents and children
- Services for everyone
- Flexible at the point of delivery
- Starting very early
- Respectful and transparent
- Community driven and professionally coordinated
- Outcome driven

---

parents/carers and children that involved the contribution of cross-agency partnerships, statutory and voluntary agencies, community groups and, most importantly, local parents/carers. The aims and objectives they were based on are listed in Box 13.8. The ethos of the programme was to establish a bottom-up approach to localization of established services underpinned by principles identified in Box 13.9.

Each SSLP area covers 750–1000 children and offers a range of services that include home visiting, quality play and child care, and enhanced health advice and workers to achieve the following governmental public health targets:

- information and guidance on breast feeding, nutrition, hygiene and safety made available to all families in the SSLP;
- a 10 per cent reduction of children aged 0–4 years admitted to hospital with gastroenteritis, lower respiratory tract infection or severe injury;
- antenatal advice and support for all pregnant women and their families.

In addition many SSLPs offer targeted, timely, preventive home visiting support by a multiagency, multiskilled outreach team that may include specialist community public health nurses, nursery nurses, family support workers, oral health educators, literacy advisors, experts in the management of difficult childhood behaviour, speech and language therapists and social workers. These professionals are, in turn, supported by a programme that may offer any remit of services based upon the needs of the local community (Box 13.10).

13.10 Evaluation of Public Health Initiatives

The evaluation of all health and social care interventions is important in identifying what works well and what is not effective. Smith *et al.* (2005, p. 7) state that 'evaluation is the critical assessment of the value of an activity'. Citing Jenkinson (1997), Smith *et al.* (2005) go on to suggest that evaluation is important within any public health initiative or intervention to inform the evidence base for such interventions and influence decisions regarding practical and cost-effective service provision. In this,

---

BOX 13.10

Example of programmes offered within a Sure Start local programme.

- Holiday play schemes
- Oral health scheme
- Enhanced home safety check scheme
- Teenage pregnancy support group
- Breastfeeding support group
- Maternal depression group
- Domestic violence/abuse support group
- Parent/carer forums
- 'Drop in' centres
- Additional toy libraries
- Early literacy schemes
- Flexible respite
- Child health/well child clinic
- Adult training with crèche support
- Antenatal and postnatal groups
- Parenting and behaviour workshops

---

the Sure Start initiative is no exception and is subject to an independent evaluation. The National Evaluation of Sure Start (NESS) is led by a team of researchers from the Institute for the Study of Children, Families and Social Issues, Birkbeck, University of London. This evaluation is a longitudinal study that compares and contrasts children aged 9 months, 3 years and 5 years from non-SSLP areas and SSLPs. The preliminary findings from the evaluation in November 2005 demonstrated that SSLP households were generally 'less chaotic' within the 9-month age range and that mothers of children within the 3-year age range were, in general, more accepting of their children's behaviour. The 3-year-old children of non-teenage mothers demonstrated reduced behavioural problems and increased social competence. However, disappointingly, the 3-year-old children of teenage mothers (14 per cent of sample) demonstrated a higher incidence of behavioural problems and lower social competence. These findings indicate that SSLPs are currently benefiting moderately disadvantaged parents/families, i.e. those perceived as having a 'greater human capital', but not those parents/families with 'less human capital' (e.g. teenage parents, lone parents, workless households). The findings also suggest that programmes led by health agencies fared moderately better in the outcomes for children and their families than those led by local authorities and/or education (Belsky *et al.* 2005).

The NESS findings raise two important issues: the Sure Start programme is not reaching some of the most disadvantaged families and the service provision in some local programmes is not working as well as it should. This may be, in part, due to the difficulties professionals face when introducing a community development programme, including community suspicion and indifference. The most recent national evaluation report (DfES 2006b, p. 8) suggests that:

> Outreach and home visiting represent the gateway between families and integrated services. Creating relationships with families to gain their trust and interest was essential for SSLPs but that it was a delicate business requiring sensitivity and persistence. In the best practice examples parents felt equal partners, 'inviting' the programme to work with them.

By the end of 2006, Sure Start 'individual' programmes were phased out and underwent metamorphoses into Children's Centres, which will continue to be situated in areas of greatest need. The government aims to provide one for every community – 3500 centres by 2010 (National Audit Office 2006). The vision is that the Children's Centres will truly integrate health, education and social services to provide comprehensive services for children, young people and their families. They will incorporate the Sure Start 'brand' and ethos, working to the same targets and objectives of achieving community-driven, professionally led, health, education and social support services that meet the needs of vulnerable children, young people and their families.

Case Study Example

Early on a cold winter morning a woman with a small child and pushing a toddler in a buggy came into the local Sure Start centre reception asking to see her health visitor. Mary, her 4-year-old son Davy and 2-year-old daughter Sasha were well known to the health visitor. Four years previously, Mary was estranged from her parents and heavily pregnant with her first child Davy, when there had been a severe incident of domestic abuse, perpetrated by Mary's partner and father of the unborn child. A case conference was convened and Davy's name was placed upon the local authority Child Protection Register (CPR) as being 'at risk of physical abuse and neglect'. Following registration, a comprehensive, multiprofessional child protection plan was drawn up and initiated, which involved intensive visiting by all health and social care services involved with the family; these included a named social worker, the midwife, the health visitor and a probation officer, as Mary's partner had not long been out of prison for previous offences including drugs and violence. It was also decided in light of this information that the family would be subject to a 'no lone visiting' policy in order that visiting professionals would be safeguarded. As part of the plan, the health visitor arranged regular joint visits with the social worker and other members of the multiprofessional team, gradually building up a professional working and supportive relationship with the family.

Both health and social services were keen that the family should access local groups within the area; however, despite frequent encouragement and facilitation by offering to accompany the family, both Mary and her partner avoided attending any groups or local services. Over a period of 12 months there were no further reported incidents of domestic abuse and it was clear to all professionals involved that Davy was thriving and was adored by both his parents. Mary's partner had completed a workshop on anger management arranged through the probationary services, and the situation and relationship with professionals was such that the 'no lone visiting' policy was lifted; 14 months after initial registration, Davy's name was removed from the CPR.

Regular health visitor and social work contact with the family continued. Six months following 'de-registration' the social worker contacted the health visitor to inform her that the domestic abuse had re-occurred and that Mary was expecting a second child. What was most alarming for the professionals involved was that Mary stated that the domestic abuse had never really stopped, it had just lessened and been mostly verbal in nature.

A further initial case conference was convened and both Davy and Sasha, the unborn baby, were again placed upon the CPR. A further child protection plan was put in place and this time it was made clear to the family that unless they were prepared to be open and honest with the professionals involved then care proceedings would be taken in order to ensure the children were fully protected. Intensive support of the family recommenced. By this time the local area had an SSLP, and as part of the services provided by Sure Start a combined antenatal and postnatal group had been established in the Sure Start centre for all parents in the locality. Mary was encouraged to attend the group, along with other expectant mothers and new parents/carers with children up to 6 months of age. Crèche facilities were provided for Davy, which enabled Mary to relax and chat to other mothers who lived locally. Unfortunately Mary's partner was unable to attend the group as he was now working long hours. The group enabled Mary to make friends locally and grow in confidence; when Sasha was born she was delighted to attend the group and show off her baby to the other mothers.

Mary continued to attend the group regularly until Sasha was 6 months old, by which time Davy was well settled in the local Sure Start nursery and both children were thriving. Both parents denied any re-occurrence of domestic abuse and both children's names were removed from the CPR. The health visitor maintained regular contact with Mary, formally through child health checks and also opportunistically at local groups and in the local area. At each contact Mary was questioned as to her wellbeing and about the relationship between herself and her partner; each time Mary stated that all was well. However, on one occasion the health visitor saw Mary out with both children in the local shopping precinct and noted that Davy's behaviour was difficult for Mary to manage. When the health visitor asked Mary how she was, Mary complained that she did not know how best to manage Davy's increasingly difficult and aggressive behaviour. The health visitor arranged with Mary to visit her at home with the Sure Start child behavioural specialist the following week. However, on the date

(Continued)

> **Case Study Example (Continued)**
>
> arranged the health visitor was surprised when Mary contacted her stating that Davy's behaviour had improved and she no longer needed anyone to visit. It was 2 days later that Mary came into the Sure Start reception, and on seeing the health visitor she broke down in tears, 'it's started again, and I can't stay' was all she said.
>
> The health visitor was able to contact the Sure Start domestic abuse advisor who immediately came to see Mary at the centre and informed Mary of her options, while emergency crèche facilities were utilised for the children so that Mary could talk without distraction and so that the children would not be distressed by their mother's emotional state. Immediate legal advice was arranged by the domestic abuse advisor who was able to arrange refuge accommodation in another Sure Start area. With Mary's permission the health visitor contacted Social Services to inform them of the situation and it was decided that as Mary had acted to safeguard herself and her children by accessing appropriate support, then no further action would need to be taken at that time.
>
> On leaving the centre, Mary commented that the centre with which she had become so familiar with had given her 'a chance to cry for help' before the situation at home had escalated further. She now had the confidence to break the cycle of abuse. Mary is now in regular contact with her parents, is rehoused in another Sure Start area and with the support of Sure Start is taking her GCSEs. Mary hopes to become a midwife.

Conclusion

This chapter has considered the concept of risk and risk management associated with the vulnerability of children, young people and their families, poverty and deprivation, and personal safety. Approaches to changing, improving and evaluating health and social provision for children, young people and their families have been discussed.

The principles and interventions discussed here are also applicable in a broader context to other vulnerable groups in society. For example, some towns like those along the Sussex coast have high populations of older people – the principles of Sure Start could be applied locally in order to meet the health and social care needs of older persons.

What is hoped to be made clear from these discussions is that, used in isolation, no single approach can revolutionise risk assessment, risk management and identify necessary health and social care provision. What is needed from all service providers and professionals working within public health is a flexible, partnership approach to working with vulnerable clients that initiates positive change and that, in turn, will produce a healthier and more productive society.

References

Beck U. (2002) *Risk Society. Towards a new modernity*. London: Sage Publications.

Beckett C. (2005) *Child Protection: an introduction*. London: Sage Publications.

Belsky J., Melhuish E., Barnes J., Leyland A.H., Romaniuk H. (2005) *Early Impacts of Sure Start Local Programmes on Children and Families*. London: HM Stationery Office. http://www.surestart.gov.uk/_doc/P0001867.pdf.

Benner P. (1982) From novice to expert. *American Journal of Nursing* 82 (1), 402–7.

Chalmers K.I. (1993) Searching for health needs; the work of health visiting. *Journal of Advanced Nursing* 18, 900–11.

Christensen P. (2004) The health-promoting family: a conceptual framework for future research. *Social Science and Medicine* 59, 377–87.

Clarke A. (1999) *Community Nurses and the Law*. London: CPHVA Publications.

Collins Reference Thesaurus (1993) *Collins Reference Thesaurus*. Godalming: Ted Smart Publishers.

Concise Oxford English Dictionary (2006) *Concise Oxford English Dictionary*, 4th edn. Oxford: Oxford University Press.

DEE (Department of Education and Employment) (1999) *Sure Start: making a difference for children and families.* Sudbury: DEE Publications.

DfES (Department for Education and Skills) (2003) *Every Child Matters.* London: HM Stationery Office.

DfES (Department for Education and Skills) (2004) *Every Child Matters: change for children.* Nottingham: DfES Publications.

DfES (Department for Education and Skills) (2006a) *Every Child Matters: change for children. Making it happen, working together for children, young people and families.* www.emc.gov.uk.

DfES (Department for Education and Skills) (2006b) *National Evaluation Report. Outreach and home visiting services in Sure Start local programmes.* Nottingham: DfES Publications.

DH (Department of Health) (2004) *Choosing Health: making healthier choices easier.* London: HM Stationery Office.

DH (Department of Health), DEE (Department for Education and Employment), Home Office (1999) *Working Together to Safeguard Children.* London: HM Stationery Office.

DH (Department of Health), DEE (Department for Education and Employment), Home Office (2000) *Framework for the Assessment of Children in Need and their Families.* London: HM Stationery Office.

Gillies V. (2006) Parenting, class and culture: exploring the context of childrearing. *Community Practitioner* 29 (4), 114–17.

Great Britain Home Office (1998) *Supporting Families.* London: HM Stationery Office.

Griffiths P. (2002) Understanding effectiveness for service planning. In: *Public Health in Policy and Practice: a source book for health visitors and community nurses* (ed. Cowley S.), pp. 146–61. London: Bailliere Tindall.

Hall D.M.B., Elliman D. (2003) *Health for all Children,* 4th edn. Oxford: Oxford University Press.

Haralambos M., Heald R.M. (1985) *Sociology: themes and perspectives.* Slough: University Tutorial Press.

Health and Safety Executive (2006) *Violence at Work: a guide for employers.* Sudbury, Suffolk: HSE Books.

HM Government (2006) *Working Together to Safeguard Children: a guide to interagency working to safeguard and promote the welfare of children.* London: HM Stationery Office.

Houston A.M., Cowley S. (2002) An empowerment approach to needs assessment in health visiting practice. *Journal of Clinical Nursing* 11, 640–50.

Jenkinson C. (1997) Assessment and evaluation of health and medical care: an introduction and overview. In: *Assessment and Evaluation of Health and Medical Care* (ed. Jenkinson C.). Buckingham: Open University Press.

Kemp P., Bradshaw J., Dornan P., Finch N., Meyhew E. (2004) *Routes Out of Poverty: a research review.* York: Joseph Rowntree Foundation.

Kemshall H. (2002) *Risk, Social Policy and Welfare.* Buckingham: Open University Press.

Lamplugh D. (1999) Take care of yourself (preventing violence at work). *Nursing Standard* 13 (23), 24.

Lamplugh D., Woods M., Whitehead J. (1993) *Working Alone – surviving and thriving.* London: Pitman Publishing.

Lord Laming (2003) *The Victoria Climbie Inquiry.* London: HM Stationery Office.

Lucas K., Lloyd B. (2005) *Health Promotion: evidence and experience.* London: Sage Publications.

Luker K., Chalmers K. (1990) Gaining access to clients: the case of health visiting. *Journal of Advanced Nursing* 15, 74–82.

Marcellus L. (2005) The ethics of relation: public health nurses and child protection clients. *Journal of Advanced Nursing* 51 (4), 414–20.

Mayhew C., Chappell D. (2001) *Occupational Violence: types, reporting patterns, and variations between health sectors.* No. 139. University of New South Wales. Department of Industrial Relations. ttp://wwwdocs.fce.unsw.edu.au/orgmanagement/WorkingPapers/wp139.pdf (accessed 1 Sept 2006).

Morrison T. (2000) Working together to safeguard children: challenges and changes for inter-agency co-ordination in child protection. *Journal of Professional Care* 14 (4), 363–73.

Naidoo J., Wills J. (2000) *Health Promotion: foundations for practice,* 2nd edn. London: Bailliere Tindall.

National Audit Office (2003) *A Safer Place to Work. Protecting NHS hospital staff from violence and aggression. Executive summary.* London: HM Stationery Office. http://www.nao.org.uk/publications/nao_reports/02-03/0203527.pdf (accessed 1 Sept 2006).

National Audit Office (2006) *Sure Start Children's Centres. Executive summary.* London: HM Stationery Office.

Neligan G.A., Purdam D., Stiener H. (1974) *The Formative Years.* Oxford: Nuffield Provincial Hospitals Trust/Oxford University Press.

NMC (Nursing and Midwifery Council) (2004) *Code of Professional Conduct: standards for conduct, performance and ethics.* NMC Standards 07.04. London: Nursing and Midwifery Council.

Orr J. (1992) Assessing individual family health needs. In: *Health Visiting. Towards community health nursing* (eds Luker K., Orr J.). London: Blackwell Publishing.

Plough A., Krimsky S. (1987) The emergence of risk communication studies: social and political context. *Science, Technology and Human Values* 12 (3/4), 4–10. (Special issue on the technical and ethical aspects of risk communication.)

Ruckelshaus W.D. (1985) Risk, science and democracy. *Issues in Science and Technology* 1 (3), 19–38.

Rutter M., Giller H., Hagell A. (1998) *Anti-social Behaviour by Young People.* London: Cambridge University Press.

Sandel M., Wright R. (2006) When home is where stress is: expanding the dimensions of housing that influence asthma morbidity. *Archives of Diseases in Childhood* 91, 924–48.

Saunders K. (2001) *Using Evidence to Assess Vulnerability in Health Visiting: developing and implementing the family health assessment. Final report*. Winchester: Winchester and Eastleigh NHS Trust.

Shelter (2006) *Children and Families Policy*. http://england.shelter.org.uk/policy/policy-967.cfm (accessed 21 Aug 2006).

Smith S., Sinclair D., Raine R., Reeves B. (2005) *Understanding Public Health: Health care evaluation*. Maidenhead: Open University Press/McGraw-Hill Education.

Stuart-Brown S. (2005) Promoting health in children and young people: identifying priorities. *Journal of the Royal Society for the Promotion of Health* 125 (5), 61–2.

Utting D. (1995) *Family and Parenthood: supporting families, preventing breakdown*. York: Joseph Rowntree Foundation.

Wanless D. (2004) *Securing Good Health for the Whole Population. Final report*. Norwich: HMSO Publications.

Wilkinson R., Marmot M. (2006) *Social Determinants of Health: the solid facts*. New York: World Health Organization.

CHAPTER 14

Developing Programmes, Services and Reducing Inequalities

Xena Dion

Public Health Skills: Developing programmes and projects

- Programme and project planning: development, implementation, management, evaluation and review
- Developing existing skills and essential new skills: community development, project management and effective leadership
- Four steps to developing public health programmes and services

Introduction

Contemporary public health is no longer the science and medically focused specialism that emerged from the 19th century primarily to combat contagious diseases. It now encompasses the wider determinants of health and takes a more 'artistic' approach to improving health and reducing health inequalities through developing programmes and services that engage local communities (DH 1999a, 2003a, 2004a). Nurses and midwives are not only expected to contribute to this agenda but to lead initiatives that make real improvements to people's lives (DH 1999b, 2002a, 2003b). This work, although informed by the science of medicine and epidemiology, demands high levels of interpersonal, creative, management and leadership skills rather than those of clinical medicine and nursing. Many of them are not simply learnt but developed through an ongoing and intelligent synthesis of theoretical and experiential learning by the practitioner.

Taking a realistic and practical approach, this chapter serves to explain the skills needed to work with other professionals, agencies and lay people to make real differences to local people. A case study example is used to demonstrate the application of these skills to the planning, implementation, management, evaluation and review of a comprehensive multiagency public health project. The emphasis in this chapter is on *skills* and the *application* of those skills rather than the theoretical and policy framework that underpins public health, which is discussed in other parts of this book.

14.1 Context

Put simply and briefly, the UK can not afford to fund the health care of a population that is living longer and has increasing long-term demands on its health service (Wanless 2004). Unless, as Wanless candidly explains, the public are prepared to take a greater interest in and responsibility for maintaining good health, the country's health care system faces collapse. Health professionals are now being asked, with increasing urgency, to work together and in partnership with other agencies to make real inroads in helping people to maintain good health or improve it, particularly the most disadvantaged (DH 1999a, 2003a, 2004a). Moreover, as the wider determinants of health and the cycle of decline that affects disadvantaged populations are better understood (Marmot & Wilkinson 2005; Prime Minister's Stategy Unit 2005), the ways in which health professionals engage in tackling health inequalities has to be more imaginative and creative than ever before. This, as seen from the case study example, may take them far away from their 'traditional' professional boundaries and activities as they work in partnership with others to tackle the root causes of poor health.

14.2 Developing Existing Skills

Developing community programmes demands a quite different way of thinking than hospital and community-based nursing and midwifery and quite different skills. It means considering the impact of poor health, in the widest sense of the term, on the community as a whole and looking for the very long-term gains that may not be noticeable for a generation or even beyond. It pulls away from focusing on immediate problems of acute ill health and sickness and from interventions to help one individual or one family. Without this cognitive shift, the more tangible skills will be weak as effective leadership needs vision, belief in the work and enthusiasm (Antonakis *et al.* 2004; Verzuh 2005).

Whilst many of the practical skills needed in developing programmes and services (such as project management, marketing and financial management) are not included in undergraduate nurse education, training, coupled with effective learning from professional experience, does provide a solid foundation on which to develop essential new skills (DH 2004b). For example, nurses and midwives are mostly good communicators, work effectively in teams and have basic management skills. They share and pass information backwards and forwards between people all the time and learn to encourage and motivate patients and colleagues to do well. They plan and 'project manage' their day's work, delegate, monitor and evaluate the effectiveness of interventions. They assess and manage risks both to patients and to themselves and colleagues and apply existing skills to new situations all the time (Benner *et al.* 1996). Is it possible then that all that is needed to develop new programmes and services is for these skills to be further advanced to deal with new challenges that arise from working in new ways?

If that were simply the case there would be no shortage of people from a nursing and midwifery background to progress the public health agenda. But, as Ball (2002, p. 4) found, the skills needed are so complex and advanced that:

> the pool of people with the skills to manage complex local initiatives such as Sure Start is small (and growing smaller).

The scope, complexity and sophistication of skills needed to develop new programmes and services to improve health and reduce health inequalities must not be underestimated. The practitioner needs high levels of competency (levels three to four) in a large percentage of the core dimensions described in the NHS Knowledge and Skills Framework (KSF) (DH 2004b). The acquisition of this breadth and depth of skills relies as much on the practitioner's self-motivation and ability to develop and synthesise their existing skills from new experiences as on theoretical learning. Theoretical learning from project management, leadership, health needs assessment for example are essential to public health practice, but the real skills lie then in the practitioner's ability to aptly and astutely adapt and apply them to the dynamic challenges of developing new programmes and services in local communities.

14.3 Essential New Skills: Community Development, Project Management and Effective Leadership

For even the most experienced clinical nurses and midwives, developing new programmes and services in the community demands many additional skills and learning. Understanding the dynamics of population groups and community development, for example, is essential, as is project management and *effective* leadership. Self-learning workbooks such as *Developing Healthier Communities* (HDA 2004) provide a valuable tool from which to acquire the necessary new skills to aid developing new services and facilities. However, actually making things happen demands essential skills from the field of project management.

Organizing a normal day's activities either at work or home involves basic elements of project management such as meeting time deadlines and utilizing resources. However, when things get complicated and different things need to happen at different times, with different people and resources being reliant on each other, things can easily become muddled. Project management helps the leader to plan systematically, identifying critical pathways through a complex process and ensuring that one area is successfully completed in time for the next part to progress. The skills learnt through project management include estimating timeframes, planning, scheduling events, critical path analysis, costing and organizing resources and stakeholder analysis. These skills are underpinned by several formal project management tools, which demand further skills in their use and application. Collectively, project management skills enable the project to finish on time, within the estimated budget and with the end result intended (Verzuh 2005).

Developing community-based public health programmes and services require many additional and sometimes unusual project management skills. Some, for example, are described in reports from Sure Start, a national public health initiative (DfES 2005). Programme managers are expected to:

- manage staff, project volunteers and buildings;
- continue consultation and the development of projects with local residents;
- evaluate services to ensure they meet local needs;
- respond effectively to any new situations as they arise, whatever they may be!

> I could never have imagined doing some of the things I've done in this job; I've actually commissioned a bus. (DfES 2005, clause 2.13)

The Sure Start experience highlights the complexities of developing new programmes and services to improve health and help reduce health inequalities at local levels. It is not surprising that finding skilled people to lead the work is challenging:

> At the beginning we had difficulties finding the right kind of person; it takes management and negotiating skills, knowledge of finance, vision for service delivery and political diplomacy. This is a new breed of manager. (DfES 2005, clause 2.13)

In addition to these skills, practitioners leading public health initiatives need to 'know the community', have a good knowledge and understanding of the 'science' of public health (epidemiology, demography, causes of ill health, etc.) and public health policy, and knowledge and understanding of the roles and responsibilities of different agencies. Equally, they need effective leadership skills to move the work forward and make it happen (DH 1999b, 2002b, 2004b).

Effective leadership is not a collection of tangible skills that are simply taught and then put into practice like a series of movements in a given situation. Leadership skills and the characteristics that make a good leader are extremely complex. It involves some element of personality and a large amount of 'emotional intelligence' and maturity (Performance and Innovation Unit 2001; Goleman *et al.* 2002; Salovey *et al.* 2004). Effective leadership needs skills and emotional intelligence to show self-confidence, motivate and manage oneself as well as others, negotiate, share decision making, and take responsibility when things go wrong – to name but a few abilities. Undoubtedly leadership is an essential, fundamental and huge part of developing new programmes or services successfully.

Activity

If you would like to explore this further, before proceeding with this chapter try reading Chapter 9, which concentrates specifically on strategic leadership skills.

```
┌─────────────────────────────────────────┐
│        STEP 1 – getting started          │
│  • What is the population group?         │
│  • What are the big concerns?            │
│  • Who are the professionals and key lay │
│    people in the local community that can│
│    help make it happen?                  │
│  • Getting people on board               │
│  • Organizing the first meeting          │
└─────────────────────────────────────────┘

┌──────────────────────────────────┐   ┌──────────────────────────────────────┐
│  STEP 4 - Evaluation and review   │   │   STEP 2 – Gathering information       │
│  • How effective is the           │   │  • Who has what data?                  │
│    programme/service              │   │  • What has been done before?          │
│    to those using it?             │   │  • Consulting people: who and how?     │
│  • How efficient is that          │   │  • Putting it into action – setting    │
│    effectiveness in               │   │    deadlines                           │
│    terms of the resources being   │   │  • Bringing data back to the group and │
│    used?                          │   │    making sense of it                  │
│  • Who is using it and who isn't  │   │                                        │
│    and why?                       │   │                                        │
│  • How can it be improved?        │   │                                        │
└──────────────────────────────────┘   └──────────────────────────────────────┘

        ┌──────────────────────────────────────────────┐
        │      STEP 3 – Planning and implementing        │
        │  • What can be achieved?                       │
        │  • Who will it help and how?                   │
        │  • How will it work? i.e. who will run it,     │
        │    administer it, fund it, attend it, be       │
        │    responsible for it?                         │
        │  • Who will lead and project manage it?        │
        │  • Set short- and long-term goals and be clear │
        │    about who is responsible for them           │
        │  • Project manage the work – make it happen    │
        └──────────────────────────────────────────────┘
```

Figure 14.1   The four steps to developing programmes, services and reducing inequalities.

14.4   Steps to Developing Public Health Programmes and Services

Nurses and midwives may develop the skills necessary to develop programmes and services aimed at improving health and reducing inequalities, but how are those skills *applied* to make it happen? Based on a case study experience, Figure 14.1 summarises the sequential, logical and common sense steps taken to develop the new programme of activities and services. These are explained in greater detail with reference to the associated skills needed and their application to practice. The questions within the boxes are by no means definitive or complete. There are huge numbers of questions to be asked at every stage of the process and more between. Questioning, analysis and reflection form an essential part of the 'planning cycle', which keeps the process moving and improving and is also an integral part of project management, ensuring the project progresses systematically, within expected timeframes and to its optimum quality level (Verzuh 2005).

14.4.1   Step 1: getting started

> **Key skills**
>
> Knowledge of national and local public health policy; knowledge of community development; utilizing theoretical frameworks; developing vision; self-development and awareness.

Before starting down the path there has to be, as stated earlier, a *belief* in the public health ethos and its process. It is this belief that underpins genuine enthusiasm and commitment to public health practice, which are key elements of effective leadership and help towards developing a vision for the way forward. This key skill in public health work does not mean having in mind a final goal as a *fait accompli*. Instead it demonstrates a clear and expert understanding of the potential that can be realised by professionals from different disciplines and agencies working together and with local people in

Section 4

equal partnership to improve health and wellbeing. Having vision is a 'skill' in itself, which is not learnt through study or practice but, again, comes from several skills grounded in experiential learning and self-development. Developing a vision relies on the person's skills to interpret, understand and utilise information. This includes public opinion, particularly amongst those hardest to reach, as well as the scientific knowledge that forms the theoretical framework for public health. It also means having a sound knowledge and understanding of community development within a public health context (HDA 2004) and of public health and related government policy to ensure the work is compatible with the aims and objectives of the many different agencies and organizations involved.

Knowing the community

Key skills

Critical analysis; communicating – asking and listening; cultural awareness; knowledge of, but thinking beyond, existing professional territories; local history.

Just as it makes no sense to plan a big expensive party without taking into consideration the age range and cultural tastes and values of the guests, it makes no sense to develop a new programme or service without considerable knowledge of the local population. This starts with identifying the different population groups, particularly – if health inequalities are to be effectively tackled – black and minority ethnic groups and vulnerable groups such as unsupported young mothers, rough sleepers, asylum seekers and vulnerable older people (DH 2003a). This is not as straightforward as it sounds. Some minority ethnic groups struggle for recognition despite having very different cultures. The gypsy traveller population, for example, although one of the largest minority ethnic groups in the UK (CRE 2004) are not identifiable through the system of ethnic 'grouping' used by the Office for National Statistics (ONS). They are categorised together with 'white British', 'white Irish' or 'white other'. This system is not only used for the national census held every 10 years (ONS 2001) but is also widely adopted as a means to identify minority groups by many other agencies and organizations. Consequently, they and other such population groups are frequently under-represented through the collection of formal statistical data. Public health practitioners need the skills, therefore, to appraise such data critically and look beyond it if they are to gain a more insightful and accurate profile of the local community.

Once the community's minority and/or most marginalised groups are accurately identified, if health inequalities are to be effectively tackled specific cultural values and norms must be better understood. The academic skills to do this at any depth are rooted in social anthropology, through which the student learns to study and understand population groups with sensitivity to their cultural and social differences. Although it would bring an invaluable perspective to public health practice the subject area is too great to explore further in this text. Nurses and midwives can, at least, better understand different cultural values through good interpersonal and communication skills. This entails building relationships, particularly amongst more marginalised groups, asking the right questions in a manner that elicits open and honest responses and, above all, listening. These skills are also integral to wider public consultation discussed later, which makes a vital contribution to the wider picture of 'knowing the community'.

Initiating partnership working: getting others on board

Key skills

Communication and interpersonal skills; networking; motivating others; leadership.

Developing programmes and services aimed at improving health and wellbeing and reducing inequalities is a huge and complex task. It is simply not possible to do it alone; working effectively as part of a multiprofessional team is an essential public health skill. The success of building such a team, which includes lay people as well as professionals, lies in the leadership skills and ability of the person initiating the work to enthuse and gain the commitment of others (Hudson & Hardy 2002). To this end it is advantageous to 'network' and take the time to visit key people working in the community individually. This enables the programme developer to find out the perspectives of different agencies and individuals; their role and aims; the issues and challenges they face; their vision for the future and what they would like to change, etc. Importantly, it provides an opportunity to identify the professionals who see themselves as part of the bigger picture and are keen to work with others to achieve similar goals. Making use of networks at this stage to locate additional people that could contribute to the project in the future may save a great amount of time later in the project.

Current government strategy for tackling inequalities includes public services working together with other agencies and organizations to make a real difference (DH 1999a, 2003a). Professionals from all public agencies are extremely busy, pressured and underresourced, and have to prioritise their work. Communication, marketing, and leadership skills, particularly in motivating others and having clarity and vision for what can be achieved is essential to gaining their commitment. It is also a useful skill to recognise when people are creating barriers to collaborative working! Working with those who are equally enthusiastic and who share the vision of what can be achieved is conducive to progress, as can be seen from the following case study.

Case Study Example

Developing a programme of activities and outreach services in a disadvantaged community.

A large town on the south coast of the UK boasts some of the most expensive properties in the country and houses some of the wealthiest. Yet within 5 km there are pockets of disadvantage and social deprivation where people have significantly worse health and lower life expectancy. With a remit to 'improve health and wellbeing and reduce inequalities' in that area the author, later to become the project manager, set out to develop new programmes and services that would make a real difference to people's lives. A public health development group (PHDG) was formed to act as a planning and steering group and included representatives from: Social Services, the youth services, the police, the Alcohol and Drug Advisory Service, education, housing, elderly care, the Environmental Agency, churches, leisure services, health promotion, adult learning, the emotional and behaviour problems team from the local comprehensive school, local residents (× 3), the mental health team and the Local Authority (community liaison officer).

Following the steps depicted in the main text of this chapter, the PHDG made their decision about what new services and facilities could be provided by weighing the needs expressed (i.e. what facilities were considered most needed or wanted by local residents) with what would make the most impact (i.e. on improving health and wellbeing), with what would be most acceptable (i.e. what would be most accessible to most people), and with what was realistically achievable (i.e. within reasonable resources and physical possibility). After considerable debate the group planned to bring together several activities and services under one roof, which they believed would make a considerable difference to as many people's lives as possible. This included:

- an after-school activities facility on three afternoons a week, to include football, tag-rugby, hockey, outdoor and indoor games, arts and crafts, drama, dance and music, and a coffee shop;
- a drop-in session for women, with an emphasis on mental health problems;
- a coffee morning for older people to include activities (bingo, games, outings, etc.);
- outreach services provided weekly by several agencies from housing, the Citizens Advice Bureau, the Drug and Alcohol Advisory Service, family planning and benefits advice.

The programme opened with a highly successful 'launch' day covered by the local media. Several local dignitaries attended, including the local member of parliament, local councillors and a local celebrity. Over 300 people attended and free refreshments complimented the taster sessions for the activities.

(Continued)

Case Study Example (Continued)

The project's potential was to make real improvements to the lives of local people in many ways, for example:

- widening access to sports and physical activities designed to improve health and prevent obesity and related chronic diseases in later life;
- increasing physical activity in adults through encouraging the parents/carers to participate in the sports and physical activities;
- raising self-esteem through achievements in the above activities and in participating in arts and crafts, music, drama and dance;
- developing a sense of community through bringing local people into regular contact with each other in an informal and participatory setting;
- creating an opportunity to develop further community projects by providing a living example of what can be achieved when professionals work together and with local residents.

The project was supported by a strong volunteer element. Several local women volunteered to help supervise the sessions to enhance the safety and wellbeing of the children attending (although the primary responsibility lay with the parents/carers) and to run the coffee shop. These women not only participated in, but led, some of the planning and development of the ideas and activities prior to the launch of the project, which helped give the local community a sense of ownership.

Volunteers were also forthcoming from the local university. Two senior physical education students gave time each week to coach football. Hockey coaching was provided by two local business men who volunteered their time due to their passion for the game and to look out for potential future recruits to their teams. The enthusiasm of these local volunteers for the project highlighted the potential people saw in it.

Organizing the first meeting

Key skills

Chairing meetings; administration; organizing; leadership; interpersonal skills; delegation; team building.

The efficiency with which the first meeting is organised is critical to the success of future partnership working with others. With so much rapid and profound change in public services, professionals may be wary of meetings without very pertinent and defined purposes and outcomes. The multitude of organizational skills required to administer and chair effective meetings are described and explained more fully on easily accessible internet resources.

Activity

Visit the websites www.meetingwizard.org and www.effectivemeetings.com, and explore them to find out more about conducting meetings.

But not all the key skills involved in running effective meetings are 'taught'. They, again, rely on a foundation of excellent communication, interpersonal skills and emotional intelligence (Salovey *et al.* 2004) and demand a focused and motivating manner that ensures everyone is heard, their opinions and contribution are valued, yet commands action.

14.4.2   Step 2: gathering information

Data collection (informing the vision)

> **Key skills**
>
> Searching for information; networking; understanding statistics.

The rationale behind developing new programmes or services is normally to address unmet health needs – but first they need to be identified. An essential function of the steering group would be to organise an extensive population profile and health needs assessment (NICE 2005). These form part of the process of 'knowing the community' and, although laborious, underpin public health practice as they provide a formal framework and evidence base to inform decisions regarding community development. The assessment should include mapping existing services and facilities to identify gaps, as well as building a profile of health conditions and determinant factors (NICE 2005). The profile also provides the evidence needed when bidding for funding for local initiatives – another key public health skill!

The amount of work involved in a health needs assessment or community profile would be prohibitive for one professional or agency alone. By working collaboratively, representatives from different agencies have the potential to build a comprehensive, insightful and extremely valuable profile of a community. The skills needed to undertake such a profile are numerous and diverse and include many of those needed to develop new programmes and services. Project management skills are needed to plan and execute the process, and good leadership skills are essential to delegate work and motivate others (NICE 2005). As with 'knowing the community', the public health skill in data collection and profiling is to interpret and make sense of the available information whilst also heeding its limitations and looking beyond what is actually presented.

Public consultation

> **Key skills**
>
> Communication and interpersonal skills; networking; questionnaire design; interviewing.

In developing new programmes and services, data would not be complete without including the opinions of local people. It brings an essential lay perspective and improves relationships between professionals and service users and improves access to and involvement in services (NICE 2006). The term includes several 'formal' methods of consultation such as focus groups, questionnaires, interviews, opinion panels and workshops (NHS Executive 1999a, 1999b). Although these are important in obtaining public views they are greatly enhanced by the use of less formal methods. Valuable insight into the real issues that contribute to health inequalities can be most effectively obtained by informal discussions between community leaders and workers and the hardest to reach members of the community. This relies on 'knowing the community' and networking and interpersonal skills to secure the help of professionals, volunteers and church and community leaders who have an established relationship with the most marginalised and disengaged residents. The opinions and views obtained then must be made to count by ensuring they are considered in the decision-making forum.

The skills needed for public consultation are wide and varied. They begin with advanced communication and interpersonal skills, the lack of which presents one of the greatest barriers to effective consultation (NHS Executive 1999a). The practitioner needs open and honest responses from those consulted, which demands sophisticated communication and interpersonal skills (both verbal and non-verbal) – as questioner and active listener (Hartley 1999). But they must also be skilled in designing succinct and appropriately worded questionnaires, conducting effective and efficient interviews, both with groups and individuals, and/or organizing and facilitating larger scale consultation events such as workshops and conferences to secure a wide scope of opinion (NHS Executive 1999a, 1999b).

Making sense of information

> **Key skills**
>
> Epidemiology knowledge; appraisal; critical analysis of data; knowledge of public health theory.

The collected data provide a solid basis on which to inform collective decision making within the steering group. But the data have to be critically examined and interpreted within the context of the community and public opinion. Skills in critical analysis and appraisal of data are essential to ensure the data are accurately evaluated and effectively utilised. However, to understand and make *sense* of the information collected, particularly the views and opinions of local people, a sound knowledge and consideration of public health theory is needed to appreciate the relationship between health, its wider determinants – education, housing, cultural values, the environment etc. – and the real effects they have on individuals (HDA 2004; Marmot & Wilkinson 2005). A particularly pertinent listening skill during public consultation is that of 'not evaluating what you have heard until you *understand* it' (Hartley 1999, p. 59). An example of this in context is provided by the project to which the case study refers. Whilst seeking public opinion as part of the information-gathering process, several women from the gypsy traveller community disclosed their very strong belief that their health significantly deteriorated when living in houses as they felt 'dried out', 'closed in' and 'trapped'. Their primary health 'need' was to be travelling. Without some understanding of the travelling culture ('knowing the community') and the wider determinants of health, the relationship between travelling and health would not have been appreciated by the non-traveller professionals. Consequently they would be pursuing fruitless 'health improving' activities with a significant waste of time and other resources. Cultural sensitivity, however, does not guarantee needs will be more readily met and it would be inappropriate to suggest this. But it makes the way more negotiable.

14.4.3   Step 3: planning and implementation

> **Key skills**
>
> Creativity; leadership; shared decision making; risk taking; knowledge of national and local health policy; bidding for funds.

Deciding the new programme or service

From the information available, the steering group behind the project must decide on the new programme or service to be initiated. To be effective this should be shared with the population group to which the project is being targeted. Sharing the decision-making process with lay people is, perhaps, the ultimate submission of power by professionals and the agencies they represent. This may sound dramatic but the dominance by professionals over lay people creates some of the toughest barriers to effective community development (NESS 2005; NICE 2006). If local residents believe that their opinions have not been considered and/or that professionals are still forging ahead in pursuit of meeting their own needs and priorities, they may be unlikely to engage in any new services and facilities they perceive as being provided *for* them rather than *with* them (NICE 2006). Consequently, little progress would be made in improving health and reducing health inequalities.

Decision making involves considerable skills in examining, estimating and debating the benefits – improving health and reducing inequalities – against the costs involved – staff time, equipment, use of premises, etc. (Ranyard *et al.* 1997). In community development projects, however, the costs are not just financial. They include factors impossible to price and seldom mentioned such as the risks of failure, loss of trust and broken relationships between professionals and between lay people and professionals, and stress and sickness from significantly increased workloads and strained relationships (Hudson & Hardy 2002).

Decision making is such a complex cognitive process that each individual, with their own unique set of skills and experience, brings a different perspective. In developing new programmes or services those perspectives help ensure that as comprehensive as possible a consideration is given to the factors involved in the decision making, such as: its potential size and scope; identifying exactly the people most likely to benefit from it and how; the health factors and determinants to be influenced; how it will make a difference to people's lives; and the costs involved in terms of people, money and time. Exploring the potential impact on organizational priorities and targets set by the government through the Healthcare Commission and National Service Frameworks emanating from *The NHS Plan* (DH 2000) may help secure organizational support. Although meeting these targets should not, from a public health and lay person's perspective, be seen as a primary factor when deciding on new programmes and services, greater organizational support is more likely if it contributes in some way to the organization earning more funding!

How will it happen? Developing the project plan

Key skills

Project management; planning; organizing; budget management; report writing; risk assessment.

At this point in developing a new programme or initiative the person/s leading the work must be agreed by the steering group. It is essential they have protected time in keeping with the scale of the project or existing work pressures will impede progress. One of their first tasks is to develop a plan of action. Accurate, organised information is essential to make sense and bring order to the most complex project. A well-designed and structured project plan that addresses the 'what, why, when, how, where and who' of the proposed new service or programme is the cornerstone for success (Verzuh 2005). Project management skills are needed to plan the project exactly; the plan needs to include summarily:

- costing the project;
- identifying funding sources;
- creating a Gantt chart or detailed schedule of events and activities for the project;
- risk analysis;
- identifying roles and responsibilities of staff and stakeholders.

Activity

Supportive computer package tools such as PRINCE 2 (www.prince2.com), widely used in health and other public sector organizations, can support the development of a project plan effectively, but demand additional skills in their use and application. Visit the website and assess your project management skills.

Implementation

Key skills

Project management; action planning; networking; organizing; delegation; policy and report writing; financial/budget management; managing staff and people; marketing; management; leadership; communication and interpersonal skills; risk management; problem solving; trouble shooting; creativity; community capacity building.

In order for the project plan to be implemented and the goals achieved, the project manager must act as the catalyst to lift the words of the page and turn them into action or they remain mere rhetoric. The 'science' of public health coupled with that of project management provides that person with a powerful toolkit with which to develop new programmes and services to improve health and reduce health inequalities. But however good the tools may be, implementaion relies on the person's skill or 'art' of applying the skills to achieve the goals set and execute the project plan. The essential skills in this phase of the project, therefore, are more reliant on the leader's personal attributes and abilities acquired through experiential learning and considerable self-development than merely on academic education. This is a time of intense activity. The person needs self-confidence, self-motivation, creativity and sheer determination to make the project happen, as well as excellent interpersonal, organizational and trouble-shooting skills and the ability to delegate, motivate and manage others (Goleman *et al.* 2002; Verzuh 2005).

An example of the intense amount of work to be done in the implementation phase, taken from the project to which the case study relates, follows below. Between them the tasks demand high level (i.e. levels 3–4 in the NHS KSF; DH 2004b) key skills, as noted above:

- find and recruit the team of helpers, including paid and/or session staff and volunteers;
- find teachers, coaches and/or other appropriate skilled professionals to lead the sessions;
- locate and arrange the premises;
- market the new service/programme to key stakeholders (e.g. Citizens Advice Bureau, Age Concern) if they are not already involved in the multiagency steering group, to establish outreach services;
- bid for funding: numerous statutory, corporate and charitable organizations fund community initiatives and have their own internet sites.

Activity

Useful starting points to seek funds are: Community Development Xchange (www.cdx.org.uk), the Home Office (www.homeoffice.gov.uk), Department for Communities and Local Government (www.communities.gov.uk) and Volunteer Resource (www.volresource.org.uk).

Many funding organizations have a particular interest, such as sport, community development, young people, minority ethnic groups, particular disabilities, etc. They normally ask that several criteria are met before considering a grant, which means further work and includes:

- forming a committee consisting of, and preferably led by, local residents, including a chair, secretary and treasurer;
- having a written constitution;
- having written policies for health and safety, safeguarding children;
- doing risk assessments and taking action to reduce risk;
- opening a bank account specific to the project;
- financial management (setting up a bank account and budget/accounts system);
- sourcing equipment and other goods;
- planning a detailed timetable or schedule of activities for the service/facility;
- organizing the management of refreshments;
- advertising and 'marketing' the new service to the target user group and those that are in a position to recommend the service/programme;
- planning the public relations, e.g. liaising with the press to cover the launch of the new service;
- organizing the opening or launch event, including further advertising.

Successfully 'marketing' the new programme or service is essential to secure the support of key stakeholders and potential users. Although this takes many previously mentioned skills, marketing involves a specific ability to encourage people through several processes, many of which are included in the KSF (DH 2004b), to access or support new services. This is such a complex interaction and process that volumes of material have been written on that subject alone. However, in public health terms, if the new service or programme has been developed in true partnership with the community and the need has been accurately identified through effective community profiling and public consultation, there should be a need only to advertise, not sell it!

To do this productively, creativity and excellent writing skills are essential to design flyers, posters and other material that will catch people's attention and explain the new programme or service in just a few words. The organiser also needs to write a succinct article to submit to local newspaper editors. By doing this the chances of publication are increased as it saves on reporter time and travel. Good interpersonal and communication skills are needed to approach local radio stations to report on the launch or open day and to invite local public figures to attend or visit, which may give added credence and interest to the event.

Opening a new programme or service with an event or launch day marks the occasion appropriately. Its real worth, however, lies in the power of word of mouth. If people are impressed with what they see and experience they will spread the message more effectively than any other type of advertising, especially among the hardest to reach population groups (DfES 2005). But the event demands a multitude of skills from the person/s behind it. Firstly, it involves the challenge of accommodating and catering for an unpredictable number of people and, secondly, it means preparing for any type of occurrence that could happen when large numbers of people gather together. Although good risk assessment and planning skills pay off to a large extent, unforeseen situations may still arise such as the arts and crafts facilitator not turning up, the car park flooding or children being dropped off unattended – as happened during the project cited in the scenario in the case study. Handling these types of situations requires skills in complex problem solving, managing conflict, making effective decisions quickly, taking responsibility and maintaining an overall vision of the aims and objectives of the project or initiative (Verzuh 2005). In addition, creativity for stepping in to provide ideas for arts and crafts may also be needed!

14.4.4   Step 4: evaluation and review

> **Key skills**
>
> Knowledge of epidemiology; data collection; data analysis; report writing.

Evaluating a new service or programme serves several purposes. From an ethical perspective it is important to account for and justify the money spent to those who have funded the project. Whether they are tax payers, lottery ticket buyers, charity donators or people at fund raising events, feedback of how effective the initiative is in contributing to improving health and reducing health inequalities should be provided.

Money aside, the evaluation of practice, services or facilities provides nurses and midwives with an opportunity for personal learning and development that is integral to contemporary practice (DH 2004b). In addition there is a professional obligation to contribute to the evidence base needed to shape and improve future programmes and services:

> Local level evaluation is crucial for service development and remains an essential element of programme improvement structures. (NESS 2005, p. 4)

Evaluating a new programme or service is simply questioning its value in terms of effectiveness, efficiency, accessibility, equity, social acceptability and relevance to needs (NHS Executive 1999b). Comprehensive and detailed guidance for evaluating public health initiatives, particularly targeted towards the most disadvantaged population groups, is found, among others, on the Public Health Electronic Library (www.phel.gov.uk), the National Institute for Health and Clinical Excellence (www.nice.org.uk) and the National Evaluation of Sure Start (www.ness.bbk.ac.uk) websites. There are also numerous local evaluation reports posted on these sites, particularly the last, that illustrate the different methods and formats used to collect, analyse and present data.

Section 4

Activity

Access the National Evaluation of Sure Start website www.ness.bbk.ac.uk and explore this aspect of services development further.

Collecting data to evaluate new programmes or services as explained earlier takes specific skills. But just as with 'knowing the community' and 'making sense of information', the true skills of evaluation lie in how *effectively* data are collected and how *intelligently* they are processed and interpreted. This means, for example, collecting information and views not only from those that use the facility but from those of the target population who do *not* use it. For it is the latter group of people that remain marginalised and yet have the greatest health needs. For as long as such people are not benefiting from a new initiative there are improvements to be made in all areas (effectiveness, efficiency, accessibility, equity, social acceptability, relevance to needs) if health inequalities are to be effectively tackled.

14.5   Missing Skills

Invaluable lessons learnt from public health projects considered unsuccessful are often lost as the professionals involved seldom write about them for publication. However, the learning from experiences within the project in the case study, particularly from why it was unsuccessful, is extremely valid. Although the project manager had relevant and significantly developed skills from previous experience, experiential and academic learning and self-development, several factors contributed to the project failing.

One of these factors was concerned with the reasons why parents of young children did not take up the new programme of activities. Although the need for such a facility was accurately identified, some of the finer details were planned without further consultation – such as the actual timing and days on which the activities were scheduled. When it came to actually attending, parents felt the potential benefits did not outweigh the logistics of getting there. A further failing was in not securing the commitment of the local residents who volunteered to help run the after-school activities. This would have been better managed if the amount of time and work involved had been made clearer to them from the outset rather than it becoming apparent to them at the eleventh hour.

A contributing factor to the lack of uptake of outreach services was a lack of effective 'marketing'. Although this was the responsibility of the agencies involved, the fact was not made clear by the project manager and thus the services were not widely publicised. These factors provide an example of just how much detail is involved in developing new programmes and services. If any are overlooked or mishandled the overall success, despite an overwhelming amount of other work and effort, can be jeopardised.

Case Study Example

Developing a programme of activities and outreach services in a disadvantaged community – learning from the failures!

The project described in the case study above opened after a highly successful 'launch' day, but after 6 months the project was clearly failing and subsequently closed. All that remains and thrives is the coffee morning for older people.

Here was a situation where an interprofessional and multiagency initiative had come together in response to what local people had clearly expressed as highly needed. Moreover, as directed by public health policy, several local people were not just consulted but wholly involved in the project from the beginning and several more volunteered to help run the facilities following the consultation. So what went wrong? More importantly, what lessons can be learnt from this case study about the

(Continued)

> **Case Study Example (Continued)**
>
> skills needed in such initiatives, when this project, to all intents and purposes, followed established guidance for improving health and tackling inequalities, but still failed?
>
> The step by step process depicted in the main text was, undoubtedly, sound. It resulted in the setting up of a (potentially) highly successful and comprehensive project that had the ability to make real inroads in improving health and reducing health inequalities in a disadvantaged area. It was at the point of implementation that the project started to falter and ultimately fail. This was as a result of several key factors, which, with greater development skills, the project manager may have avoided:
>
> 1. At the point of opening, five of the six volunteers suddenly backed out, daunted by the amount of work involved. As the project had gone too far to abort it, the project manager and a small team of regular staff had to run the work-intense after-school activities on all three afternoons, putting huge pressure on them due to existing workloads.
> 2. The football coaches (physical education students from the local university) often just did not show up leaving the children disappointed. When they did, poor weather conditions often meant playing indoors, which was not as good from the children's perspective.
> 3. The attendance at new facilities and programmes in disadvantaged areas may be more reliant on word of mouth than any other marketing 'tool' and more people will attend if they hear something is good. Football was clearly the most sought after activity and yet its 'failings' would have been passed on and hindered other people attending.
> 4. The professionals staffing the outreach services did not 'market' their services, expecting this to be done by the project manager. As the numbers seen were small, they cut their services. People who then turned up to see them found they were no longer there that day and gave up trying to use the facilities.
> 5. In retrospect it was apparent that there was a discrepancy between the *perceived* and *actual/ genuine* needs of local people.

Conclusion

Developing programmes and services to improve health and reduce inequalities demands a greater range and depth of skills than perhaps any other area of nursing or midwifery. Many of them form an integral part of advanced clinical practice – high level communication, interpersonal, management and appraisal skills, for example. But there are many other skills to learn such as community development, profiling, project management and effective leadership. The skills of contemporary public health practice stem from an intelligent synthesis of theoretical learning – the 'science' – with practical application and experience – the 'art'.

To make real inroads in reducing health inequalities the public health practitioner must have an insightful knowledge of the community, its population groups and views of local people. This means making sense of, yet looking beyond, the data collected to form an accurate and culturally sensitive picture of the local community. From this the *real* issues of local people, particularly the most disadvantaged and hardest to reach population groups, can be better understood and therefore more effectively addressed.

Equally important, the practitioner must be prepared to learn from both successful and 'failed' projects as has been illustrated in this chapter. The lessons learnt from mistakes are invaluable yet are often hidden away behind the lack of confidence in sharing them with others. All too often professional journals are full of projects that are portrayed as successful and little is written of what can be learnt from situations that could have gone better. Contemporary public health practice for nurses and midwives is laced with risk taking and experimentation. The crime is not in making mistakes or 'failing' but in not sharing those experiences (however painful or embarrassing) and watching others perpetuate the same mistakes.

References

Antonakis J., Cianciolo A., Sternberg R. (2004) *The Nature of Leadership*. Thousand Oaks, CA: Sage Publications.

Ball M. (2002) *Getting Sure Start Started*. National Evaluation of Sure Start (NESS) Report No. 2. London: NESS

Benner P., Tanner C., Chesla C. (1996) *Expertise in Nursing Practice: caring, clinical judgment and ethics*. New York: Springer Verlag.

CRE (Committee for Racial Equality) (2004) *Gypsies and Travellers: a strategy for the CRE, 2004–7*. London: Committee for Racial Equality.

DfES (Department for Education and Skills) (2005) *Sure Start. Implementing Sure Start local programmes: an in-depth study*. Nottingham: Department for Education and Skills.

DH (Department of Health) (1999a) *Saving Lives: our healthier nation*. London: HM Stationery Office.

DH (Department of Health) (1999b) *Making a Difference: strengthening the nursing, midwifery and health visiting contribution to health and healthcare*. London: Department of Health.

DH (Department of Health) (2000) *The NHS Plan*. London: HM Stationery Office.

DH (Department of Health) (2002a) *Shifting the Balance of Power: next steps*. London: Department of Health.

DH (Department of Health) (2002b) *Liberating the Talents: helping primary care trusts and nurses to deliver the NHS Plan*. London: Department of Health.

DH (Department of Health) (2003a) *Tackling Health Inequalities: a programme for action*. London: Department of Health.

DH (Department of Health) (2003b) *Public Health in England*. London: HM Stationery Office. www.dh.gov.uk.

DH (Department of Health) (2004a) *Choosing Health: making healthier choices easier*. London: HM Stationery Office.

DH (Department of Health) (2004b) *The NHS Knowledge and Skills Framework (NHS KSF) and the Development Review Process*. London: HM Stationery Office.

Goleman D., McKee A., Boyatzis R. (2002) *Primal Leadership: realizing the power of emotional intelligence*. Boston, MA: Harvard Business School.

Hartley P. (1999) *Interpersonal Communication*, 2nd edn. London: Routledge.

HDA (Health Development Agency) (2004) *Developing Healthier Communities*. London: Health Development Agency.

Hudson B., Hardy B. (2002) What is a 'successful' partnership and how can it be measured? In: *Partnerships, New Labour and the Governance of Welfare* (eds Glendinning C., Powell M., Rummery K.). Bristol: Policy Press.

Marmot M., Wilkinson R. (eds) (2005) *Social Determinants of Health*, 2nd edn. Oxford: Oxford University Press.

NESS (National Evaluation of Sure Start) (2005) *Implementing and Managing your Sure Start Local Evaluation Programme*. London: HM Treasury. www.ness.bbk.ac.uk/documents/GuidanceReports/1139pdf.

NHS Executive (1999a) *Patient and Public Involvement in the New NHS*. Leeds: NHS Executive.

NHS Executive (1999b) *Public Health Resource Pack*. London: NHS Executive.

NICE (National Institute for Health and Clinical Excellence) (2005) *Health Needs Assessment: a practical guide*. London: NICE.

NICE (National Institute for Health and Clinical Excellence) (2006) *An Assessment of Community Engagement and Community Development Approaches to Health Improvement, Including the Use of Collaborative Methodology and Community Champions*. Draft Guidance Document. London: NICE. www.nice.org.uk.

ONS (Office for National Statistics) (2001) *Count Me In: census 2001*. London: Office for National Statistics.

Performance and Innovation Unit (2001) *Strengthening Leadership in the Public Sector. A research study by the PIU*. London: Performance and Innovation Unit.

Prime Minister's Strategy Unit (2005) *Improving the Prospects of People Living in Areas of Multiple Deprivation in England*. London: Prime Minister's Strategy Unit.

Ranyard R., Svenson O., Crozier W. (1997) *Decision Making: cognitive models and explanations*. London: Routledge.

Salovey P., Brocken M., Mayer J. (2004) *Emotional Intelligence: key readings on the Mayer and Salovey model*. New York: National Professional Resources.

Verzuh E. (2005) *The Fast Forward MBA in Project Management*, 2nd edn. Princeton, NJ: John Wiley & Sons.

Wanless D. (2004) *Securing Good Health for the Whole Population. Final report*. London: HM Treasury Office.

CHAPTER 15

Programme Planning for Health Education

Chris Griffiths

Public Health Skills: Programme planning

- Preparation for programme planning
- Delivery, management and evaluative skills in programme planning for health education: children and young people's health, public health and inequalities
- Ideology and strategy in the 'Healthy schools' initiative, accessing health services and planning framework for a health fair

Introduction

The main focus of this chapter is on the public health skills required to plan, deliver, manage and evaluate programmes designed to improve the health and wellbeing of children and young people. It therefore contains a very practically based scenario demonstrating the five key steps undertaken by a school nursing team in planning health education targeted at young people within a school environment. The example is a multiagency venture resulting in the delivery of a health fair coordinated by a school nursing team together with their education partners.

15.1 Children and Young People's Health

The importance of promoting health and wellbeing in this group is well documented (Madge & Franklin 2003; Chambers & Licence 2005). The aim is to enable them to make the transition to adulthood and to achieve their maximum potential in terms of education, health, development and wellbeing. Aynsley Green (2000) stated that children and young people are the nation's most precious resource; they deserve the best care as they are the life blood of the nation and are vital for our future economic survival and prosperity. Childhood should be a time of happiness and good health. Whilst it is acknowledged that children and young people in Britain enjoy a higher standard of health than their predecessors, there are still many factors that conspire against the achievement of optimal health and wellbeing for children and young people (DH 2004a). For example, individual lifestyle factors have an important influence on health as do socioeconomic, cultural and environmental aspects, often outside the control of the child or young person and which can affect their health and access to health services. These wider determinants of health include poverty, social exclusion, employment, housing, education and environment (Dalgren & Whitehead 1991).

> **Activity**
>
> Revisit Chapter 13 to remind yourself of the impact of the wider determinants of health on children's health and wellbeing.

15.2   Public Health and Inequalities

Public health improvement to tackle health inequalities is a major national concern today and is written into policy directives on children and young people's health. Many of the issues identified in these policies have been raised over the last 25 years. It was in 1980 that the Black report (Black 1980) identified inequalities in health that were further highlighted in *Health Divide* (Townsend & Davidson 1988). As identified in earlier chapters, Acheson's (1988) definition of public health formed the cornerstone for public health practitioners to develop strategies for dealing with these inequalities. In 2004 Wanless published a way forward for government departments to address the public health issues through identifying the financial frameworks required for moving the public health agenda on (Wanless 2004). Whilst there have been some improvements in the health of children and young people since the Black report of 1980, there is still a need to address current issues of inequality and access to good health for all children and young people.

This is the most prominent theme of *Choosing Health* (DH 2004b) in which the ideology for dealing with the health of children and young people is based on the premise that individuals are ultimately responsible for their own and their children's health and that healthy children become healthy adults. However, there is mounting evidence to suggest that much adult disease has its origins in early life, and events in childhood and young adulthood have long-term consequences that determine adult wellbeing (Wright *et al.* 2001; WHO 2003). For young people facing the transition to adulthood from childhood it is a time of great change. Parents become less influential with the young person; peer pressure becomes more manifest and risk taking more ubiquitous. Piaget (1972) advocated that for the young person this is a time of egocentrism (self-centredness), which suggests that they believe they are above mundane risks and demands. Part of growing into adulthood is about risk taking but, as Bagnall and Dilloway (1996) suggested, young people are unaware of the scale of the risk involved.

Some examples to illustrate the reason for concern about the health and wellbeing of young people include the following:

- Britain has the highest rate of teenage conceptions and sexually transmitted infections in Western Europe (Metcalfe 2004);
- the Mental Health Foundation (1998) suggests that at any particular time, up to 20 per cent of school-age children and young people may suffer from mental health problems that translate into preventable mental illness such as depression, self-harm, eating disorders and drug misuse;
- it has been estimated that if the current increase in childhood obesity continues, children will have a shorter life expectancy than their parents (Crowther *et al.* 2004);
- being overweight in childhood is also associated with poor psychological wellbeing, including low self-esteem and negative body image (Hall & Elliman 2003).

15.3   Ideology into Strategy

Nevertheless, government policy supports the ideology that young people should be supported in taking responsibility for their own health and making informed choices and decisions regarding their emotional and social development, and health and wellbeing both now and in the future (DH 2004a, 2004c, 2005a). The transference of this ideology into practice can be seen in some of the emerging strategies to make healthier choices easier choices. Not surprisingly, schools have been identified as one of the key settings for promoting the health of children and young people (DH 1992; WHO 1997; Moon *et al.*

1999; Rowlings & Jeffreys 2000; Sinkler & Toft 2000). The length of time spent by children and young people in school in industrialised countries has changed very little since 1979 when it was estimated that this was 15 000 hours (Rutter *et al.* 1979).

A school can provide the ideal environment for delivering a planned and coordinated programme of personal, social and health education to children and young people on a large scale (Downie *et al.* 1990; Hagquist & Starrin 1997). As Lightfoot and Bines (1998) suggested, those that attend school are a captive audience placed within a child-centred, educational environment. However, it is important to acknowledge that those who do not attend school should not be forgotten.

Since the introduction of the school national curriculum (Kelly 1990) and regular pupil assessment, excessive demands have been made on teaching staff that has seen health promotion sidelined and often dismissed from the school agenda. Indeed, there is no statutory provision for health promotion in the national curriculum. In secondary schools most health promotion is taught by teachers, without necessarily specific knowledge of the health issues discussed. Visiting health professionals are given brief timetabled sessions, which are often cancelled due to pressures from the national curriculum. It is hardly surprising then, that children and young people cannot remember the sessions being held and their content (Madge & Franklin 2003).

15.4   Healthy Schools Initiative

In an attempt to address this issue, the 'Healthy schools standard' was introduced in 1999 (DEE 1999) and developed in 2005 into the 'Healthy schools' programme (DH 2005a). It is the government's intention that all schools should be working towards national 'Healthy schools' status by 2009 (DfES 2004, 2005a; DH 2004b, 2004c). The 'Healthy schools' programme comes at a time when health policy is focusing on negative aspects of health like obesity, substance misuse and poor sexual health. The 'Healthy schools' programme reflects the government's commitment to address the lack of health promotion in the national curriculum and put measures in place to achieve a healthy population of children and young people. The vehicle for this is seen as the adoption of a whole school approach that involves not only the children and young people but the whole community (DH 2005a).

Children and young people know what their health needs are and these are not always in line with government policy directives. However, as Humphries (2002) suggested, there are parallels between the views that young people hold about their health and those held by professionals. This is an important observation as professionals have been criticised for deciding the content and format of health promotion programmes. Aggleton *et al.* (1998) have identified that young people think health topics such as sexual health and drugs are too narrow, and do not meet their needs. Government policy has attempted to address this issue by proposing children and young people should be asked for their views (DH 2004a).

Activity

The importance of partnership working and user involvement in service development is discussed in Chapters 4, 5 and 6. Revisit these chapters to refresh your understanding of this important public health skill.

If the ideology of government advocates supporting young people in making healthier choices, easier choices and encouraging them to take responsibility for their own actions and decisions, then it would seem appropriate to ask them what resources they need to achieve this goal. The question for public health nurses is, therefore, what do children and young people want from the NHS?

15.5   Accessing Health Services

There is no clear picture of the number of children and young people who access the range of services offered by the NHS or the value they put on those services. There is also some question about attitudes that young people have towards their own health. Balding (2001) suggested that nine out of 10 young people surveyed felt they were in control of their health while at least a quarter of those surveyed did not think they could influence their health through their own efforts. Barron (2005) has identified that young people are a difficult group to attract to health services because access to services may not meet their needs. For example, if they receive disapproval by health professionals and are worried about the possible lack of confidentiality they will not seek help. Evidence from a number of studies suggests that young people rarely visit their GP and those that do tend to visit with physical complaints rather than for sensitive issues (Bagnall & Dilloway 1996; Bunack 2000; Coleman & Schofield 2001). Young people would, however, choose to see a 'teenage health specialist' at a drop-in facility for their health care, which could be provided at school as well as in other community settings (Jones *et al.* 2000; Hall & Elliman 2003; Flint 2006). Access to services has traditionally been led by girls (Madge & Franklin 2003), who tend to talk to someone about their difficulties. Boys and young men on the other hand have always been considered more difficult to engage in health services, and consideration needs to be given to tackling this issue, especially as males generally have higher morbidity than females (Williamson 1995; Osborne 2000). Madge and Franklin (2003) suggested boys are more likely to turn to help lines or the internet for support, an avenue addressed in recent government recommendations for children and young people (DH 2004a, 2004b).

School nurses are arguably the most appropriate health professional to run a confidential drop-in service as they have the knowledge and skills to provide general health information, advice and support about health issues such as diet and nutrition, physical activity, emotional wellbeing, puberty, smoking and sexual health (DH 2004a, 2004b, 2004c, 2006; NMC 2004). School nurses occupy a unique position to deliver on health goals as their service is located within the NHS but operationalised within an educational setting – the school being the focus of the nurse's work (Bagnall & Dilloway 1996).

The following case study example demonstrates one school nursing team's approach to planning health education targeted at young people within a school environment. The example is a multiagency development and delivery of a health fair, coordinated by a school nursing team with their education partners. It followed consultation with young people in order to identify their specific needs and adapted Ewles and Simnett's (1999) health promotion model to provide a framework in which to describe the planning process undertaken (Box 15.1). The Ewles and Simnett (1999) planning framework allowed flexibility for the case study example, and allows the reader to follow a step by step approach to the development and implementation of a multiagency health fair for a cohort of young people within a given locality.

BOX 15.1

Planning framework for the health fair: *Source*: Adapted from Eweles and Simnett (1999).

Stage 1 Identifying needs and priorities
Stage 2 Setting aims and objectives
Stage 3 Identifying the resources required
Stage 4 Planning evaluation methods
Stage 5 Planning action
Stage 6 Evaluating its effectiveness and reset goals

Case Study Example

Using a planning framework

Stage 1: identifying needs and priorities

The decision to run a health fair followed a discussion with a school nurse and a senior member of teaching staff at a mixed ability senior school of 1400 children and young people (age 12–18 years). The school staff and school nurses had built a sound working relationship with the children and young people in the school and this enabled them to target identified needs in a supportive manner.

(Continued)

Case Study Example (Continued)

The children and young people in the school had identified several unmet health needs that had not been addressed. The teachers and school nurse felt that these issues could not be ignored as it had come to light that some of the children and young people were engaging in risk-taking behaviour involving highly risky encounters with their health. It was jointly agreed that the best way to address these needs was to consult the children and young people collectively within the school and ask them what they saw as their priority in health needs, and how they would like these addressed. The health needs appeared particularly relevant to the senior school population (age 15–18 years) where it has been suggested there is less parental influence over the decisions, including risk taking, that young people make (Piaget 1972; Bagnall & Dilloway 1996).

The young people were encouraged to become involved as suggested by the Green Paper *Youth Matters* (DfES 2005b) and, if interested, to identify themselves to a recognised member of staff. The young people were then asked to identify key areas of health concern, gaps in their knowledge and how these could be addressed. The information was supplied through the completion of a confidential questionnaire. Parahoo (1997) asserted that questionnaires are one of the few methods of data collection that potentially keeps respondents anonymous. Four main health needs were identified (Figure 15.1).

The highest number of responses reflected health needs related to mental health and associated factors. These were identified by 48 per cent of all respondents. Drug- and alcohol-related behaviours were identified as an issue by 19 per cent of all respondents. Sexual health was identified by 11 per cent, whilst identification of suspicious lumps attracted 9 per cent. The remaining responses were for less specific health needs such as healthy eating, exercise, housing, personal and fire safety, immunizations and first aid.

It was interesting to note that mental health was identified as the highest need along with drugs, alcohol and sexual health as these needs are consistent with government ideology identified in the National Service Framework for children, young people and maternity services (DH 2004a), *You're Welcome, Quality Criteria* (DH 2005b), *Choosing Health: making healthy choices easier* (DH 2004b) and the Chief Nursing Officer's review of the contribution of nursing, midwifery and health visiting to vulnerable children and young people (DH 2004c). Following analysis of the health needs, the young people suggested that the best way of addressing these issues would be through a health fair.

Stage 2: setting aims and objectives

The aim was to support young people in meeting their identified health needs by encouraging them to take responsibility for their own health, both now and into adulthood. This was to be achieved by giving information, advice and support to enable them to make informed choices about their health and wellbeing and to know where to access services within the community in which they live.

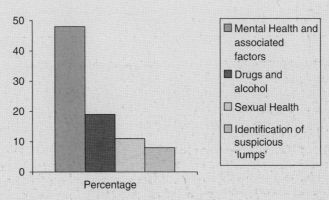

Figure 15.1 The four main health needs identified in the case study.

(Continued)

Case Study Example (Continued)

The objectives were specific and included statements that defined what the young people would have achieved by the end of the health fair; they included:

- an increased level of knowledge for young people to be able to make informed decisions;
- an awareness of where and how to access services;
- enhanced partnership links between health and education.

To ensure the objectives were met it was felt essential to involve a range of expertise from each of the identified areas of health need. A cross-section of service providers and service users and a focus group to include six young people (three male and three female), the school nurse, a senior member of teaching staff and the student support advisor from the school was therefore recruited.

Other agencies were invited to join the focus group but all declined due to other work commitments. The school nurses were particularly well placed to build effective relationships with a wide range of individuals, groups and communities and to provide a clear leadership focus for the health fair. Their particular strengths lay in working with school staff – although their relationships with others such as Connexions workers, social care staff, voluntary agencies, mental health workers, community leaders, parents, carers, children and young people were key in the development of the health fair.

Stage 3: identifying the resources required

Following the setting of aims and objectives, the focus group met to identify what resources would be required to make the health fair a success. The young people were crucial in the progression of the health fair as there were time constraints on the school staff and other agencies. The National Service Framework for children, young people and maternity services (DH 2004a) and *Youth Matters* (DfES 2005b) both encourage this approach to involvement and the commitment shown by the young people to the project was to be commended.

The methods adopted for promoting health and engaging the young people during the health fair were identified by the services available to participate in the event. Most of the statutory agencies were contracted to improve the health and wellbeing of young people and their involvement was provided at no extra cost. Agencies in the voluntary and private sectors required payment, although a local supermarket offered to provide a token community voucher to support the event. This had to be considered in the overall objectives. The inclusion of all relevant agencies would augment existing partnership arrangements and had the potential to demonstrate multiagency health promotion, which could only enhance multiagency links for the school-age community.

The school was agreed as the venue at no extra cost. The school premises had adequate toilet facilities, disabled access and appropriate storage and were acceptable for health and safety purposes. There was also adequate car parking outside the building to ensure ease of carrying in equipment. Provision was made for disabled school staff, pupils and visitors in accordance with the Disability Discrimination Act 1995 to provide adequate access, toilet facilities and health information in appropriate format and language.

It was therefore agreed that a multiagency health fair would be set up for 1 day on the school premises. The format of the day would be structured information stands incorporating a wide spectrum of professionals and agencies. Car parking and refreshments would be provided by the school. Consequently, to meet all the identified needs of the young people, agencies providing information on the following areas were invited to attend:

- early intervention team (mental health);
- young people's sexual health team;
- smoking awareness/smoke stop (school nursing team);
- young people's drug and alcohol services;
- local sports centre representatives;
- healthy eating (school nursing team);
- young people's advice service (to include housing);
- health professional (breast and testicular awareness);

(Continued)

Case Study Example (Continued)

- school physical education department;
- connexions;
- alcohol awareness (school nursing team);
- fire prevention service;
- general information (school nursing team);
- first aid (school medical room staff).

All agencies were either approached by school staff or the school nurse to ascertain their willingness to attend and their confirmed availability. Letters of confirmation and details were sent by the school. Posters were positioned on the school site by the young people and information was given to young people by school staff. Agencies were able to set up their stand the night before if they so wished and car parking was reserved to ensure easy transition of resources to the building. An area of the car park was cordoned off for the fire service to position the fire engine and safety demonstration equipment. Each individual agency was responsible for the resources they provided.

Each agency was given an information stand appropriate to their profession or agency and they provided a wide range of services. Each stand offered leaflets on specific health concerns, information on local specialist services, relevant national websites and help lines and an opportunity to arrange appointments if appropriate. Individuals who needed confidential help on the day were accommodated and appointments could be made for all agencies at the general information stand, which was manned by school nurses. The use of leaflets and posters as a health resource has long been debated; however, Russell *et al.* (1979) suggests that leaflets add a couple of percentage points to the effectiveness of the verbal advice given by health professionals.

Stage 4: planning the evaluation methods

Gathering information beforehand and evaluation of an activity is important in order to understand and judge the worth of the activity (Peberdy 2002). It is also key in determining whether an intervention has been effective and successful (Tones & Green 2006). The focus group discussed whether or not to use formal or informal evaluations and all members accepted that evaluation was important as it is often necessary for agencies to provide data to inform future services. The group considered that a simple, randomised questionnaire was the most appropriate form of data collection required for this first event.

Although the evaluation was planned, it was not thought worthwhile to follow this up at a later date as some of the young people attending the health fair would have left school, thus invalidating the data. It was also thought that these young people were of senior school age and as mentioned earlier in the chapter their priorities change in a short period of time (DfES 2005b).

Stage 5: planning the action

At this stage it was imperative to write a detailed plan bringing the whole event into focus. This included who was responsible for each part of the event and an events programme for the day. Once completed, this was sent to all parties by letter and email to ensure delivery. A timescale and follow-up meeting was arranged to ensure all targets were being achieved, the day was going according to plan and that the evaluation process was in place.

The health fair day arrived and the education representatives, school nurses and young people commenced their day early to ensure all was in place. The stands were well positioned, bright and inviting, and the fire safety staff were introduced to other agencies at the start of the day to ensure they were not excluded from the main event by being positioned in the car park. The stands were fully staffed by a variety of multiagency staff who had no difficulty getting to know each other and arranging future meetings. There was a vast assortment of enthusiastic staff and information for young people to take away and read at their leisure. The young people who had volunteered to help were eager to assist in any way that was needed. One in particular assisted a young man with disability in his quest to

(Continued)

Case Study Example (Continued)

undertake a smoking awareness assessment, which she did with great humour. The flow of young people continued over several hours and the day was looking to be a great success. The staff and young people were very grateful for the refreshments supplied as all were exhausted at the end of the session. Virtually all leaflets and information were taken by young people, along with a wealth of knowledge supplied by the staff present. All appeared to have enjoyed the day and felt it worthwhile.

As planned (in stage 4), the young people had developed a randomised questionnaire as a way of evaluating the day. This asked the following key questions:

1. *Did you find the health fair valuable?* One hundred and nineteen responses were received and the results can be seen in Figure 15.2.
2. *Have you learnt anything today that you will change to improve your health?* One hundred and four responses were received and the results can be seen in Figure 15.3.
3. *Is there anything you would like to see more of in future events?* The qualitative responses to this question indicated that the young people were very positive and enjoyed the health fair overall. The vast majority wanted the health fair to become an annual event. The topics in general had met their needs, although several young people had requested the event to become more interactive. There had also been a specific request by a group of young people to include blood pressure monitoring and fitness testing, which would now be considered.

Stage 6: evaluate effectiveness and reset goals

Information from the evaluations collated by the young people was a positive outcome to the day, helping to inform future events. In addition the event was very positively evaluated by all professionals, who had also made good multiagency links on the day of the health fair. This favourable outcome would go a long way towards improving partnership working with children and young people in the future.

All parties were keen to repeat the event in the next school year and to open it up to all children and young people at the school, together with their parents. However, the health need assessment questionnaire was considered to be too simplistic and would need to be developed and refined for future events. This would go some way to ensuring that all identified needs and topics could be addressed adequately as young people may have very different health needs in the future and these would need to be assessed accordingly.

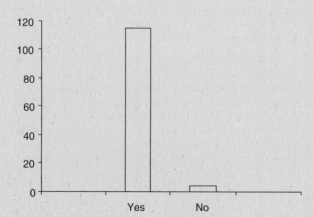

Figure 15.2 Response to question 1: 'Did you find the health fair valuable?'

(Continued)

Case Study Example (Continued)

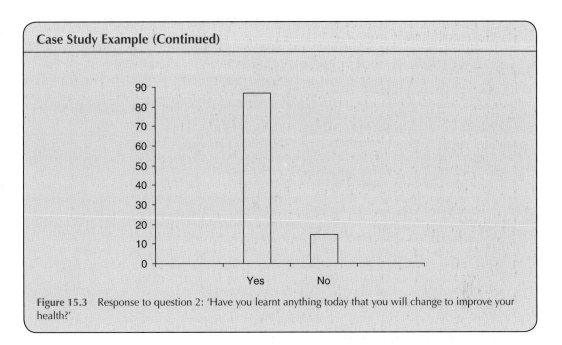

Figure 15.3 Response to question 2: 'Have you learnt anything today that you will change to improve your health?'

Conclusion

This chapter has discussed and offered a worked example of how school nurses work in partnership to plan health education with and for children and young people. The case study example offered the experience of a health fair, produced within existing school nurse resources and incorporating service providers and users in its delivery to attempt to fulfil the health needs of young people.

This successful health fair is a good example of partnership working where the agenda is set, managed and evaluated with the children and young people themselves.

References

Acheson D. (1988) *Public Health in England*, London: Department of Health.

Aggleton P., Whitty G., Knight A., Prayle D., Warwick I., Rivers K. (1998) Promoting young people's health: the health concerns and needs of young people. *Health Education* 6, 213–19.

Aynsley Green A. (2000) Who is speaking for children and adolescents and their health at policy level? (Education and debate). *British Medical Journal* 321 (7255), 229–32.

Bagnall P., Dilloway M. (1996) *In a Different Light*. London: Queen's Nursing Institute.

Balding J. (2001) *Young People in 2000*. Exeter: School Health Education Unit.

Barron S. (2005) Sexual health of adolescents. *Primary Health Care* 15 (5), 37–41.

Black D. (1980) *Inequalities in Health: report of a research working group*. London: Department of Health.

Bunack R. (2000) Young teenagers' attitudes towards general practitioners and their provision of sexual health care. *British Journal of General Practice* 40 (456), 550–4.

Chambers R., Licence K. (2005) *Looking after Children in Primary Care. A companion to the Children's National Services Framework*. Oxford: Radcliffe Publishing.

Coleman J., Schofield J. (2001) *Key Data in Adolescence 2001*. Trust for the Study of Adolescence, www.tsa.uk.com.

Crowther R., Rolfe L., Morgan S., Rutter H., Watson J. (2004) *Indications of Public Health in the English Regions 3: lifestyle and it's impact on health*. Stockton on Tees: South East Public Health Observatory on behalf of the Association of Public Health Observatories.

Dalgren G., Whitehead M. (1991) *Policies and Strategies to Promote Social Equity in Health*. Stockholm: Stockholm Institute of Future Studies.

DEE (Department of Education and Employment) (1999) *National Healthy Schools Standard Guidance.* London: Department of Education and Employment.

DfES (Department for Education and Skills) (2004) *The Evaluation of the Extended Schools Pathfinder Project.* Nottingham: HM Stationery Office.

DfES (Department for Education and Skills) (2005a) *Higher Standards, Better Schools for All: more choice for parents and pupils.* London: HM Stationery Office.

DfES (Department for Education and Skills) (2005b) *Youth Matters Green Paper.* London: DfES Publications. http://www.dfes.gov.uk/publications/youth/ (accessed 3 July 2006).

DH (Department of Health) (1992) *The Health of the Nation – a strategy for health in England.* London: HM Stationery Office.

DH (Department of Health) (2004a) *Core Document, National Service Framework for Children, Young People and Maternity Services. Core standards.* London: Department of Health.

DH (Department of Health) (2004b) *Choosing Health: making healthier choices easier.* London: Department of Health.

DH (Department of Health) (2004c) *The Chief Nursing Officer's Review of the Nursing, Midwifery and Health Visiting Contribution to Vulnerable Children and Young People.* London: Department of Health.

DH (Department of Health) (2005a) *National Healthy School Status: a guide for schools.* London: Department of Health.

DH (Department of Health) (2005b) *You're Welcome, Quality Criteria: making health services young people friendly.* London: Department of Health.

DH (Department of Health) (2006) *School Nurse: practice development resource rack.*, Nottingham: Department of Health/Department for Education and Skills.

Downie R.S., Fyfe C., Tannahill A. (1990) *Health Promotion: models and values.* Oxford: Oxford University Press.

Ewles L., Simnett I. (1999) *Promoting Health: a practical guide*, 4th edn. Edinburgh: Bailliere Tindall.

Flint C. (2006) Launching the teenage health demonstration sites programme. In: *Health Challenge for England: next steps for choosing health* (Department of Health). London: HM Stationery Office.

Hagquist K., Starrin B. (1997) Health education in schools – from information to empowerment models. *Health Promotion International* 12 (3), 225–32.

Hall D., Elliman D. (2003) *Health for All Children*, 4th edn. Oxford: Oxford University Press.

Humphries J. (2002) The school nurse and health education in the classroom. *Nursing Standard* 16/17, 42–5.

Jones R., Coleman J., Dennison C. (2000) *Community Health Initiatives for Young People: a working paper.* Trust for the Study of Adolescence, www.tsa.uk.org.

Kelly A.V. (1990) *The National Curriculum: a critical review.* London: Sage Publications.

Lightfoot J., Bines W. (1998) Promoting young people's health: the health concerns and needs of young people. *Health Education* 6, 213–19.

Madge N., Franklin A. (2003) *Change, Challenge and School Nursing.* London: National Children's Bureau.

Mental Health Foundation (1998) *The Big Picture: promoting children and young people's mental health.* London: Mental Health Foundation.

Metcalfe T. (2004) Sexual health: meeting adolescents needs. *Nursing Standard* 18 (46), 40–3.

Moon A.M., Mullee M.A., Rogers L. (1999) Helping schools to become health-promoting environments: an evaluation of the Wessex Healthy Schools Award. *Health Promotion International* 14 (2), 111–22.

NMC (Nursing and Midwifery Council) (2004) *Proficiencies for Specialist Community Public Health Nursing.* London: Nursing and Midwifery Council.

Osborne N. (2000) Children's voices: evaluation school drop-in health clinic. *Community Practitioner* 72 (3), 516–18.

Parahoo K. (1997) *Nursing Research, Principles, Process and Issues.* London: Macmillan Press.

Peberdy A. (2002) Evaluating community action. In: *The Challenge of Promoting Health: exploration and action*, 2nd edn (eds Jones L., Sidell M., Douglas J.), 85–101. London: Palgrave.

Piaget J. (1972) Intellectual evolution from adolescence to adulthood, *Human Development* 15 (1), 1–12.

Rowlings L., Jeffreys V. (2000) Challenges in the development and monitoring of health promoting schools. *Health Education* 100 (3), 117–23.

Russell M.H., Wilson C., Taylor C., Baker C.D. (1979) Effects of general practice against smoking. *British Medical Journal* 2, 231–5.

Rutter M., Maughan B., Mortimore P., Ouston J. (1979) *Fifteen Thousand Hours.* London: Open Books.

Sinkler P., Toft M. (2000) Raising the national healthy school standard (NHSS) together. *Health Education* 100 (2), 6–7.

Tones K., Green J. (2006) *Planning and Strategies for Promoting Health.* London: Sage Publications.

Townsend P., Davidson N. (1988) The Black report. In: *Inequalities in Health* (ed. Black D.). London: Penguin.

Wanless D. (2004) *Securing Good Health for the Whole Population. Final report.* London: HM Treasury Office. www.hm-treasury.gov.uk/wanless (accessed 6 July 2006).

Williamson P. (1995) Their own worst enemy. *Nursing Times* 91 (48), 25.

WHO (World Health Organization) (1997) *Promoting Health through Schools: report of a WHO Expert Committee on school health education.* Geneva: World Health Organization.

WHO (World Health Organization) (2003) *Global Strategy for Infant and Young Child Feeding.* Genevea: World Health Organization.

Wright C.M., Parker L., Lamont D. (2001) Implications of childhood obesity for adult health: findings from thousand families cohort study. *British Medical Journal* 323, 1280–4.

CHAPTER 16

Ethically Managing Self, People and Resources to Improve the Health and Wellbeing of Patients and Clients in the Community

Neil Jackson and Lynda Rogers

Public Health Skills: Managing self, people and resources ethically

- Ethical theories, ethical principles and their application
- Concepts of ethics: utilitarianism and deontology as applied to the client and practice
- Legal and professional frameworks and their application
- The role of advocacy and reflections on practice and dilemmas raised

Introduction

This chapter considers some of the ethical and legal issues that nurses working in the field of public health need to understand. The ethical and legal issues relate to the management of self and others as well as resources. The chapter should enable the nurse to become aware of and apply legal and ethical frameworks that guide and inform practice. A scenario is developed, in the form of a case study, to provide examples of ethical and legal issues: these are examined through a hypothetical example assignment, written by Sunita Ranj, a registered nurse undertaking a unit of learning on ethical and legal concepts at her local university. Sunita demonstrates her learning through the case study and raises ethical and legal issues around a patient (Mrs Hammond) who is being cared for in her own home by a multiagency team. Discussion points are raised during the chapter in order to explore some of the dilemmas faced within everyday practice.

Sunita Ranj has been qualified as a registered nurse for 10 years. She has been working in the community for the past 5 years and works across a number of community nursing and multiagency teams. Sunita has not undertaken any formal professional study for 4 years and is currently studying a module of learning on ethics and law. Undertaking this module, she feels, will help her current nursing practice by developing her knowledge and skills in relation to managing the health needs of patients with chronic diseases such as asthma, diabetes or chronic obstructive pulmonary disease (COPD).

The assignment, given below in Section 16.1, that Sunita is undertaking is part of the ethics and law module and takes the form of a case study exploring her current clinical practice. The assignment learning outcomes are outlined in Box 16.1. Sunita is going to present her assignment using a case study that reflects the nursing care and professional interactions experienced with a patient cared for in the home and supported by the family and a multiagency team.

By following the arguments in Sunita's case study the reader will not only be able to examine aspects of the ethical, legal and professional theories but will also be able to apply them to frameworks that

---

BOX 16.1

Learning outcomes for assignment on ethics and law module.

Students are required to:
- Present and evaluate ethical, legal and personal value systems and the ways in which they relate within a practice environment
- Demonstrate a knowledge and understanding of ethical theories
- Demonstrate an understanding of legislation that relates to professional practice
- Illustrate a knowledge and understanding within the case study of ethical principles and standpoints

---

BOX 16.2

Structure of the case study.

- Introduction and patient history
- Ethical theories
- Ethical principles and their application to the case study
- Legal and professional frameworks and their application to the case study
- The role of advocacy
- Reflections on practice and dilemmas in care provided to Mrs Hammond and her family
- Case study conclusions

---

guide and inform practice. The reader will also be able to see how Sunita constructs and develops arguments within the case study. The structure of the case study can be seen in Box 16.2.

16.1 Sunita's Case Study

16.1.1 Introduction and patient history

This case study will explore the ethical and legal issues related to a patient who has COPD. A multi-agency approach to care is adopted as part of the package of care designed to enable the patient to remain in her home. Although there are many aspects of care and intervention related to this patient's assessed needs, the assignment will focus on her wish to remain in her home.

The case study will present and discuss selected ethical theories and consider how they relate to nursing. The case study will also explore issues related to advocacy, autonomy, beneficence, non-maleficence and justice. Where appropriate, the presentation and critical discussion of ethical standpoints and principles will be given. Confidentiality will be maintained as required by the Nursing and Midwifery Council (NMC) *Code of Professional Conduct: standards for conduct, performance and ethics* (NMC 2004). Therefore, the names and places will be changed and the patient will be referred to by the pseudonym of Mrs Joyce Hammond. The case study will focus on the wish of Mrs Hammond to be nursed at home with her family supported by health and Social Services. Possible dilemmas that could arise will also be explored and analysed.

Mrs Joyce Hammond's *medical history* indicates that she has smoked since 13 years of age and has a history of a persistent cough followed by pains in her chest for the past 3 years. An eventual diagnosis of COPD was revealed and she now has very limited capacity to walk and is continuously breathless. This has led to restricted physical activity as her condition deteriorates. Despite her deterioration she has expressed a wish to be cared for at home.

Socially, Mrs Hammond, who likes to be called Joyce, is 45 years of age and has lived with her partner Nigel, aged 49, for 10 years. They each have adult sons from previous relationships. Mrs Hammond was working as an administrator until she became ill 3 years ago and is now unable to work. She is in receipt of disability benefit. Nigel continues to work full time as an electrician but realises that he will need some time off work to be with Joyce as her condition deteriorates.

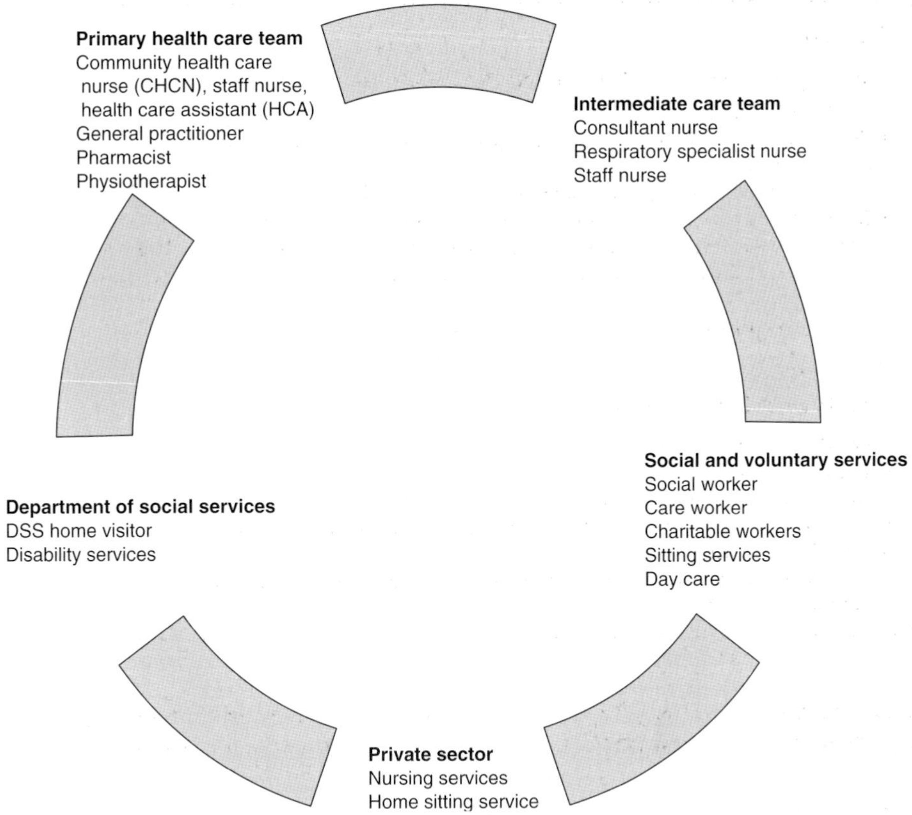

Primary health care team
Community health care
 nurse (CHCN), staff nurse,
 health care assistant (HCA)
General practitioner
Pharmacist
Physiotherapist

Intermediate care team
Consultant nurse
Respiratory specialist nurse
Staff nurse

Social and voluntary services
Social worker
Care worker
Charitable workers
Sitting services
Day care

Department of social services
DSS home visitor
Disability services

Private sector
Nursing services
Home sitting service

Figure 16.1   Multiagency team involved in the care of Mrs Hammond.

Joyce has discussed her diagnosis and prognosis with her family and considers herself to have been reasonably cheerful since her diagnosis. However, in the past few weeks she is complaining of feeling tired and 'a bit flat'. *Psychologically*, she has no previous history of mental ill health.

Joyce feels very comfortable with her social and *spiritual beliefs* and she does not feel the need to discuss them in depth. She has stated that she cannot see the significance of this aspect of care to her nursing intervention. Joyce is a practising Roman Catholic and her religion is very important to her.

Joyce has become very comfortable with the visits by her GP and the main nursing team. However, as Joyce's condition has deteriorated the multiagency team has become more involved in her care and she now has contact with many services and individuals (Figure 16.1). The GP takes the view that although he is sympathetic to Mrs Hammond's request to be cared for at home, the services and resources to support her and her family are limited and this could result in her having to have periods of hospitalization or respite care in a local nursing home. The multiagency team respect the explanation that the doctor has given to Mrs Hammond but feel that the patient has a right to choose where to be cared for. As a nurse, I feel it is important for me to be an advocate for Mrs Hammond to promote her wishes. In doing this I shall be demonstrating respect for her autonomy (Beauchamp & Childress 2004). This is something I shall do at the monthly review meetings that take place at the health centre. It is at these meetings that the multiagency team will review the health and social care needs for Mrs Hammond and her family.

The outcome of the first review meeting with the multiagency team resulted in agreement that Mrs Hammond should remain at home but if circumstances change, either with her health, family support, home conditions or the ability of the multiagency team to provide the services and resources that are required, then the situation would be reviewed and a new direction of care developed.

Section 4

16.1.2   Ethical theories

Ethics in the context of health care is concerned with the practical application of norms and values to discover what ought or ought not to be done in any given health care situation. It is concerned with determining principles that might be applied to situations and with virtues that an individual might need in order to choose the right course of action to take (Beauchamp & Childress 2004). Among the stances explored are deontology, utilitarianism and virtue ethics.

Deontology (Beauchamp & Childress 2004) suggests that the *moral worth of an act is in its intent* so that, providing that the intention is genuinely good, we have done the right thing. To follow this theory I would need to discover my duty to Mrs Hammond, perform that duty, and that in the same circumstances I and others would take the same actions, thus turning one's actions into universal law as outlined by Kant (Gillon 2003).

Utilitarianism (Beauchamp & Childress 2004) suggests that the *moral worth of an act is in its consequences* for the majority, so that if the outcome is good the act was good. To follow this theory I should consider the best consequences (i.e. the best outcome) for the majority in relation to Mrs Hammond and follow either a rule or act in a particular way in order to bring about positive consequences. As the nurse it may be useful for me to take the same actions as when following the theory of deontology, but the reasons for doing so would be different.

Virtue ethics (Crisp & Slote 1997) suggest that in order *to act morally one must be a virtuous person* and have, or strive for, a key set of characteristics such as temperance, courage, justice and prudence (Gillon 2003). In order to follow this theory I need to decide, according to my conscience, what I believe to be the right course of action and follow it with strength of will.

16.1.3   Ethical principles and their application to the case study

Ethics is concerned with rights, wrongs and what ought to be (Rumbold 2000). Ethics is not just about factual information or personal emotions alone (Seedhouse 2001). Each person has their own view-point but from an ethical perspective arguments are often developed from these ideas and coupled with principles and beliefs that come from a variety of influences (Beauchamp & Childress 2004).

Utilitarianism is based on the philosophy of the greatest happiness for the greatest number (Beauchamp & Childress 2004). Actions (the things we do) are identified as 'right' if the outcome is best for the greatest number (Beauchamp & Childress 2004). 'Rightness' is dependent on the consequences of the actions, which is why this theory is sometimes referred to as consequentialist theory (Seedhouse 2001; Beauchamp & Childress 2004). Actions are judged right or wrong on the basis of whether they tend to promote 'pleasure and happiness' and diminish 'pain and unhappiness'. Bentham (1748–1832) and Mill (1806–1873) are two major theorists of this ideology (Gillon 2003).

Deontology is based on the principles of duty and laws. Unlike utilitarianism, deontologists argue that the concepts of 'good' and 'right' actions are not exclusive to 'good consequences' alone but if the intentions and thoughts were good then the actions and outcomes based on these thoughts and actions are right and good (Beauchamp & Childress 2004). It must be remembered that when we act we often cannot predict outcomes, so in fact all we have is our analysis of a situation and our action based on that analysis. Good intent based on knowledge must be a key component of good practice.

Deontology is often considered to be based on the ideas of duty and rules that should be obeyed and adhered to regardless of the outcome. Kant (1734–1804), who developed this ideology, argued that what is right for one must be right for all people (Gillon 2003). This is called the 'universal law'. He further argued that laws that are valid for all should compel obedience and be binding. This he referred to as the categorical imperative. There are four principles that are referred to in contemporary ethics: *autonomy, justice, beneficence* and *non-maleficence* (Beauchamp & Childress 2004).

Concepts of ethics, utilitarianism and deontology as applied to the care of Mrs Hammond

The first and perhaps most important concept to be discussed in relation to the care of Mrs Hammond is that of autonomy (Gillon 2003; Beauchamp & Childress 2004). Autonomy refers to the notion that people own themselves and have a fundamental right to self-government. It is not therefore possible to give autonomy or to take it away; it can only be present, absent, respected, disrespected or overridden. As a nurse, I first need to decide whether or not Mrs Hammond seems to be competent and rational. As she does appear so, it follows that she is currently autonomous and as a nurse I am required to respect this. Autonomy is the concept that underpins the need to gain the consent of patients before commencing treatment. The importance of autonomy was realised following the 1949 Nuremberg trials of Nazis who used humans for experiments. The declaration of Helsinki (World Medical Association 2001) related to research but is applicable to all aspects of practice. This declaration demanded that all those involved in prescribing or carrying out treatments gain the patient's informed consent. It is not possible to respect autonomy without adhering to basic principles in ethics such as telling the truth (veracity), free participation of the individual, giving the individual information relating to the procedure, an honest discussion of risk and the absence of coercion. Mrs Hammond's autonomy has been respected so far in that she has been involved in honest discussions about her future care. This included discussion with the multiagency team about the possibility they may not be able to meet her wishes on the basis of limited services and resources.

There are circumstances in which autonomy can and should be overridden – if the person is unconscious, under the influence of drugs or mentally incompetent. In these circumstances the nurse should respond to the wishes of the person (if known) before the current circumstances come about. In the situation that I find myself in with Mrs Hammond, autonomy is an important question to consider. Mrs Hammond has made a decision about the context in which she wants to be cared for and has made it at a time when she is competent. Given that this is a request from an autonomous person, I have a duty to respect it, thereby respecting the autonomy of Mrs Hammond.

However, this is not the only duty I have. There is also the duty to the multiagency team and to the health services to manage resources ethically and to work within a team that is itself managed ethically. I also have an equivalent duty to all patients to meet their needs as far as is possible, in accordance with their wishes. My duty in relation to a deontological approach (Gillon 2003) would be to respect Mrs Hammond's wishes because duty to the patient is paramount. A utilitarian standpoint (Beauchamp & Childress 2004) argues that the nurse's caseload be seen as a whole and that nurses organise themselves as a resource in such a way that they bring about the greatest good for the greatest number. Depending on other calls on the nursing services duty a nurse might behave in exactly the same way towards a patient but for different reasons.

This raises questions about the second major principle that underpins the ethical management of self, resources and others in practice, that of justice (Beauchamp & Childress 2004). Justice in this case refers to the fair distribution of resources to those who are entitled to receive them. It would be wrong for the nurse to think that their duty to one patient must be fulfilled at the expense of duty to the multiagency team and other patients. As a nurse working across health and social care there are often situations that present the nurse with multiple and conflicting roles. This situation has to be resolved in such a way that the nurse distributes their expertise (as a resource) as fairly as possible.

The following discussion is an example of how nurses can manage resources, others and self and illustrates the ethical stance that a nurse could hold in relation to practice.

Discussion of concepts of ethics, utilitarianism and deontology as applied to practice

If the nurse sees duty to the individual as all-pervading (deontological), which the NMC code of conduct implies (NMC 2004), then the nurse will conceptualise their caseload as a series of individual patients that the nurse owes an equal duty to. If, however, the nurse takes the view that they must balance their duty to some with their duty to others (utilitarian) they will conceptualise the caseload as one in which goods and harms, or potential harms, have to be weighed.

Public health is, of itself, a utilitarian concept, suggesting as it does that health care and practitioners working in the field of public health should seek to maximise good and minimise harm for as many as possible through policy and practice. For these practitioners, justice relates to the fair distribution of resources and the prime resource that must be allocated fairly is the practitioner himself or herself. This suggests a number of things: effective time management so that resources are not lost, good clinical judgement about the need to intervene, the length of the intervention and when to end the intervention or withdraw the care. This takes the stance of working with patients towards self-care and independence and not engaging in futile treatment. Justice, in this case, asks the question, 'are the right resources (the nurse's knowledge, skills and time) being used for the right care delivered in the right way at the right time and being distributed equitably?' The incorporation of the principle of justice into clinical practice does not imply that there is a predetermined right answer or formula that can be followed. It is rather the case that in each situation the nurse has to ask the question, 'what is fair in this set of circumstances?' If a nurse responds to need 'a', what implications does it have for needs 'b', 'c' and 'd', etc.?

Beneficence (Beauchamp & Childress 2004) is concerned with doing good. In seeking to do good in relation to the care of Mrs Hammond I must come to some conclusion about what good would look like in this set of circumstances. Having accepted that the patient is an autonomous person and having further decided to respect her autonomy, the decision about good in this case study has already been decided. Mrs Hammond clearly wishes to be cared for at home. I have a duty to explain to Mrs Hammond the implications of such a decision and to work through with her and the multiagency team the likely path that the illness will take. This will include an estimation of pain and the extent to which that pain can be controlled, and an estimation of the services required to deliver personal care at home as and when required. In doing this I am respecting Mrs Hammond's autonomy by giving full disclosure about the proposed course of action, thereby allowing Mrs Hammond to make an informed decision. To withhold information at this point would be to deny Mrs Hammond the right to make decisions about herself and thereby through the use of paternalism (Gillon 2003) subtly undermine her autonomy.

The care that will take place must strike a balance between doing good (beneficence) and avoiding harm (non-maleficence). The process of being cared for at home with a long-term condition may be more physically distressing than that of being cared for in hospital, but the psychological pain may be greater. The possible psychological comfort of being at home may counterbalance the physical distress experienced within her long-term care trajectory. Part of good practice is to ensure good communication and information giving. I need to be honest with Mrs Hammond about the extent to which support can be given from the multiagency team. Honesty is a key theme in relation to the maintenance of autonomy, beneficence and non-maleficence, as dishonesty (including withholding information) is paternalistic behaviour on the part of the practitioner (Beauchamp & Childress 2004). In respecting the person's autonomy I must allow for the possibility that Mrs Hammond will make a decision with which they disagree. The nurse must remember that as a professional they must seek to serve the public and not make them obey them because 'nurse knows best'. This is not to say that the nurse should agree with decisions made. The nurse can and should point out the negative consequences of a course of action but should stop short of manipulating information, and thereby the actions of a person, to avoid them taking a course of action with which the nurse disagrees. Mrs Hammond's decision to be cared for at home may cause her and her partner more distress and pain at times than electing to spend time in hospital. Nevertheless it is an informed choice that they make and must be respected as such. The uncomfortable conclusion here is that autonomous people have the right to make decisions that practitioners (and others) think are not in their best interest. However, in taking this view the nurse needs to remind himself or herself that their views are not necessarily that of the patient, and although the patient may take a course of action which may be harmful to them they do so with full knowledge and acceptance of the consequences of their actions.

In practice, nurses come across issues where it is difficult to understand the decisions that are made, indeed some issues seem to have no easy answer. These are referred to as *dilemmas*. A dilemma is a situation in which a choice has to be made between two courses of action which each have undesirable elements (Thompson *et al.* 2006). It is suggested that an understanding of law and ethics can help health care professionals to work through these decisions. Utilizing ethical theories in practice can help us make sense of the problems even if we find the outcomes difficult.

Rumbold (2000) argues that before a nurse can undertake good practice they must have explored the question 'what is ethics?' It is suggested here that this complex question is not one that can be easily answered. Indeed, Rumbold himself acknowledges that 'there can be no clear cut answers to every day questions'. However, nurses are expected to undertake professional intervention based on a body of knowledge that is both legally and professionally sound. Implicit in this practice is that practitioners will practice in such a way as to not knowingly or intentionally do harm based on the principles of professional practice, such as those set out within the NMC *Code of Professional Conduct* (NMC 2004).

As mentioned earlier in the case study, ethics is concerned with concepts such as right and wrong as well as duty and considerations of what one ought to do. Whatever the practice decision, it must be acknowledged that decisions are often influenced by an individual's personal beliefs (morals) as well as the legal and professional obligations to act in a way that is acceptable to a professional body and to society. Komaromy (2001) argues that although the health service was established to provide care at the point of need and to 'universalise the best' (Bevin 1948, cited by Komaromy 2001) individual practitioners are often faced with dilemmas in practice that force them to make a decision based on best practice and the best interest of the patient. Seedhouse (2001) argues that ethics enables us to conduct life (both personal and professional) in such a way as to produce a good outcome.

16.1.4   Legal and professional frameworks and their application to the case study

Montgomery (2003) argues that we are obliged both by national and international (European Union) legislation to take measures to ensure that members of our society (the public) have improved health (Montgomery 2003). He also contends that as health becomes the responsibility of the individual as well as the nation, three trends have emerged that have influenced the way public health is perceived. These are:

- individual rights to health care based on equal service;
- equal access to service;
- equality of care.

Montgomery (2003) is clear, however, that although the individual may perceive themselves as having a right to health care based on equal service, equal access and equality of care (DH 2000), we need to understand that this right is not universal and can only be provided based on what resources are available at the point of delivery (Plant 1989, cited in Montgomery 2003). Dimond (2005) is clear that although no one is above the law and ignorance is no defence, practitioners working in the field of public health must remain aware that their practice is not only empowered through the law but that the law also has expectations that practice is not undertaken when competency is not to an acceptable standard.

The NMC *Code of Professional Conduct* (2004) is a set of rules that all nurses are expected to adhere to within the course of their work. Hedrick (2004) argues the codes set standards that enable, whilst Dimond (2005) describes how the NMC code translates the legal framework that the nursing profession is expected to work within. It is important that nurses understand the professional as well as society's expectations of conduct and practice and this is best translated by demonstrating good practice in all aspects of care and intervention for a patient.

In the case of Mrs Hammond it was particularly important that I listened to her needs and wishes with regard to being cared for at home. After the multiagency team had explained that Mrs Hammond would be cared for at home it was acknowledged that there may come a time when this was no longer possible. Mrs Hammond was anxious and distressed about the possibility of hospitalization or nursing home care so I spent time listening to her concerns. Clause 2 of the *Code of Professional Conduct* (NMC 2004) states that each person should be respected and treated as an individual with clause 2.4 specifying that the practitioner should promote the interest of the patient. Because of the requirement to maintain confidentiality (clause 5), permission was sought from Mrs Hammond to discuss her case and advocate for her wishes during the first meeting with the multiagency team.

Montgomery (2003) is clear that although the public may have a perception that care in the community can be provided whenever and as required, this is not always the case. Social Services and Primary Care Trusts (PCTs) have finite budgets that they are expected to work within; this is a stance relating to the concepts of justice and utilitarianism (Gillon 2003). Although a duty of care is mandatory as far as safety and health care intervention is concerned, these do not necessarily have to be provided where the patient requests. Therefore, if there are insufficient funds to provide staff such as health and social care assistants, night sitters or extra visits from primary care staff during weekends, or Mrs Hammond's condition is such that her health needs cannot be provided by the multiagency team, then she may not be able to stay at home on a permanent basis.

Multiagency teams have to make decisions on a daily basis with regard to how much intervention they can provide for patients in order to facilitate care at home. These decisions should be taken within a knowledgeable, professionally accountable framework. Komaromy (2001) argues that despite government legislation, care in the community is still reliant on considerable input by informal carers. The constraints of sufficient and appropriate staffing as well as the ability of the family to support Mrs Hammond's wishes could influence the level and quality of care provided. It is at these junctures of conflict that the nurse can advocate for the hopes and wishes of the patient.

16.1.5   The role of advocacy

Rumbold (2000) suggests that advocacy is concerned with promoting and safeguarding the well being and interest of patients and clients, whilst Tschudin (2005) argues that although a nurse needs to be aware of their role as an advocate, they should also be cognisant of their own rights and need for support as well. The Patient Advisory Liaison Services (PALS) suggest that because a nurse has close contact with the patient and their family they may not be the best person to speak on behalf of the patient and that an independent person or representative, such as a member of staff from PALS, may be more effective and therefore of more use to the patient.

Having listened to Mrs Hammond and her partner I felt it was important to ensure that their views were heard and understood, not only because of a duty of care but also because Mrs Hammond may not have been able to articulate her needs and rationale for staying in her home without appearing to the team to be subjective and emotional. To disregard the patient's subjective experience of illness would amount to a disregard of autonomy. Therefore I decided to discuss Mrs Hammond's concerns and views at the first meeting with the multiagency team. I was able to represent her views whilst acknowledging the constraints within the services on offer. Honesty with Mrs Hammond helped in this process, as I had not made any unrealistic promises to her. As such, I was demonstrating the principle of fidelity thereby acknowledging Mrs Hammond's autonomy (Beauchamp & Childress 2004).

16.1.6   Reflections on practice and dilemmas in the care provided to Mrs Hammond and her family

Benner (1984) and Benner and Wrubel (1989) intimate that *reflection* is a recounting of an experience and can be presented in a number of ways. Dewey (1933), one of the earliest exponents of reflection, states that the review process enables a learning of the experience and further questioning of the phenomena to be achieved. Schon (1987) developed his own theory based on Dewey's work and alludes to aspects of reflection – that of reflecting on and reflecting in action. Schon considers that *reflecting in action* is a process whereby the individual recognises a problem exists and thinks about their actions during and throughout the problem situation. Whereas he suggests that *reflecting on action* is a retrospective contemplation of practice which is undertaken in order to understand the issues related to the problem. By reflecting or thinking about the problem after the event, a development of knowledge takes place and change can occur (perhaps doing things differently if the situation should occur at another time). Burnes and Bulman (2000) claim that reflection is a useful tool for nurses to use and that they should be aware of the value of reflection in their practice so that they can develop an understanding of their experience(s). With this in mind, set out below are my reflections on Mrs Hammond's care and interventions.

Mrs Hammond was cared for in the place she felt most comfortable and the multiagency team, including myself, was glad that this outcome was possible. On reflection, the four major principles of ethics provided a useful structure for having a dialogue about dilemmas in practice.

1. Did the multiagency team respect Mrs Hammond's autonomy? The evidence in the case study suggests they did and would have done so even had Mrs Hammond been admitted to hospital at some time during her long-term care. The key to this process was honesty at all stages, including honesty about the distribution of resources.

2. Did the multiagency team seek to do good (beneficence)? The evidence from the case study identifies that this happened, and the nature of the good was negotiated with the patient, although it was not necessarily my idea of good. Pain control was difficult at times and could have been better in hospital but Mrs Hammond felt that the psychological benefits of being at home with her partner outweighed the negative aspects of pain.

3. Did the multiagency team avoid harm (non-malifence)? Mrs Hammond experienced greater physical discomfort than she would have done in hospital and this troubled the team. However, the team had to remind themselves that their role is to serve and respect the autonomous wishes of Mrs Hammond as a competent person.

4. Did the team act in a way that led to the just distribution of resources? The evidence in the case study suggests they did but only because the pressure on the team from outside influences was not too heavy at that point. This is one of the most difficult principles to follow. The stance taken on justice can relate closely to personal thoughts about deontology, utilitarianism and virtue. If the team are deontologists and perceive the caseload as serial (and equivalent) duty, the question arises as to how the time of the team gets distributed. Is it first come, first served or sickest first – who gets less of my time and why? There are no right or wrong answers to this question. A utilitarian stance fits better with the way of working in the community, but if the nurse follows this dictum they might find themselves uncomfortable in relation to the *Code of Professional Conduct* (NMC 2004) and the real sense of duty felt to all patients. Virtue ethics would ask the question, 'what would a good person do?' If this stance were taken, I would strive to resolve to do the best I could with the resources available to me so as to ensure the best possible outcome.

Ethics does not provide all the answers but provides a framework that we can use to consider the options before taking action. Nurses will continue to struggle with dilemmas that are presented as in this case study. Yet Beauchamp and Childress (2004) argue that it is moral reasoning itself that drives practitioners to seek to find resolution, if not answers. Therefore ethics is not simply about finding answers but feeling comfortable in the knowledge that one's practice is appropriate, professional, legal and enables one to 'feel comfortable' with the actions taken within a professional, legal and personal framework. All practitioners, in whatever sphere of practice, need to utilise ethical theories as well as legislation to ensure safe and appropriate practice. Beauchamp and Childress (2004) argue that this can be achieved by 'facing dilemmas'. The multiagency team certainly faced the dilemmas presented by Mrs Hammond's care; not all were resolved but, most importantly, the wish that she remain in her home was achieved, which was the main purpose of my advocacy.

16.1.7 Case study conclusions

The incorporation of ethical thinking and analysis into practice is not particularly difficult to do. Nurses have always thought through cases within an ethical framework but always need to acknowledge or appreciate the process attached to this. Being more aware of the process of ethical decision making will sharpen up the questions a nurse needs to ask himself or herself. Prior to studying the module on law and ethics, my view was that ethics was about grand questions for others to deal with, but I now appreciate that ethics is also about the everyday aspects of nursing practice.

Conclusion

The ethical and legal issues relating to the management of self and others as well as resources have been explored in this chapter using a case study, 'staff nurse and client' approach. Ethical, legal and professional theories have been considered and discussed in relation to the case study but also applied to frameworks that guide and inform practice for nurses. These frameworks have also been applied so as to demonstrate issues that can arise in practice and how they can be addressed from a practice perspective.

The rights of the patient client is central to good practice and underpins the requirements set out in the NMC *Code of Professional Conduct* (NMC 2004). However, it has also demonstrated how difficult this can be for the professional nurse when decisions have to be made when encompassing the needs of self and the management of others.

References

Beauchamp T.L., Childress J.F. (2004) *Principles and Practice of Medical Ethics*. Oxford: Oxford University Press.

Benner P. (1984) *From Novice to Expert: excellence and power in clinical nursing practice*. San Diego, CA: Addison-Wesley.

Benner P., Wrubel J. (1989) *The Primary of Caring*. Menlow Park, CA: Addison Wesley Press.

Burnes S., Bulman C. (eds) (2000) *Reflective Practice in Nursing: the growing of the professional practitioner*, 2nd edn. Oxford: Blackwell Publishing.

Crisp R., Slote M. (1997) *Virtue Ethics*. Oxford: Oxford University Press.

Dewey J. (1933) *How We Think*. Boston: C. Heath.

DH (Department of Health) (2000) *The NHS Plan: a plan for investment. A plan for reform*. London: HM Stationery Office.

Dimond B. (2005) *Legal Aspects of Nursing*. Upper Saddle River, NJ: Pearson Education.

Gillon R. (2003) *Philosophical Medical Ethics*. Chichester: John Wiley & Sons.

Hedrick J. (2004) *Law and Ethics*. Foundations in Nursing and Healthcare Series. Cheltenham: Nelson Thorns.

Komaromy C. (ed.) (2001) *Dilemmas in UK Health Care*. Buckingham: Open University Press.

Montgomery J. (2003) *Health Care Law*. Oxford: Oxford University Press.

NMC (Nursing and Midwifery Council) (2004) *Code of Professional Conduct: standards for conduct, performance and ethics*. London: Nursing and Midwifery Council.

Rumbold G. (2000) *Ethics in Nursing Practice*. London: Balliere Tindall.

Schon D. (1987) *Educating the Reflective Practitioner*. San Francisco: Jossey-Bass Publishers.

Seedhouse D. (2001) *Ethics, the Heart of Health Care*. Chichester: John Wiley & Sons.

Thompson I.E., Melia K., Boyd K.M., Horsburgh D. (2006) *Nursing Ethics*, 5th edn. Edinburgh: Churchill Livingstone.

Tschudin V. (2005) *Ethics*. London: Balliere Tindall.

World Medical Association (2001) *Declaration of Helsinki (Edinburgh revision)*. Ferney Voltaire, France: World Medical Association.

Glossary of Terms

This glossary offers definitions of key terms used throughout the book. The majority of these terms come from recognised and authoritative sources. The majority of definitions used are those offered by the Department for Education and Skills (DfES), the National Library for Health (NLH), the Nursing and Midwifery Council (NMC), the Public Health Electronic Library (PHEL), Skills for Health and the World Health Organization (WHO).

access the extent to which people are able to receive the services, information or care they need. Issues involved in accessibility include physical access, distance of travel, communication (e.g. interpreters) and the provision of culturally appropriate services so that people are not discouraged from seeking help (PHEL).

advocacy a combination of individual and social actions designed to gain political commitment, policy support, social acceptance and systems support for a particular health goal or programme. Such action may be taken by and/or on behalf of individuals and groups to create living conditions which are conducive to health and the achievement of healthy lifestyles. Health professionals have a responsibility to act as advocates for health at all levels of society (WHO 1998; NMC 2004a).

antidiscriminatory practice this actively removes barriers that may prevent people or groups engaging in community activity or accessing or using services.

assessment of health need a process that helps inform planning of health care for individuals and their families, communities and the wider population.

autonomy taking responsibility for one's own actions.

capacity all the resources available to an organization, service or community including people, equipment, money, skills, expertise and information (PHEL).

capacity building developmental work and activities that increase the ability of a community to take action or provide a service. Chapter 4 of the book explores this in the context of helping a community to take part in the social and economic regeneration of their area by encouraging and developing people's skills and confidence, building up an infrastructure by setting up and strengthening networks (PHEL).

care for the purposes of this book the term is used to denote children being looked after by a local authority or adults and children being looked after by the health services.

Care order a court order made under the Children Act 1989 section 31 that places a child in the care of a designated local authority and enables the local authority in whose favour the order is made to share parental responsibility with the parent(s). The court may only make the order if it is satisfied that the child is suffering or likely to suffer 'significant harm'; and that the harm is attributable to the care given to the child.

Child the Children Acts 1989 and 2004 state a child is anyone who has not yet reached their 18th birthday. Children therefore means children and young people.

Child and Adolescent Mental Health Services (CAMHS) this refers to the broad concept of services that contribute to the mental health care of children and young people, whether provided by statutory services (health, social services or education) or by voluntary services (e.g. National Society for the Prevention of Cruelty to Children, NSPCC). It encompasses services provided by school nurses and general practitioners as well as more specialised services dedicated solely to the treatment of children with mental health problems.

child protection process of protecting individual children identified as either suffering, or at risk of suffering, significant harm as a result of abuse or neglect.

Children's Trust Children's trusts bring together all services for children and young people in an area, underpinned by the Children Act 2004 duty to cooperate, to focus on improving outcomes for all children and young people.

clinical governance a statutory duty placed on the NHS to ensure high-quality health care. Section 4 of the book deals with this specifically. The aim is to ensure high standards of care, safeguarding patients against poor performance and reducing variations between providers of services.

collaborative working includes working with others in health and social care, those working in social security, benefits, education, housing and the environment. It also includes those working in advice, guidance and counselling services, and employers and employees in a range of different sectors, or example voluntary agencies, community networks and legal and judicial agencies.

Commission for Social Care Inspection (CSCI) launched in April 2004, this is a single, independent inspectorate for all social care services in England, including the children's services. It has three main functions: regulating care services, assessing and inspecting local authority services, and helping support improvements in those local authority services.

commissioning a systematic process by which local authority and health services identify local needs for services and assess them against the available public and private sector provision. Priorities are decided and services purchased from the most appropriate providers through contracts and service agreements. As part of the commissioning process, services are subject to regular evaluation (PHEL).

common assessment framework (CAF) this can be used as an assessment tool by the whole children's workforce to assess the additional needs of children and young people at the first signs of difficulties. The framework provides a mechanism that any practitioner working with children can use (or have access to) to identify unmet needs, so as to prevent a child's needs becoming more serious.

community this is a group of people living or working in a geographically defined area (geographical community) or who have a characteristic cause, need or experience in common (community of interest). A community is one form of group (PHEL).

community development work with people on a neighbourhood or community basis that promotes self-help, mutual support and collective action. The underlying idea is finding new and imaginative solutions to problems and better use of existing resources (PHEL).

community involvement this entails both consultation and participation, with local people participating in the development of policies to improve the health of their community as well as having a say in the prioritizing, planning and delivery of services. It involves the voluntary sector and wider public being included in higher strategic planning levels as well as lower levels of decision making and input (PHEL).

deprived areas areas characterised by significantly low social and economic levels measured on a range of indices such as unemployment and lower rates of income per head or agreed indices compared with the national average (PHEL).

determinants of health the wide range of personal, social, economic and environmental factors that determine the health status of people or communities. They include health behaviours and lifestyles, income, education, employment, working conditions, access to health services, housing and living conditions and the wider general environment (PHEL).

Director of Children's Services every top tier local authority in England is required to appoint a Director of Children's Services under section 18 of the Children Act 2004. Directors are responsible for discharging local authority functions that relate to children in respect of education, social services and children leaving care.

disease prevention   measures to prevent the occurrence of disease and also arrest its progress and reduce its consequences (WHO 1998).

Early years foundation stage (EYFS)   this provides the statutory framework to deliver improved outcomes for all children across every area of learning and development and to help close the achievement gap between disadvantaged children and others. All EYFS providers must register with Ofsted, and for independent, maintained and non-maintained, and special schools with provision for children from birth to the end of the August after their fifth birthday (DfES 2006a).

electronic learning or e-learning   learning and teaching utilizing electronic media, in particular the internet (the world wide web), access to extensive databases connected to national and international computer networks, and the use of email to communicate.

empowerment   a process through which people gain greater control over decisions and actions affecting their health. It may be a social, cultural, psychological or political process through which individuals and social groups are able to express their needs, present their concerns, devise strategies for involvement in decision making, and achieve political, social and cultural action to meet those needs (WHO 1998).

enable   taking action in partnership with individuals or groups to empower them, through the mobilization of human and material resources, to promote and protect their health (WHO 1998).

epidemiology   the study of the distribution and determinants of health states or events in specified populations, and the application of this study to control health problems (definition used by Health UK; Last 2001).

equality   the degree to which a resource is equally distributed (PHEL).

equity   concerned with how fairly resources are distributed throughout a group of people according to population, not individual, need. Initiatives to address health equity try to distribute resources, opportunities, access, etc. fairly (according to need) not equally (PHEL).

evaluation   assessing if an intervention (e.g. a service, project or treatment) achieves its aim and objectives. Process evaluation is an ongoing examination of the processes, activities, methods of planning and implementation of an intervention and includes staff performance, quality, client satisfaction and cost-effectiveness. Impact evaluation measures the immediate or mid-term effects of an intervention. Outcome evaluation is an assessment of the long-term effects of an intervention or some aspect of an intervention (PHEL).

evidence-based practice   the best current research information available based on a systematic analysis of the effectiveness of a treatment, service or any other intervention and its use in order to produce the best outcome, result or effect (PHEL). Chapter 11 takes a close look at the whole process of evidence-based practice in public health activity.

extended schools   these offer a range of services and activities, often beyond the school day, to help meet the needs of children and young people, their families and the wider community. Example of this includes support for family learning, breakfast clubs and after school clubs (DfES 2006a).

factors that affect health and wellbeing   these are a range of personal, social, economic and environmental factors that determine the health status of individuals and populations.

health   a state of complete physical, psychological and social wellbeing – not merely the absence of disease or infirmity. Health is a resource for everyday life and not the object of living. It is a positive concept emphasizing social and personal resources as well as physical capabilities. A comprehensive understanding of health implies that all systems and structures that govern social and economic conditions and the physical environment should take account of the implications of their activities in relation to their impact on individual and collective health and wellbeing (WHO 1998).

health development   the process of continuous, progressive improvement of the health status of individuals and groups in a population (WHO 1998).

health education   communicating information and fostering the motivation, skills and confidence (self-efficacy) necessary to take action to improve health. Health education includes the communication of information concerning the underlying social, economic and environmental conditions impacting on health, as well as individual risk factors and risk behaviours and use of the health system (WHO 1998). An example is offered in Chapter 15, which develops a health education programme in schools.

health gain   a measured improvement in the health of an individual person or population group. This method of expressing improved health outcomes can be used to show the relative advantage of one treatment or intervention (e.g. drugs, screening, vaccination or change in diet) over another in producing the greatest health gain (PHEL).

health impact assessment   a process that determines how a proposal will affect health and can be used as a practical way to influence decision makers. The process involves developing screening criteria to select policies or projects for assessment, profiling the areas and communities affected, applying a predefined model of health to predict potential impacts, evaluating the options, and making recommendations for action (PHEL).

health improvement   the main function of health improvement is to find ways of preventing ill health, protecting good health and promoting better health – it is closely linked to the quality of life and the concept of wellbeing.

health inequalities   the gap in health status and in access to health services between different social classes, ethnic groups and between populations in different geographical areas (PHEL).

health policy   a formal statement or procedure within institutions (notably government) which defines priorities and the parameters for action in response to health needs, available resources and other political pressures (WHO 1998).

health promotion   the process of enabling people to increase control over and improve their health. As well as covering actions aimed at strengthening people's skills and capabilities, it also includes actions directed towards changing social and environmental conditions to prevent or to improve their impact on individual and public health (PHEL).

health-promoting schools   these can be characterised as schools constantly strengthening their capacity as a healthy setting for living, learning and working (WHO 1998).

health protection   activities that protect health, identify and manage risk and prevent ill health. These include communicable disease control, control of environmental hazards to health, management of public health emergencies, and population immunization and screening programmes (DfES 2006a). Chapter 10 provides clear examples of working in this field of public health.

health needs assessment   a systematic method for reviewing health needs and issues facing a given population. It leads to agreed priorities and the allocation of resources that will improve health and reduce inequalities in a given population. The three chapters in Section 1 of the book cover this area.

healthy public policy   an explicit concern for health and equity in all areas of policy and by accountability for health impact. The main aim of healthy public policy is to create a supportive environment to enable people to lead healthy lives. Such a policy makes healthy choices possible or easier for citizens. It makes social and physical environments health-enhancing (WHO 1998).

individuals   community public health practice is directed at individuals, families, groups and communities in a population undifferentiated by diagnosis, including the child, young person, person of working age and older person.

interprofessional education   occasions when two or more professions learn from and about each other to improve collaboration and the quality of care.

intersectoral collaboration   a recognised relationship between part or parts of different sectors of society, which has been formed to take action on an issue to achieve health outcomes or intermediate health outcomes in a way that is more effective, efficient or sustainable than might be achieved by the health sector acting alone (WHO 1998).

life skills   the skills necessary for coping with everyday life. In particular the groups of psychological and interpersonal skills which can help people make informed decisions, communicate effectively, and develop coping and self-management skills that may help them to lead a healthy and productive life (PHEL). Chapter 7 examines communication skills in this context.

lifestyle   a way of living based on identifiable patterns of behaviour which are determined by the interplay between an individual's personal characteristics, social interactions and socioeconomic and environmental living conditions (WHO 1998).

Local authorities (LAs)   these can take any number of forms: a county council in England, a metropolitan district council, a non-metropolitan district council for an area where there is no county council, a London borough council, the Common Council of the City of London, and the Council of the Isles of Scilly (DfES 2006a).

mediation in health promotion, a process through which the different interests (personal, social, economic) of individuals and communities, and different sectors (public and private), are reconciled in ways that promote and protect health (WHO 1998).

network a grouping of individuals, organizations and agencies organised on a non-hierarchical basis around common issues or concerns, which are pursued practically and sympathetically, based on commitment and trust (WHO 1998).

needs assessment systematic processes by which organizations use information to judge the health of their population and then decide what services should be provided to meet local needs. The aim is to identify unmet needs that can affect health (e.g. access to services, untreated diseases) and make recommendations about ways to address these needs (PHEL).

participation people having the opportunity to fully contribute to and share in the decision-making process.

partnership a partnership for health is a voluntary agreement between two or more partners to work cooperatively towards a set of shared health outcomes (WHO 1998). Chapters 5 and 6 explore different and complimentary approaches to partnership working.

practice-based commissioning designed to provide services based on the identified health needs of a local community and tailored to those needs.

practice/work base setting any institutional or non-institutional environment in which students gain and/or demonstrate the skills, knowledge and attitudes needed for successful practice.

Primary Care Trust (PCT) local, freestanding NHS statutory bodies responsible for planning, providing and commissioning health services for the local population. The government sees these as the cornerstone to delivering the NHS. Established under the provisions of the Health Act 1999, they provide local GP, community and primary care services and commission hospital services from other NHS trusts.

primary health care health care made accessible at a cost the country and community can afford with methods that are practical, scientifically sound and socially acceptable (WHO1998).

public health in this book, public health is defined as 'the science and art of preventing disease, prolonging life and promoting health through the organised efforts and informed choices of society, organizations, public and private communities and individuals' (Wanless 2004).

Public services agreements these are 3-year agreements, negotiated between each of the main departments and HM Treasury, which set out a department's high level aims, priority objectives and key outcome-based performance targets.

risk behaviour specific forms of behaviour that are proven to be associated with increased susceptibility to a specific disease or ill health (WHO 1998).

risk factor social, economic or biological status, behaviours or environments which are associated with, or cause, increased susceptibility to a specific disease, ill health or injury (WHO 1998).

safeguarding and promoting the welfare of children the process of protecting children from abuse and neglect, preventing impairment of their health and development, and ensuring they are growing up in circumstances consistent with the provision of safe and effective care that enables children to have optimum life chances and enter adulthood successfully.

screening this involves carrying out tests either to identify a treatable disease at a very early stage before it has caused symptoms or damage, or to identify a risk factor which can lead to a disease (NLH).

service users/consumers a consumer or the interrelated term service user is a person who uses or has used health, social services or other services.

settings these are the place or social context in which people engage in daily activities in which environmental, organizational and personal factors interact to affect health and wellbeing.

social capital this represents the degree of social cohesion that exists in communities. It refers to the processes between people that establish networks, norms and social trust and facilitate coordination and cooperation for mutual benefit (WHO 1998).

socioeconomic status a description of a person's position in society which uses criteria such as income, level of education achieved, occupation and value of property owned (PHEL).

social exclusion   describes people or areas suffering from a combination of linked problems such as poor health, unemployment, inadequate skills, low incomes, poor housing, lack of educational opportunities, family breakdown, etc. which prevent accessing services, participating in social activities, obtaining the support and standards of living enjoyed by the majority, and being able to become integrated into the local community (PHEL).

stakeholders   people who have an interest in an organization, project or activity, e.g. service users, partners, employees, shareholders, the government, the voluntary sector, the local community, the NHS, local government, schools and businesses (PHEL).

strategic working   working collectively to an agreed plan towards common goals within a perspective that is wider than the individuals or the group themselves. Chapter 9 explores strategic leadership as the focus of strategic working.

substance misuse   the updated National Drug Strategy and 'Every child matters' programme (DfES 2006b) 'be healthy' outcome both use the term 'drugs', which refers to controlled drugs within the meaning of the Misuse of Drugs Act 1971. Reducing the use of these drugs by children and young people will often involve broader education, assessment and intervention covering a wide range of substances. Early use of these substances is a recognised risk factor for problem drug use in later life.

surveillance   the collection, collation and analysis of data to provide useful information about the distribution and causes of health and diseases and related factors in populations. These activities form the basis of epidemiology, which is the diagnostic backbone of public health practice (NLH). It is fully discussed with worked examples in Chapter 3.

sustainable development   development that meets the needs of the present without compromising the ability of future generations to meet their own needs.

Specialist community public health nursing (SCPHN)   used in relation to the SCPHN pathway of the award. The definition of SCPHN is taken from the Nursing and Midwifery Council *Standards of Proficiency for Specialist Community Public Health Nurses* (NMC 2004b) and refers to the NMC registration of specialist community public health nurses. This form of practice has distinct characteristics that require public protection. These include the responsibility to work with both individuals and a population, which may mean taking decisions on behalf of a community or population without having direct contact with every individual in the community.

voluntary sector   the range of groups whose activities are carried out on a not-for-profit basis and which are not public or local authorities. These organizations are normally formally constituted and employ professional and administrative staff. They may or may not use volunteer help (PHEL).

wellbeing   everyone deserves the opportunity to achieve their full potential. *Every Child Matters: next steps* (DfES 2004) sets out five outcomes that are key to children and young people's wellbeing: stay safe, be healthy, enjoy and achieve, make a positive contribution, and achieve economic wellbeing.

References

DfES (Department for Education and Skills (2004) *Every Child Matters: next steps*. London: HM Stationery Office.

DfES (Department for Education and Skills) (2006a) *Care Matters: transforming the lives of children and young people in care*. London: HM Stationery Office.

DfES (Department for Education and Skills) (2006b) *Working Together to Safeguard Children: every child matters; change for children*. London: HM Stationery Office.

Last J.M. (2001) *Dictionary of Epidemiology*. New York: Oxford University Press.

NLH (National Library for Health) http://www.library.nhs.uk.

NMC (Nursing and Midwifery Council) (2004a) *Code of Professional Conduct: standards for conduct, performance and ethics*. London: Nursing and Midwifery Council.

NMC (Nursing and Midwifery Council (2004b) *Standards of Proficiency for Specialist Community Public Health Nurses*. London: Nursing and Midwifery Council.

PHEL (Public Health Electronic Library) http://wwwphel.gov.uk/glossary/glossary.asp.

Skills for Health (2004) *Standards/Competencies for the Practice of Public Health Glossary*. London: Skills for Health.

Wanless D. (2004) *Securing Good Health for the Whole Population. Final report*. London: HM Treasury Office.

WHO (World Health Organization) (1998) *Glossary of Health Promotion*. Report No. WHO/HPR/HEP98.1. http://www.qlibdoc.who.int/hq/1998/who_HPR_HEP_98.1.pdf.

Index